1986/87 Nursing Events

APRIL

8-12
American Nephrology Nurses' Association National Symposium. Hyatt Regency Hotel, New Orleans. Contact: ANNA National Office, (609) 589-2187.

10-11
"The Destiny of Nursing: Interaction of the Discipline with Society." Vanderbilt Plaza Hotel, Nashville, Tenn. Contact: Vanderbilt University Hospital Department of Nursing, (615) 322-2081.

13-17
American Association of Neuroscience Nurses' Annual Meeting. Denver. Contact: AANN, (312) 823-9850.

14
"Pulmonary Update: PCP in AIDS, Ventilator Management, and ABGs." Maimonides Medical Center, Brooklyn, N.Y. Contact: New York City Chapter AACN, P.O. Box 690, Gracie Station, New York, N.Y. 10028.

20-24
Cardiac Critical Care Nursing Symposium. Stouffer's Inn on the Square, Cleveland. Contact: Center for CME, the Cleveland Clinical Educational Foundation, (800) 762-8172 or 8173.

27-5/2
American Occupational Health Conference. Currigan Convention Center, Denver. Contact: AAOHN Department of Professional Affairs, (404) 262-1162.

30-5/3
Oncology Nursing Society's Annual Congress. Los Angeles Convention Center. Contact: ONS, (412) 344-3899.

MAY

15-16
National Nursing Symposium on Home Health Care. Ann Arbor, Mich. Contact: University of Michigan School of Nursing, (315) 763-3210.

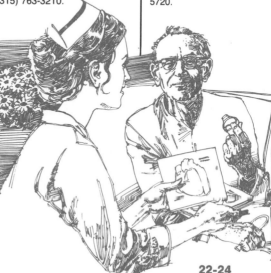

19-20
"Multiple Trauma: Advanced Topics for Nurses." Suburban Hospital, Bethesda, Md. Contact: Maryland Institute for Emergency Medical Services Systems, (301) 528-3930.

20-23
American Association of Critical Care Nurses National Teaching Institute. Anaheim, Calif. Contact: AACN National Office, (714) 644-9310.

27-31
Society of Critical Care Medicine's Annual Educational and Scientific Symposium. Washington, D.C. Contact: SCCM, (714) 870-5243.

JUNE

13-19
ANA Annual Conference, "Planning for Tomorrow: Securing Nursing's Future." Anaheim, Calif. Contact: ANA, (816) 474-5720.

22-24
American Diabetes Association's Annual Meeting and Scientific Sessions. Anaheim Convention Center, Anaheim, Calif. Contact: ADA, (212) 683-7444.

22-25
Canadian Nurses Association's Annual Meeting and Convention. Regina, Saskatchewan. Contact: CNA, (613) 237-2133.

23-25
New York City Chapter of the American Association of Critical Care Nurses Annual Symposium and Research Day. Barbizon Plaza Hotel, New York. Contact: New York City Chapter AACN, P.O. Box 690, Gracie Station, New York, N.Y. 10028.

27-7/1
National Association of School Nurses Annual Conference. Sheraton Hotel/Copley Plaza, Boston. Contact: NASN National Office, (303) 850-9033.

Yearbook86/87

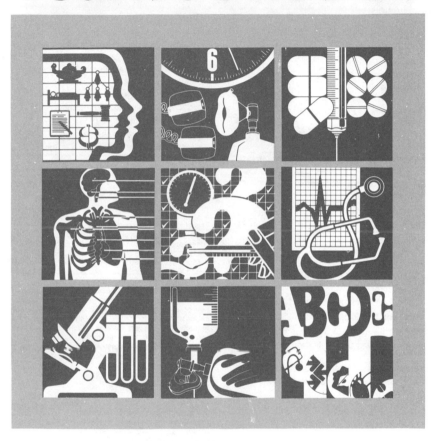

NURSING86 BOOKS™
SPRINGHOUSE CORPORATION
Springhouse, Pennsylvania

NURSING86 BOOKS™

SPRINGHOUSE CORPORATION BOOK DIVISION

Chairman
Eugene W. Jackson

President
Daniel L. Cheney

Vice-President and Director
Timothy B. King

Vice-President, Book Operations
Thomas A. Temple

Vice-President, Production and Purchasing
Bacil Guiley

Program Director, Reference Books
Stanley E. Loeb

YEARBOOK86/87

Editorial Director
Helen Klusek Hamilton

Clinical Director
Minnie Bowen Rose, RN, BSN, MEd

Art Director
Sonja E. Douglas

Staff for this volume

Editors: Kevin J. Law, Nancy J. Priff

Clinical Editor: Sandra Ludwig Nettina, RN, BSN

Acquisitions: Margaret L. Belcher, RN, BSN

Drug Information Manager: Larry Neil Gever, RPh, PharmD

Editorial Services Supervisor: David R. Moreau

Copy Editors: Traci Deraco, Diane M. Labus, Doris Weinstock

Production Coordinator: Sally Johnson

Designers: Linda Jovinelly Franklin, Christopher Laird

Illustrators: Michael Adams, Dimitrios Bastas, John Cymerman, Harry Davis, Len Dawson, Sam Dion, Jack Freas, Marie Garafano, Tom Herbert, Robert Jackson, Robert Jones, Adam Mathews, Robert Phillips, George Retseck, Dennis Schofield, Dan Sneberger

Art Production Manager: Robert Perry III

Art Assistants: Donald Knauss, Mark Marcin, Sandy Sanders, Joan Walsh, Robert Wieder

Typography Manager: David C. Kosten

Typographers: Elizabeth A. DiCicco, Amanda C. Erb, Ethel Halle, Diane Paluba, Nancy Wirs

Senior Production Manager: Deborah C. Meiris

Production Manager: Wilbur D. Davidson

Production Assistant: Tim A. Landis

Indexer: Barbara Hodgson

Researchers: Barbara Buggey, Susan Howard

Editorial Assistants: Maree E. DeRosa, Marlene C. Rosensweig

Special thanks to Rose Foltz and Jill Lasker, who assisted in preparation of this volume.

The clinical procedures described and recommended in this publication are based on research and consultation with medical and nursing authorities. To the best of our knowledge, these procedures reflect currently accepted clinical practice; nevertheless, they can't be considered absolute and universal recommendations. For individual application, recommendations must be considered in light of the patient's clinical condition and, before administration of new or infrequently used drugs, in light of latest package-insert information. The authors and the publisher disclaim responsibility for any adverse effects resulting directly or indirectly from the suggested procedures, from any undetected errors, or from the reader's misunderstanding of the text.

NRLYB-010386
ISBN 0-87434-031-4

Yearbook86/87

This volume is the first of an annual series conceived by the publishers of *Nursing86*® magazine. Gathered with the aid of a panel of experts from every area of nursing and medical practice, information in each volume will provide an annual update of the most significant developments in health care. Covering all areas of nursing practice, from clinical information to career and professional considerations, this new series brings today's nurse the timely information she needs to practice nursing with skill and confidence.

Other publications:

NURSES REFERENCE LIBRARY®
Diseases
Diagnostics
Drugs
Assessment
Procedures
Definitions
Practices
Emergencies
Signs & Symptoms

NEW NURSING SKILLBOOK™ SERIES
Giving Emergency Care Competently
Monitoring Fluid and Electrolytes Precisely
Assessing Vital Functions Accurately
Coping with Neurologic Problems Proficiently
Reading EKGs Correctly
Combatting Cardiovascular Diseases Skillfully
Nursing Critically Ill Patients Confidently
Dealing with Death and Dying
Managing Diabetes Properly
Giving Cardiovascular Drugs Safely

NURSING PHOTOBOOK™ SERIES
Providing Respiratory Care
Managing I.V. Therapy
Dealing with Emergencies
Giving Medications
Assessing Your Patients
Using Monitors
Providing Early Mobility
Giving Cardiac Care
Performing GI Procedures
Implementing Urologic Procedures
Controlling Infection
Ensuring Intensive Care
Coping with Neurologic Disorders
Caring for Surgical Patients
Working with Orthopedic Patients
Nursing Pediatric Patients
Helping Geriatric Patients
Attending Ob/Gyn Patients
Aiding Ambulatory Patients
Carrying Out Special Procedures

NURSING NOW™ SERIES
Shock
Hypertension
Drug Interactions
Cardiac Crises
Respiratory Emergencies
Pain

NURSE'S CLINICAL LIBRARY™
Cardiovascular Disorders
Respiratory Disorders
Endocrine Disorders
Neurologic Disorders
Renal and Urologic Disorders
Gastrointestinal Disorders
Neoplastic Disorders
Immune Disorders

***Nursing86* DRUG HANDBOOK™**

MediQuik Cards™

CLINICAL POCKET MANUAL™ SERIES
Diagnostic Tests
Emergency Care
Fluids and Electrolytes
Signs and Symptoms
Cardiovascular Care
Respiratory Care
Critical Care
Neurologic Care
Surgical Care

NURSE REVIEW™ SERIES
Cardiac Problems
Respiratory Problems
Gastrointestinal Problems
Neurologic Problems

Contents

Emergency care

Diagnostic tests

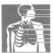

Diseases

Drugs

Law, ethics, and professional practice

Nursing procedures

Advisory board, clinical consultants, and contributors

At the time of publication, the advisors, clinical consultants, and contributors held the following positions:

Advisory board

Debra C. Broadwell, RN, ET, PhD, Associate Professor, Emory University School of Nursing, Atlanta

Karin M. Byrne, RN, MS, CS, JD, Director of Nursing Staff Development, Mount Auburn Hospital, Cambridge, Mass.

A. Bruce Campbell, MD, PhD, Attending Physician, Hematology/Oncology, Corippo Memorial Hospital, La Jolla, Calif.

Brian B. Doyle, MD, Clinical Professor of Psychiatry and of Family and Community Medicine, Georgetown University School of Medicine, Washington, D.C.

Stephen C. Duck, MD, Director, Endocrinology and Metabolism, Milwaukee Children's Hospital; Associate Professor of Pediatrics, Medical College of Wisconsin, Milwaukee

John J. Fenton, PhD, DABCC, Professor of Chemistry, West Chester (Pa.) University; Director of Chemistry, Crozer-Chester Medical Center, Chester, Pa.

Mary Lillian "Lillée" Gelinas, RNC, MSN, Director of Nursing, Memorial Hospital of Burlington County, Mount Holly, N.J.

A. Hadi Hakki, MD, FRCS, Assistant Professor of Surgery, Hahnemann University Hospital, Philadelphia; Associate Attending Surgeon, Bryn Mawr (Pa.) Hospital

Nancy M. Holloway, RN, MSN, CCRN, Critical Care/Emergency Nursing Consultant, Nancy Holloway & Associates, Oakland, Calif.

Ruth S. Kitson, RN, BAAN, MBA, Director of Nursing, Critical Care Services, Toronto Western Hospital

Brenda Marion Nevidjon, RN, MSN, Providence CancerCare Manager/Clinical Nurse Specialist, Providence Medical Center, Seattle

John J. O'Shea, Jr., MD, Senior Staff Fellow, Cell Biology and Metabolism Branch, National Institute of Child Health and Human Development, National Institutes of Health, Bethesda, Md.

Susan Jane Rumsey, RN, BSN, MPH, Perinatal Outreach Education Coordinator, Wake Area Health Education Center, Raleigh, N.C.

Barbara L. Solomon, RN, C, DNSc, Research Associate, Walter Reed Army Medical Center, Washington, D.C.

June L. Stark, RN, BSN, CCRN, Critical Care Instructor/Renal Nurse Consultant, New England Medical Center Hospitals, Boston

John K. Wiley, MD, FACS, Associate Clinical Professor of Surgery, Wright State University School of Medicine, Dayton, Ohio

Clinical consultants

John M. Bertoni, MD, PhD, Associate Professor of Neurology, Thomas Jefferson University, Philadelphia

Marlene M. Ciranowicz, RN, MSN, Independent Nurse Consultant/Nursing Instructor, LaSalle University, Philadelphia

Thaddeus P. Dryja, MD, Assistant Professor of Ophthalmology, Harvard Medical School, Massachusetts Eye and Ear Infirmary, Boston

Betsy Elmer, RN, BSN, Infection Control Practitioner, Buffalo (N.Y.) General Hospital

Sheila Glennon, RN, MA, CCRN, Chief, Critical Care Nursing, Norwalk (Conn.) Hospital

A. Hadi Hakki, MD, FRCS, Assistant Professor of Surgery, Hahnemann University Hospital, Philadelphia; Associate Attending Surgeon, Bryn Mawr (Pa.) Hospital

William M. Keane, MD, FACS, Surgeon, Pennsylvania Hospital, Philadelphia

Janet McMenamin, RN, MSN, CCRN, Transplant Coordinator, Delaware Valley Transplant Program, Philadelphia

John J. O'Shea, Jr., MD, Senior Staff Fellow, Cell Biology and Metabolism Branch, National Institute of Child Health and Human Development, National Institutes of Health, Bethesda, Md.

Susan E. Shapiro, RN, MS, CEN, Head Nurse, Emergency Services, Hospital of the University of Pennsylvania, Philadelphia

Eric Z. Silfen, MD, Staff Physician, Georgetown University Hospital and Emergency Medicine Associates, Washington, D.C.

Lana Wilhelm, RN, BSN, Nutritional Support Nurse, St. Louis University Hospitals

Contributors

Bonnie L. Anderson, MD, Resident in Radiology, Bowman-Gray School of Medicine, North Carolina Baptist Hospital, Winston-Salem

Wendy L. Baker, RN, BSN, MS, Staff, Critical Care Medicine Unit, University of Michigan Hospitals, Ann Arbor

Patricia L. Baum, RN, BSN, Research and Clinical Consultant, Peripheral Vascular Nursing, University of Massachusetts Medical Center, Worcester

Nora Lynn Bollinger, RN, MSN, Oncology Clinical Nurse Specialist, Walter Reed Army Medical Center, Washington, D.C.

Cecilia Borden, RN, MSN, Nurse Educator, Helene Fuld School of Nursing, Trenton, N.J.

Barbara Gross Braverman, RN, MSN, CS, Psychiatric Clinical Nurse Specialist, Medical College of Pennsylvania, Philadelphia

Lillian S. Brunner, RN, MSN, ScD, FAAN, Nurse-Author, Brunner Associates, Inc., Berwyn, Pa.

Barry J. Burton, RN, BSN, CEN, Consultant in Emergency Care/ACLS and BCLS Instructor, Philadelphia

Susan Diane Chenowith, RN, BS, CEN, JD, Legal Consultant and Lecturer, Philadelphia

Barbara Walsh Clark, RN, MSN, Former Associate Professor of Nursing, Bucks County Community College, Newtown, Pa.

William M. Dougherty, BS, Manager, Technical and Customer Services, Worldwide Geometric Data, Wayne, Pa.

Sr. Rebecca Fidler, MT(ASCP), PhD, Chairperson, Health Sciences, Salem (W. Va.) College

Dawn Flowers, RN, BSN, Staff Nurse, National Institutes of Health, Bethesda, Md.

Katherine L. Fulton, RN, Clinical Supervisor, Gastrointestinal Unit, The Genesee Hospital, Rochester, N.Y.

Mary Ann Hauser Gardiner, RN, BSN, Nurse Clinician, Home Nutrition and Intravenous Therapy, Travenol Laboratories, Inc., Baltimore

Mary Lillian "Lillee" Gelinas, RNC, MSN, Director of Nursing, Memorial Hospital of Burlington County, Mount Holly, N.J.

Larry Neil Gever, RPh, PharmD, Drug Information Manager, Springhouse Corporation, Springhouse, Pa.

Shirley Given, HT(ASCP), Supervisor of Histology, Crozer-Chester Medical Center, Chester, Pa.

Marcia Goldstein, RN, BSN, CHN, Clinical Nurse Specialist, Nephrology, Albert Einstein Medical Center, Northern Division, Philadelphia

Christine Grady, RN, MSN, CNS, Clinical Specialist, Immunology, Allergy, and Infectious Disease, Clinical Center, National Institutes of Health, Bethesda, Md.

Mary Lou Hamilton, RN, MS, Assistant Professor, College of Nursing, University of Delaware, Newark

Annette L. Harmon, RN, MSN, CEN, Former Assistant Director of Nursing, Newton-Wellesley Hospital, Newton–Lower Falls, Mass.

Tobie Virginia Hittle, RN, BSN, CCRN, Head Nurse, Intensive Care Unit, The Genesee Hospital, Rochester, N.Y.

Elizabeth Johnstone, RNC, BS, Staff Nurse, National Institutes of Health, Bethesda, Md.

Joyce LeFever Kee, RN, MSN, Associate Professor, College of Nursing, University of Delaware, Newark

William E. Kline, MS, MT(ASCP), SBB, Director, Technical Services, St. Paul (Minn.) Red Cross

Clarke Lambe, MD, Clinical Assistant III, Department of Pathology, University of Arizona, Tucson

Laurel Kareus Lambe, MS, RD, Nutrition Consultant, Tucson, Ariz.

Carol A. Lindeman, RN, PhD, FAAN, Dean, School of Nursing, Oregon Health Sciences University, Portland

Vivian Meehan, RN, BA, Nurse Clinician, Eating Disorders Program, Highland Park (Ill.) Hospital; President and Founder of the National Association of Anorexia Nervosa and Associated Disorders (ANAD)

Anna P. Moore, RN, BSN, MS, Assistant Professor and Coordinator, Psychiatric Mental Health Nursing, School of Nursing, Petersburg (Va.) General Hospital

S. Breanndan Moore, MD, DCH, FCAP, Staff Physician, Blood Bank and Transfusion Service, Mayo Clinic, Rochester, Minn.

Roger M. Morrell, MD, PhD, FACP, Chief, Neurology Service, Veterans Administration Medical Center, Allen Park, Mich.; Professor of Neurology and Microbiology/Immunology, Wayne State University School of Medicine, Detroit

Sandra Ludwig Nettina, RN, BSN, Clinical Editor, Springhouse Corporation, Springhouse, Pa.

Patricia M. Orr, RN, MBA, CCRN, Head Nurse, Burn Center, Saint Agnes Medical Center, Philadelphia

Frances W. Quinless, RN, PhD, Assistant Professor, Rutgers University College of Nursing, Newark, N.J.

Frank C. Riggall, MD, Associate Professor and Head, Division of Reproductive Endocrinology, University of Florida College of Medicine, Gainesville

Carolyn Robertson, RN, MSN, Diabetes Nurse Specialist, New York University School of Medicine

Sandra Schuler, RN, MSN, Assistant Professor of Nursing, Montgomery College, Takoma Park, Md.

Eleanor Tintner Segal, RN, BS, JD, Associate, Sacks and Basch, Philadelphia

Ellen Shipes, RN, ET, MN, MEd, Clinical Nurse Specialist, Enterostomal Therapy, Vanderbilt University Hospital, Nashville, Tenn.

Jean A. Shook, RN, MS, CS, Psychiatric Clinical Nurse Specialist, Medical College of Pennsylvania, Philadelphia

Basia Belza Tack, RN, MSN, ANP, Former Clinical Nurse Educator, Allergy and Infectious Diseases Nursing Service, Clinical Center, National Institutes of Health, Bethesda, Md.

Barry L. Tonkonow, MD, Staff Physician, Doylestown (Pa.) Hospital

Sharon McBride Valente, RN, MN, CS, Adjunct Assistant Professor, Department of Nursing, University of Southern California, Los Angeles

Connie A. Walleck, RN, MS, CNRN, Clinical Nurse Supervisor/Clinical Nurse Specialist, Neurotrauma Center, Maryland Institute of Emergency Medical Services, Baltimore

Joseph B. Warren, RN, BSN, Territory Manager, Kinetic Concepts, San Antonio, Tex.

Terri E. Weaver, RN, MSN, CS, Pulmonary Clinical Nurse Specialist, Hospital of the University of Pennsylvania; Clinical Instructor, University of Pennsylvania School of Nursing, Philadelphia

Beverly A. Zenk Wheat, RN, MA, Oncology Nurse Consultant, Stanford (Calif.) University Hospital

Foreword

Social scientists have proclaimed that we're now living in an "information society." Like most catchphrases, this one's essential meaning has been obscured by trendiness and overuse. Just what exactly is this information society, and what is the nurse's place in it?

Picture this scene. You're at the nurse's station in a busy critical care unit of a major metropolitan teaching hospital. Computers, printers, monitors, telephones, and information relay systems are everywhere. One printer is running off the results of a literature search—a list of recent publications pertinent to a patient's disorder. Another is printing lists of medications scheduled for administration; still another, scheduled treatments. One computer is checking for potential chemical interactions for all patients on the unit. Another computer's video screen is displaying a list of nursing practices that must be changed in light of yesterday's research findings. The international phone is ringing incessantly, as foreign nurses seek the latest clinical information from the United States. You start toward the bedside of a patient who's desperately ringing his call bell. But as you pause for a moment to think, the nearest printer disgorges a mountain of printouts that buries you under its weight. Your scream goes unheard, masked by the din in the nurses station.

An exaggeration? Of course. But you probably recognize some bits of reality in this bizarre scenario. To a nurse, the phrase information society isn't merely a cliché—it has palpable meaning. As a nurse, you know about the rapid changes that have occurred and are continuing to occur in the workplace, because you experience them every day. You know that our information society has evolved from the ever-continuing knowledge explosion—an explosion that has changed forever the way nurses work. You've seen this knowledge explosion firsthand. You've seen textbooks proliferate, with entire books now published on topics, such as gerontology, that until recently were covered as paragraphs or chapters in other texts. You've seen more and more research publications. You've seen recent scientific advances move human physiology to the intracellular level, and have witnessed the miracle of organ transplantation. You may even have complained about the difficulty in keeping current, of staying even with the knowledge explosion.

Unfortunately, keeping current will become even *more* difficult in our evolving information society. For in this new society, information itself is the strategic resource; most new jobs directly or indirectly involve the creation, processing, and distribution of information. As you know, information is both renewable and self-generating; the results of one research study invariably spawn additional studies. For example, the discovery of a new "plaque-buster" drug will undoubtedly spur more research into the treatment of coronary disease—which will produce more information.

Consider these facts:
- Between 6,000 and 7,000 scientific articles are written each day.
- Scientific and technical information now increases at a rate of 13% per year; at this rate, the existing body of information will double every 5.5 years.
- But advances in information science brought on by new, more powerful information systems and a growing number of scientists and researchers are continuously expanding the growth rate of information; by some accounts

it soon may reach 40% per year, which means that the body of existing information will double every *20 months*.

How can a nurse possibly keep up with this information explosion? I offer three suggestions. First, the professional nurse must come to think of herself as a *knowledge worker*, rather than a *technological worker*. As a knowledge worker in the information society, the nurse uses knowledge and information as the basis for the service she provides—patient care. Although she uses technology in delivering that service, technology is only the means to an end, not the end itself. For example, when providing intravenous therapy, the nurse needs knowledge of fluid and electrolyte balance, chemical interactions, and other information pertinent to the patient's condition. This, more than the technology of venipuncture, is the nurse's real contribution to the patient's care.

Second, the nurse must become a *lifelong learner*. If, as is estimated, fully half of the knowledge transmitted in health education programs is obsolete by the time the student graduates, lifelong learning is the only viable strategy for the nurse who wants to remain current. The public expects safe care from health professionals and holds them accountable for their practice, as it should. Fulfilling that expectation requires more than just continuous practice. It requires the continuous search for knowledge that can be applied in practice. The era when the nurse could claim a degree and state certification as an adequate basis for lifelong practice is long gone, never to return.

Third, the nurse in our information society must *use every available tool* to keep up to date. Computer literacy is receiving increased emphasis in educational programs; soon, it will be expected of every practicing nurse. But beyond the ability to operate computers, today's nurse needs *access* to new information. Not graced with the time to sift through the mountains of new information created each day, she needs comprehensive, reliable, and easily assimilated sources of the information she needs to keep up to date.

This book, the first of a new annual series, fulfills all three of these needs. It presents the latest developments in emergency care, diagnostic tests, drugs, detection and treatment of disease, nursing procedures, and law, ethics, and professional practice—always with an emphasis on how these developments affect nurses and the nursing profession. Major developments, such as new trends in cardiopulmonary-cerebral resuscitation and new guidelines from the Centers for Disease Control for isolation in infectious diseases, receive detailed coverage. Essays by respected authorities explore the controversial topics of DRGs and nurses as professionals. And, in each chapter, the Tips & trends section highlights some of the most exciting and pertinent developments and discoveries.

Today's nurse can't be expected to know everything, of course. But she is expected to keep her knowledge base current, to keep abreast of the latest developments affecting her and her profession. *Yearbook86/87*, the first of a series of annual updates, is designed to provide the timely information she needs to do so. It should have a place on every nurse's bookshelf.

CAROL A. LINDEMAN, RN, PhD, FAAN

CHANGES AND CHOICES

THE YEAR IN REVIEW

"The evidence is indisputable—a health care revolution is indeed under way in this country."

BY LILLIAN S. BRUNNER, RN, Litt.D, FAAN

The evidence is indisputable—a health care revolution is indeed under way in this country. Perhaps never before have so many radical changes simultaneously affected so many areas of the health care industry. Certainly never before have they influenced nursing so profoundly. How we choose to respond to these changes will determine our professional role now and in the years to come. To make positive choices, we must clearly understand the roots of these changes—social, technologic, and economic—and their specific implications for nursing.

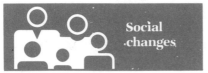

Some of the most profound trends in health care have their roots in social changes. Over the past decade or so, American society has come to value the quality of personal life more than ever. Today's challenge is to prevent illness, achieve wellness, and maintain health. Note the growing emphasis on safety, health, and fitness; the growing awareness that many health problems are lifestyle–related; and the new emphasis on correcting unhealthy habits.

Underlying and magnifying these trends is a critical population shift. The percentage of elderly persons is growing, as societal and medical advances keep increasing the life span. As a result, maintaining good health for as long as possible has become more and more important.

How are these trends affecting nursing? Historically, nurses have been concerned with only one end of the health care spectrum, caring for (usually in hospitals) the end result of unhealthy social practices, destructive life-styles, poor nutrition, and ill-planned fitness programs. But now we are beginning to break the bonds that tied us to the bedside and are responding to needs outside the hospital. We're finding ways to meet these needs in alternative care settings such as community nursing centers, urgent care centers, and ambulatory care units. We should welcome this expanded role—after all, who's better prepared than nurses to guide the public in self-care?

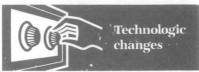

New technology has always found quick application to medicine and continues to provide almost daily progress in diagnostic and treatment methods. New techniques are the norm today—limited only by economic constraints. Fortunately, most medical technology is accessible to the average hospital, and it's changing the way nurses work. Computers have invaded the nurses' station, with software systems for tracking patient illness acuity and diagnosis, quality assurance, staffing and scheduling, performance appraisal, and cost control all demanding the nurse's understanding, flexibility, and willingness to learn new ways of working. In addition, self-regulating machines such as intravenous pumps may cut out some routine nursing tasks; however, they also require a higher level of expertise for using and monitoring the equipment.

This constant and rapid obsolescence of knowledge and techniques is causing even deeper changes in nursing. It has forced a shift in nursing education programs from content to process—emphasizing computer literacy and the ability to access new information, deemphasizing traditional nursing skills. At the same time, it has opened new opportunities for clinical and administrative specialization, creating new positions that require a high level of technical expertise. The new technology challenges nurses to blend their traditional role—as patient advocate and care-provider—with the new demands of high-tech professionalism.

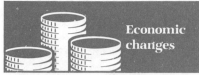

Perhaps the most radical changes in the health care industry are those resulting from the revised system of federal reimbursement for Medicare—from a retrospective to a prospective payment system based on diagnosis-related groups (DRGs).

These economic changes, designed to impose cost-containment, are exerting a profound effect on the entire health care delivery system. As a result, hospitals are admitting fewer, but often sicker, patients and discharging them earlier to avoid unrecoupable costs, increasing the need for continuing care outside the hospital.

These changes are influencing nursing in every area, from staffing to allocation of supplies. This cost-constrained hospital environment makes accurate patient assessment, careful planning, timely intervention, and precise evaluation of outcome more important than ever. It requires nurses to use advanced knowledge and skill not only to care for patients in the hospital, but also to prepare them and their families for continuing care in the community by planning for discharge and posthospital transition, including self-care teaching and use of community resources.

These economic trends have other professional implications as well. Inevitably, closer attention to costs has meant closer monitoring of nursing staff efficiency and some hospital staffing cuts. The demand for new hospital nurses has diminished slowly from the boom years of the 1970s. Some doomsayers have actually gone so far as to predict nursing's eventual demise, with nurses finally being squeezed out of the health care picture between a growing number of doctors and a legion of less-skilled but less-expensive aides and other ancillary workers. But this will

not happen. Why? For one thing, acutely ill hospital patients require highly skilled nursing care. And, for another, nursing opportunities outside the hospital are increasing. Nurses now have the opportunity to practice in nontraditional settings—home care, ambulatory care units, and independent practice. From this point of view, the economic and professional opportunities for nurses are perhaps *greater* than ever—if we adapt to these new conditions and take control of their effects on our profession. We must become a political force strong enough to influence and direct necessary changes. To accomplish this, we must learn more about health care economics. For example, all of us need to develop a keener sense of cost-benefit ratios in the areas of treatment, equipment, and supplies and to work more closely with doctors and hospital administrators in monitoring cost variables. We need to do everything possible to help administrators define the actual cost of nursing services and separate them from room and board charges. The traditional practice of burying the cost of nursing services within the daily room rate misleadingly inflates nursing costs and exaggerates the risk of staffing cuts.

The question isn't whether the health care system will continue to change—it surely will, and in ways that will have a lasting impact, both professionally and personally, on all of us. The question is *who* will influence the shape of this change. As the largest group of health care providers, we nurses occupy a uniquely powerful position in the system. But like a sleeping giant, we don't yet recognize our own power and potential influence. Will we wake up and assert ourselves or sit by and wait for a future determined and dominated by others? The choice is ours.

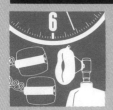

Emergency care

Life-support update—
Cardiopulmonary-cerebral resuscitation

Despite continuing refinement of cardiopulmonary resuscitation (CPR) techniques, far too many successfully resuscitated patients ultimately suffer fatal cerebral damage or, if they survive, are left with irreversible neurologic deficits. Consequently, recent research has focused on improving the neurologic prognosis in victims of cardiac arrest (and victims of other acutely life-threatening conditions, such as severe shock, focal brain ischemia, head trauma, severe hypothermia or hyperthermia, cerebral hemorrhage, and encephalitis) by developing new protocols for cardiopulmonary-cerebral resuscitation (CPCR). This research has identified three critical steps for ensuring optimum brain recovery after an ischemic episode: maximized oxygenation and improved blood flow during resuscitation, followed by meticulous brain-oriented postresuscitation management. These steps are the essentials of CPCR.

Maximized oxygenation

Of course, adequate ventilation is essential during CPCR—but too often it's not achieved. Mounting evidence suggests that the most severe cerebral damage may result not from complete cerebral anoxia but rather from *incomplete* hypoxia caused by improper resuscitation techniques. Inadequate cerebral perfusion from "trickle flow" oxygenation, as commonly results from manual ventilation, acts as a catalyst to release harmful biochemical products that eventually destroy larger masses of brain cells and produce gross cerebral edema. (See the flowchart on page 6 for a detailed explanation of this process.) Yet recent experiments have shown that maximum oxgenation of brain cells can reverse this process and restore virtually complete function, even if oxygenation is delayed for up to 1 hour.

The best way to ensure maximum oxygenation is through proper resuscitation techniques. Most rescuers outside the hospital will use the common bag-valve-mask (BVM) breathing device. To be effective, BVM requires meticulous technique. But even with perfect technique—ensuring an airtight seal between the mask and the patient's face and delivering the proper amount of air in the proper rhythm—the BVM can create problems. The airtight mask traps exhaled carbon dioxide and gives it back to the patient, possibly leading to hypercapnia and dangerous respiratory acidosis. To prevent this, rescuers should deliver oxygen—preferably 100% O_2—as soon as possible after starting CPCR. Many newer BVM devices have an oxygen reservoir or accumulator that allows direct delivery of oxygen through the mask.

But the most reliable method of oxygen delivery is through an endotracheal tube. Intubation allows precise control of oxygen delivery, minimizes airway control problems, and also enables rapid drug administration. Therefore, intubation should be done as soon as possible after initiation of basic CPR and defibrillation, and maintained throughout CPCR if necessary.

Improved blood flow

Adequate blood oxygenation itself isn't enough to prevent cerebral ischemia. To ensure adequate cerebral perfusion, cerebral blood flow must be maintained at 20% of normal, at least. Unfortunately, standard closed-chest CPR can't always accomplish this. The primary factor is time: the longer the time between onset of cardiac arrest and initiation of CPR, the less effective CPR is in maintaining the required cerebral blood flow. In the most common causes of sudden cardiac arrest, CPR is much more effective if started immediately postarrest than if delayed for even a few minutes. The reason? Circulatory stasis before CPR begins allows blood sludging and clotting with varying degrees of venous pooling, capillary leakage, and vasoparalysis. This lowers the cerebral perfusion pressure (mean arterial pressure minus cerebral venous or intracranial pressure) necessary to maintain cerebral blood flow and prevent ischemia.

"New" CPR techniques. But even when started promptly, standard closed-chest CPR often can't maintain adequate cerebral perfusion pressure. Based on the discovery that forward blood flow during closed-chest CPR is influenced as much by intrathoracic pressure fluctuations as by direct heart compressions (which are usually inadequate in closed-chest CPR), newer modified CPR techniques attempt to enhance cerebral perfusion pressure by pneumatic means. *Simultaneous ventilation-compression (SVC) CPR* involves simultaneous high pressure ventilations and closed-chest compressions. This experimental technique requires endotracheal intubation to create the extremely high airway pressures

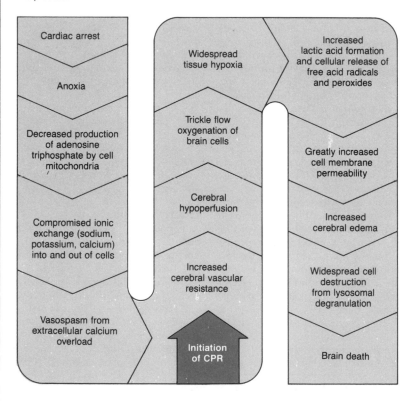

CEREBRAL ISCHEMIA DURING C.P.R.

Cardiac arrest leads to widespread tissue anoxia, setting off a complex chain of cellular reactions that eventually involve the brain. As shown below, the "trickle flow" oxygenation typically provided by manual CPR actually contributes to, rather than helps reverse, this process.

Cardiac arrest

Anoxia

Decreased production of adenosine triphosphate by cell mitochondria

Compromised ionic exchange (sodium, potassium, calcium) into and out of cells

Vasospasm from extracellular calcium overload

Widespread tissue hypoxia

Trickle flow oxygenation of brain cells

Cerebral hypoperfusion

Increased cerebral vascular resistance

Initiation of CPR

Increased lactic acid formation and cellular release of free acid radicals and peroxides

Greatly increased cell membrane permeability

Increased cerebral edema

Widespread cell destruction from lysosomal degranulation

Brain death

ESSENTIALS OF CARDIOPULMONARY-CEREBRAL RESUSCITATION

Cardiopulmonary-cerebral resuscitation comprises the ABCs of standard CPR (airway control, breathing support, and circulation support) plus measures designed to prevent or reverse the effects of cerebral hypoxia. These measures, outlined below, are only guidelines; actual steps will depend on the patient's condition and needs.

BASIC LIFE-SUPPORT TASKS	ADVANCED LIFE-SUPPORT TASKS
Airway control • Open airway using head tilt/neck lift, head tilt/chin lift, or jaw thrust method. • Attempt to inflate lungs using bag-valve-mask device or mouth-to-mouth method. • Relieve obstructed airway using finger-sweep clearing of mouth and throat, back blows, or abdominal thrusts.	• Assist with endotracheal intubation, cricothyrotomy, or tracheostomy, as necessary. • Suction airway.
Breathing support • Perform mouth-to-mouth ventilation or use bag-valve-mask device with oxygen flow.	• Assist with mechanical ventilation. • Monitor arterial blood gases.
Circulation support • Check carotid pulse. • Perform manual chest compression. • Control external hemorrhage, if severe, using tourniquets or pressure dressings. • Position patient supine with legs elevated 20° to 30°.	• Monitor cardiac rhythm through electrocardiography. • Defibrillate. • Start an I.V. lifeline. • Administer I.V. fluids and drugs (such as epinephrine, sodium bicarbonate, antiarrhythmics, and vasopressors), as necessary. • Apply medical antishock trousers (MAST suit), if necessary.
Cerebral resuscitation • Monitor level of consciousness. • Maintain optimal oxygenation and circulation during initial resuscitation, as outlined above.	• Maintain moderate hyperventilation (P_{CO_2} at 25 to 35 mm Hg), moderate hyperoxygenation (PO_2 >100 mm Hg), and physiologic pH (7.3 to 7.6) through the use of mechanical ventilation, as ordered. • Maintain normotension (mean arterial pressure 90 to 100 mm Hg and systolic blood pressure >100 mm Hg) and normal blood volume through the use of I.V. colloids and crystalloids, blood products, and vasopressors or antihypertensives, as ordered. • Prevent increased intracranial pressure by elevating the head of the bed 30°, avoiding head turning or neck constriction, minimizing suctioning, and administering corticosteroids and diuretics, as ordered. • As ordered, reduce metabolic demands by administering sedatives and by maintaining normothermia or slight hypothermia through the use of a cooling blanket and antipyretics. • Monitor blood parameters, such as hematocrit, glucose, electrolytes, osmolality, and albumin, to maintain optimal physiologic functioning.

needed. Additional asynchronous ventilations (with a BVM) are also required, as in standard CPR, to provide air exchange.

Interposed abdominal compression (IAC) CPR consists of alternating abdominal compressions and closed-chest compressions, with interposed lung inflations. The abdominal compressions, provided by hand or binder, attempt to enhance venous return to the thorax, increasing blood volume in the central circulation and helping to load the heart for its next compression cycle. But while this technique raises mean arterial pressure, it may not increase cerebral perfusion pressure and enhance blood flow to the brain. Currently, the most effective methods of augmenting blood volume are application of medical antishock trousers (MAST suit) or I.V. challenge. Both of these methods have serious drawbacks, however, chief of which is the risk of elevated intracranial pressure. The new CPR techniques, while promising, are all still experimental.

Open-chest CPR. Despite increasing evidence of closed-chest CPR's inherent drawbacks, the time-tested technique of open-chest CPR is often overlooked. Open-chest CPR provides much higher cerebral perfusion pressures than any closed-chest CPR technique. Of course, open-chest CPR can be done only by a skilled doctor in a hospital setting; but when possible, it should be considered 5 to 10 minutes after cardiac arrest.

Drugs. Drugs are often necessary to enhance blood flow during CPCR. Epinephrine is typically the first drug given. Among its many important effects is increased systemic peripheral vascular resistance (without coronary or cerebral vasoconstriction), which ultimately leads to increased perfusion pressure and enhanced cerebral blood flow.

Sodium bicarbonate, given before epinephrine (never in the same infusion), reverses acidosis by neutralizing the fixed acids released from hypoxic tissue during the borderline perfusion of CPCR. But it must be given judiciously; too much can lead to alkalosis, which *impairs* oxygen release from hemoglobin (among other effects), even at high saturation levels. Often hyperventilation alone can restore acid-base balance, particularly if begun promptly after cardiac arrest; but if sodium bicarbonate is given, further hyperventilation is necessary to enhance its effects.

Brain-oriented postresuscitation management

Cardiac arrest usually causes multiple organ failure of varying severity and duration. Common features of this post-arrest syndrome include protracted acidosis and reduced cardiac output; respiratory complications, disseminated intravascular coagulation, and hepatic and renal failure may also develop. So postresuscitation management—intensive care life support for multiple organ failure—should begin immediately after successful resuscitation and restoration of spontaneous circulation. The patient's neurologic prognosis depends on the early start and high quality of this care. While these measures can't change the initial injury, they can prevent or diminish some of the secondary systemic changes resulting from reoxygenation and reperfusion—changes that ultimately have deleterious effects on the brain.

Brain-oriented postresuscitation management focuses on stabilizing respiratory, cardiovascular, metabolic, renal, and hepatic function; slowing brain metabolism; reducing cerebral edema; and providing body maintenance. Specific steps and procedures are detailed in the chart on the previous page.

Nurses play a vital role in postresuscitation management. As chief monitors of the patient's condition, they are usually first to recognize even subtle changes that could signal a serious complication. As chief care providers, nurses can do much to promote the patient's recovery from postarrest syndrome and achieve the ultimate goal of CPCR—complete brain recovery.

BARRY J. BURTON, RN, BSN, CEN

Radiation emergencies

Barring nuclear warfare, most human radiation exposure will continue to result from medical, industrial, or laboratory accidents, as the use of radioactive materials increases. Recognizing this, the Joint Commission on the Accreditation of Hospitals (JCAH) requires all general hospital emergency rooms to have written procedures for handling victims of radiation exposure or contamination. Because these incidents are so rare, however, most medical personnel aren't familiar with the protocol for managing a radiation emergency. Use this guide to review what happens in a radiation emergency and your role in such a situation.

Prehospital care: What's been done

Usually, a person exposed to radiation displays no immediate acute effects and may not be brought to the hospital unless his exposure level is extremely high or he's also sustained associated trauma. If rescue personnel decided to transport the patient to the hospital, they would have notified emergency department (ED) personnel and ideally would have provided a brief history of the accident, including the source of radiation and any associated injuries. They would also have stabilized the patient's airway, breathing, and circulation.

What to do first

Once you've been notified that a patient with acute radiation exposure is being transported to your ED, begin to prepare for his arrival. Depending on your hospital's facilities and protocol, expect to:

• prepare a treatment room by enclosing an isolated area with lead-lined shields, or arrange to care for the patient in your hospital's X-ray room. Cover the floor of the area with newspaper or non-skid plastic.

• notify hospital maintenance personnel to shut off the air circulation system in the treatment area, if necessary.

• gather the equipment necessary to care for the patient, such as a Geiger-Müller (G-M) counter, cleansing materials (water, soap, scrub brushes), plastic or lead-lined containers for radioactive clothing and rinse water, personal dosimeters for hospital staff to wear while treating the patient, and emergency equipment, as appropriate.

• protect yourself from possible contamination by donning a surgical cap, mask, gown, gloves, and shoe coverings.

What to do next

When the patient arrives in the ED, quickly determine the extent of his contamination with the G-M counter. If you detect external contamination, cover him with a plastic sheet and move him to the treatment room. Quickly assess the patient for any serious associated injuries; treat these, as necessary, before beginning decontamination procedures.

Any open wounds or radiation burns require immediate treatment to prevent internalization of contamination. Assist with irrigation, cleansing, and debridement, as necessary; then apply waterproof dressings. Because the debrided material is radioactive, be sure to discard it into approved containers for special disposal. If the patient's burns are extensive, you may need to arrange for his transfer to a special burn unit.

Once the patient is stable, remove his clothing, shoes, and any jewelry or other metal objects. Place these items in plastic or lead-lined containers marked RADIOACTIVE: DO NOT DISCARD. Then cleanse the contaminated areas of his body with soap and water,

RADIATION FACTS

Types of radiation
Ionizing radiation exists in several forms:
• *Alpha particles* are emitted from heavy radioactive elements, such as plutonium. These positively charged particles release their energy very rapidly and can seriously damage cells in the area of contamination. However, because alpha particles don't penetrate the epidermis, they can be eliminated easily by removing contaminated clothing and washing exposed skin. Alpha particles can cause serious systemic effects only if they are ingested or inhaled or somehow penetrate the epidermis.
• *Beta particles* are emitted from the nucleus of most radioisotopes during beta decay. They're smaller and usually have less energy than alpha particles. Able to penetrate skin up to 5 mm (although clothing may block them), beta particles can burn exposed skin but are most dangerous if introduced internally.
• *Gamma rays, X-rays,* and *neutrons,* the most hazardous forms of radiation, penetrate deeply and can cause acute cellular damage in the most radiosensitive tissues—bone marrow, gonads, and gastrointestinal epithelium. Gamma rays are produced from beta decay of most radioisotopes following beta particle emission. X-rays are emitted by X-ray machines and by nuclear accelerators. Neutrons are emitted by nuclear reactors and accelerators and are found in fallout from thermonuclear weapons.

Measuring exposure
Exposure to radiation is measured in *roentgens* (R) and expressed as the *rad* (radiation absorbed dose) or the *rem* (roentgen equivalent in man). The rad is a measure of absorbed dose that varies with the type of radiation source and the tissue irradiated. The rem is a unit of

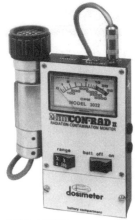

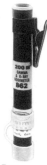

Geiger-Müller counter   **Pen dosimeter**

absorbed dose indicating the rad-equivalent effect in humans. The National Council on Radiation Protection and Measurement (NCRP) has established a maximum safe exposure limit of 500 mrem (0.5 rem) per year for nonoccupationally exposed adults; less for children and pregnant women. NCRP guidelines for emergency situations suggest a maximum safe single whole-body dose of 25,000 mrem (25 rem).

Several instruments can be used to measure radiation exposure. The Geiger-Müller (G-M) counter accurately detects low levels of radiation; an ionization chamber-type meter is more useful for high levels. A liquid or crystal scintillation isotope counter is used in the laboratory to measure radiation and identify the source element. The familiar personal dosimeter, worn as a badge, pen, or ring, registers cumulative exposure.

---

scrubbing vigorously. Pay particular attention to his feet, hands and head. Copiously rinse his eyes, ears, nose, and mouth, and wash his hair thoroughly.

Continue cleansing procedures until the G-M counter registers no external contamination. Be sure to save all wash water in plastic or lead-lined containers for safe disposal.

If cleansing doesn't reduce radiation levels, the patient may have internal contamination. Obtain blood, urine, and saliva samples, and save all body wastes in plastic bags for contamination screening. Depending on the patient's contamination level and the source of radiation exposure, you may be asked to assist with gastric lavage or to administer a cathartic or emetic

UNDERSTANDING ACUTE RADIATION SYNDROME

Whole-body exposure to gamma ray or neutron radiation can produce varied effects, depending on the total dose. Use this chart to help you identify these effects and the appropriate interventions.

SYNDROME AND WHOLE-BODY DOSE	CLINICAL MANIFESTATIONS	INTERVENTIONS
Prodromal syndrome 0 to 100 rad	Possible mild nausea and vomiting (occasionally diarrhea and anorexia) lasting only 24 hours; also transient mild decrease in leukocyte and platelet levels 4 to 5 weeks later.	Calm and reassure patient; administer antiemetic. Follow up complete blood count (CBC) on outpatient basis.
Hematopoietic syndrome (mild) 100 to 300 rad	Nausea, vomiting, and fatigue for 2 to 4 days; leukocyte and platelet depression (nadir in 3 weeks); temporary aspermatogenesis and amenorrhea; complete recovery in several months.	Monitor CBC; encourage rest; teach patient to avoid exposure to infectious agents and to avoid injury.
Hematopoietic syndrome (severe) 300 to 600 rad	Mild gastrointestinal symptoms; severe leukopenia and thrombocytopenia (nadir in 3 to 5 weeks); signs of infection (fever, chills, malaise, and pharyngitis); signs of bleeding (gingival bleeding, petechiae, and ecchymoses); epilation (loss of hair) 2 to 3 weeks after exposure.	Reverse isolation and strict aseptic technique necessary; antibiotic therapy specific for infection; blood transfusions; bone marrow transplant may be necessary.
Gastrointestinal syndrome 600 to 1,000+ rad	Severe nausea, vomiting, and bloody diarrhea occur within hours after exposure and persist; severe leukopenia and thrombocytopenia (nadir in 2 to 3 weeks); dehydration, metabolic alkalosis, and electrolyte imbalance occur within 1 week; epilation; shock, hemorrhage, and severe infection may result in 1 to 3 weeks.	Aggressive fluid and electrolyte replacement necessary; blood transfusions; reverse isolation.
Central nervous system syndrome > 2,000 rad	Immediately after exposure, severe nausea and vomiting, confusion, headache, burning sensation; within several hours, symptoms progress to ataxia, tremors, convulsions, and circulatory collapse.	Death ensues in hours to 2 days despite treatment; medicate patient for pain, treat symptomatically, and maintain comfort.

agent to help eliminate the radioactive material from the patient's gastrointestinal system. If contamination is more pervasive, you may also administer a chelating agent to absorb the radioactive material, or a blocking agent—such as potassium iodide—to prevent uptake of radioiodide by the thyroid gland.

After patient decontamination is completed, decontaminate yourself by washing with soap and water until the G-M counter readings are at acceptable levels. Remove your gown, mask, gloves, and shoe coverings and place them in plastic containers for disposal with the other radioactive materials.

SANDRA LUDWIG NETTINA, RN, BSN

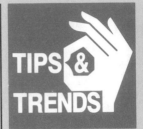

QUICK, CONVENIENT

New care centers

The fastest-growing sector of the health care delivery system, ambulatory care centers (sometimes called urgent- or immediate-care centers) are springing up all over the country, with more than 3,500 centers expected to be in operation by early 1986. Usually located in highly visible, easily accessible areas, such as suburban shopping centers, these walk-in clinics offer an alternative to hospital emergency departments and doctors' offices, providing quick, convenient medical attention at moderate prices.

Typically, the centers are staffed by a doctor, one or two nurses, and an X-ray technician, and are open 12 to 16 hours per day, 7 days per week, 365 days per year.

Although not equipped to handle major medical emergencies, most of these centers can at least stabilize emergency patients, and some offer transportation to the nearest hospital. Most often, they treat common complaints or minor trauma; they also offer routine procedures and diagnostic tests.

NEW EMERGENCY APPLICATIONS

High-frequency jet ventilation

Originally developed for use when high peak airway pressures or large intrapleural air leaks precluded conventional mechanical ventilation, high-frequency jet ventilation (HFJV) may have other important clinical applications as well. The HFJV system employs a narrow injector cannula to deliver short, rapid bursts of oxygen to the airways under low pressure. This combination of high rate, low tidal volumes, and low pressure enhances alveolar gas exchange without elevating peak inspiratory pressures and compromising cardiac output—the major drawback of conventional high volume, high pressure mechanical ventilation. Thus, HFJV is valuable for patients with hemodynamic instability and those (such as young children) at high risk for pulmonary barotrauma. It's also useful for ventilating patients during bronchoscopy, laryngoscopy, and laryngeal surgery, because its narrow cannula doesn't obstruct the operating field.

But the most exciting new uses of HFJV are in emergency situations. Because the cannula can be inserted directly into the trachea through a cricothyrotomy, HFJV may be used when upper airway trauma or obstruction precludes intubation. Use of HFJV in cardiopulmonary resuscitation enables continuous ventilation during chest compression. And its use in patients with chest trauma decreases chest wall movement and improves stability, enhancing ventilation.

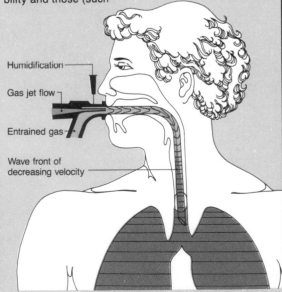

Humidification

Gas jet flow

Entrained gas

Wave front of decreasing velocity

SURFACE OXIMETRY MEASURES BOWEL TISSUE PERFUSION

A new role for oximetry

For years, researchers have tried to develop a quick, reliable method of assessing bowel tissue viability after an ischemic insult, such as mesenteric artery occlusion or bowel strangulation. They've known that accurate determination of tissue perfusion can improve the success rate of bowel resection and anastomosis, decrease postoperative complications, and lessen the need for follow-up procedures, such as laparotomy and reanastomosis. Now it appears that surface oximetry, a noninvasive method of measur-

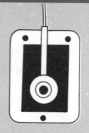

ing systemic blood oxygenation, can accurately measure perfusion in discrete areas of the bowel and possibly in other critical organs as well.

In oximetry, heated electrodes placed on the skin surface—typically on an earlobe—transmit light waves through a vascular bed and measure their resulting wavelengths;

this information is relayed to a microprocessor that calculates and displays systemic arterial oxygen saturation value.

Researchers found that by placing miniaturized oxygen electrodes directly on suspected ischemic areas of bowel tissue, they could quickly measure tissue oxygenation and, since oximetry provides constant monitoring, instantaneously detect any change. Because this promising technique precisely locates areas of ischemia, it could prove invaluable in guiding surgical intervention.

NEW SKIN COVERINGS IMPROVE BURN CARE

Artificial skin and autologous cultured epithelium

Extensive burns are among the most painful and difficult to treat of all health problems. One of the biggest difficulties is the urgent need to cover large open burn wounds to conserve body fluids and prevent infection. Until recently, autografts or allografts were the coverings of choice, despite their many inherent disadvantages, such as limited availability and susceptibility to contractures, tissue rejection, and infection. Now, two new burn coverings—artificial skin and autologous cultured epithelium—offer new hope for victims of serious burns.

Artificial skin
Artificial skin is a temporary burn covering consisting of a dermal-like lower layer, comprised of bovine hide collagen and chondroitin-6-sulfate extracted from shark cartilage, and an outer layer of medical grade Silastic, a polymeric silicone substance. As the burn wound heals, mesodermal cells migrate into the lower layer and eventually, as the artificial layer degrades, begin to form a viable dermis. Once the dermis has formed, the outer layer can be removed and replaced with an autograft.

Autologous skin
Developed at the Shriner's Burn Institute in Boston,

autologous cultured epithelium, as its name implies, is new skin grown in the laboratory from cells of the burn victim's undamaged skin. Full-thickness skin biopsies are minced and trypsinized to produce a single-cell suspension, which is cultured in test tubes. Sheets of cultured cells are then applied directly to the cleaned and debrided burn wound, forming a permanent epidermis that is resistant to contracture formation and reduces the risk of rejection. And, perhaps most significantly for victims of extensive burns, this technique can generate a virtually limitless supply of new skin.

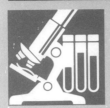

Diagnostic tests

Acetylcholine receptor antibodies

The acetylcholine receptor (AChR) antibodies test is the most useful immunologic test for confirming acquired (autoimmune) myasthenia gravis (MG). This disorder of neuromuscular transmission can affect muscles innervated by cranial nerves, such as those of the face, lips, tongue, neck, and throat, as well as other muscle groups. In normal muscle contraction, acetylcholine (ACh) is released from the terminal end of the nerve and binds to AChR sites on the muscle motor end plate. In MG, however, antibodies block and destroy AChR sites, causing muscle weakness that can be either generalized or localized to the ocular muscles.

Two test methods—a binding assay and a blocking assay—are now available to determine the relative concentration of AChR antibodies in serum. In the binding assay, purified AChRs are complexed with ^{125}I-labeled α-bungarotoxin (a molecule that binds specifically to AChRs and blocks them). A serum sample is added to this complex; after incubation, antihuman immunoglobulin is added. Antibodies bind to AChR–^{125}I-labeled α-bungarotoxin complexes, which coprecipitate with the total human immunoglobulin. The amount of radioactivity is then measured to assay the available AChR sites. AChR-binding antibodies are found in about 90% of patients with generalized MG and in about 50% of those with localized MG.

When the AChR-binding assay is negative in a patient with MG symptoms, the AChR-blocking assay may be performed. Here, the patient's serum is incubated with purified AChRs before ^{125}I-labeled α-bungarotoxin is added, to detect antibodies whose antigenic sites would otherwise be blocked. The blocking assay is relatively new, and its clinical significance is not yet fully known. However, it is specific for the autoimmune form of MG and is useful for research. Determination of AChR antibodies by either method also helps monitor immunosuppressive therapy for MG, although antibody levels do not usually parallel the severity of the disease.

Purpose
• To confirm diagnosis of MG
• To monitor the effectiveness of immunosuppressive therapy for MG.

Patient preparation
Explain to the patient that this test helps confirm MG or, when indicated, tell him the test assesses the effectiveness of treatment.

Advise the patient that he needn't restrict food or fluids. Tell him that the test requires a blood sample, who will perform the test and when, and that he may experience transient discomfort from the needle puncture and the pressure of the tourniquet. Reassure him that collecting the sample takes less than 3 minutes.

Check patient history for immunosuppressive drugs that may affect test results. Note such use on the laboratory slip.

Procedure
Perform a venipuncture, and collect the sample in a 7-ml *red-top* tube.

Precautions
Keep the sample at room temperature and send it to the laboratory immediately.

Values
Normal serum values are negative or ≤0.03 nmol/liter for AChR-binding antibodies and negative for AChR-blocking antibodies.

Implications of results
Positive AChR antibodies in symptomatic adults confirm diagnosis of MG. Patients who have only ocular symp-

HOW ACETYLCHOLINE RECEPTOR ANTIBODIES DISRUPT MYONEURAL TRANSMISSION

In myasthenia gravis, nerve impulse transmission breaks down when acetylcholine receptor (AChR) antibodies block and destroy acetylcholine receptor sites. This causes generalized or localized muscle weakness by interfering with acetylcholine's normal movement from the nerve terminal to the AChR site at the myoneural junction.

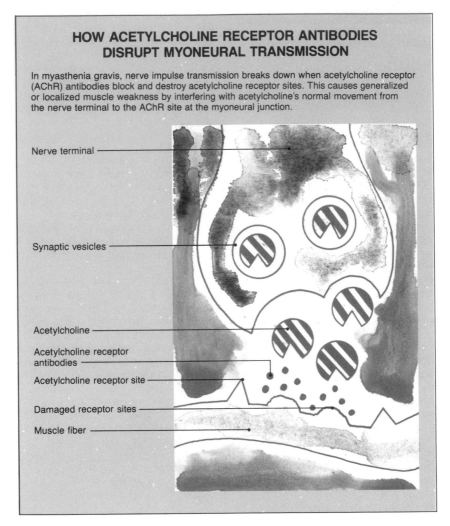

Nerve terminal

Synaptic vesicles

Acetylcholine

Acetylcholine receptor antibodies

Acetylcholine receptor site

Damaged receptor sites

Muscle fiber

toms of MG tend to have lower antibody titers than those who have generalized symptoms.

Post-test care

• Since a patient with an autoimmune disease has a compromised immune system, check the venipuncture site for infection, and report any changes promptly. Keep a clean, dry bandage over the site for at least 24 hours.

• If a hematoma develops at the venipuncture site, ease discomfort by applying warm soaks.

Interfering factors

• Failure to maintain the sample at room temperature and to send it to the laboratory immediately may affect the accurate determination of test results.

• Patients undergoing thymectomy, thoracic duct drainage, immunosuppressive therapy, or plasmapheresis may show reduced AChR-antibody levels.

• Patients with amyotrophic lateral sclerosis may show false-positive test results.

SR. REBECCA FIDLER, MT(ASCP), PhD

Androstenedione

This test helps identify the causes of various disorders related to altered estrogen levels. Androstenedione, secreted by the adrenal cortex and the gonads, is converted to estrone (an estrogen of relatively low biologic activity) by adipose tissue and the liver. In premenopausal women, the amount of estrogen derived from androstenedione is relatively small compared to the amount of the more potent estrogen, estradiol, secreted by the ovaries. Usually, estrogen derived from androstenedione doesn't interfere with gonadotropin feedback during the menstrual cycle. But in such conditions as obesity, increased adrenal production of androstenedione or increased conversion of androstenedione to estrone may interfere with normal feedback, causing menstrual irregularities.

In children and postmenopausal women, estrone is a major source of estrogen. Increased androstenedione production or increased conversion to estrone may induce premature sexual development in children and renewed ovarian stimulation, endometriosis, bleeding, and polycystic ovaries in postmenopausal women. In men, excess androstenedione may cause feminizing signs, such as gynecomastia.

Purpose

To aid in determining the cause of gonadal dysfunction, menstrual or menopausal irregularities, and premature sexual development.

Patient preparation

Explain to the patient that this test helps determine the cause of symptoms. Tell her it requires a blood sample, who will perform the venipuncture and when, and that she may experience transient discomfort from the needle puncture. If appropriate, explain that the test should be done 1 week before or after her menstrual period and that

it may have to be repeated. As ordered, withhold steroid and pituitary-based hormones. If they must be continued, note it on the laboratory slip.

Procedure

Perform a venipuncture, and collect a serum sample in a 10-ml *red-top* tube. (Collect a plasma sample in a *green-top* tube.) Label it appropriately and send it to the laboratory immediately.

Precautions

• Handle the sample gently to prevent hemolysis. If a plasma sample is taken, refrigerate it or place it on ice.
• Record the patient's age, sex, and (if appropriate) phase of menstrual cycle on the laboratory slip.

Values

Females: Premenopausal—0.6 to 3 ng/ml; postmenopausal—0.3 to 8 ng/ml; males: 0.9 to 1.7 ng/ml.

Implications of results

Elevated androstenedione levels are associated with Stein-Leventhal syndrome; Cushing's syndrome; ovarian, testicular, or adrenocortical tumors; ectopic ACTH-producing tumors; late-onset congenital adrenal hyperplasia; and ovarian stromal hyperplasia. Elevated levels result in increased estrone levels, causing premature sexual development (in children); menstrual irregularities (in premenopausal women); bleeding, endometriosis, or polycystic ovaries (in postmenopausal women); or feminizing signs, such as gynecomastia (in men). Decreased levels occur in hypogonadism.

Post-test care

• If a hematoma develops at the venipuncture site, ease discomfort by applying warm soaks.
• As ordered, resume medications discontinued before the test.

Interfering factors

• Hemolysis due to rough handling of the sample may affect test results.

• Ingestion of steroids or pituitary hormones may alter test results.

WENDY BAKER, RN, MS, CCRN

Anion gap

The anion gap reflects serum anion-cation balance and helps distinguish types of metabolic acidosis without expensive, time-consuming measurement of all serum electrolytes. This test uses serum levels of routinely measured electrolytes—sodium (Na^+), chloride (Cl^-), and bicarbonate (HCO_3^-)—for a quick calculation based on a simple physical principle: total concentrations of cations and anions are normally equal, thereby maintaining electrical neutrality in serum. Since sodium accounts for more than 90% of circulating cations, whereas chloride and bicarbonate together account for 85% of the counterbalancing anions, the "gap" between measured cation and anion levels represents those anions not routinely measured (sulfate, phosphates, organic acids such as ketone bodies and lactic acid, and proteins).

An increased anion gap indicates an increase in one or more of these unmeasured anions, which may occur with acidoses characterized by excessive organic or inorganic acids, such as lactic acidosis or ketoacidosis.

A normal anion gap occurs in hyperchloremic acidoses, renal tubular acidosis, and severe bicarbonate-wasting conditions, such as biliary fistulas and poorly functioning ileal loops.

Purpose
• To distinguish types of metabolic acidosis
• To monitor renal function and I.V. hyperalimentation.

Patient preparation
Explain to the patient that this test helps determine the cause of acidosis. Inform him that he needn't restrict food or fluids before the test. Tell the patient that the test requires a blood sample, who will perform the venipuncture and when, and that he may feel discomfort from the needle puncture and the tourniquet. Reassure him that sample collection takes only a few minutes.

Check the patient's history for recent use of drugs (such as diuretics, corticosteroids, and antihypertensives) that may influence sodium, chloride, or bicarbonate blood levels. If they must be continued, note it on the laboratory slip.

Procedure
Perform a venipuncture, and collect the sample in a 10- to 15-ml *red-top* tube.

Precautions
Handle the sample gently to prevent hemolysis, which can interfere with accurate determination of test results.

Values
Normally, the anion gap ranges from 8 to 14 mEq/liter.

Implications of results
A normal anion gap doesn't rule out

HOW ANION GAP RESULTS DISTINGUISH CAUSES OF METABOLIC ACIDOSIS

Metabolic acidosis with a *normal anion gap* (8 to 14 mEq/liter) occurs with conditions characterized by loss of bicarbonate:
• Hypokalemic acidosis, caused by renal tubular acidosis, diarrhea, or ureteral diversions
• Hyperkalemic acidosis, caused by acidifying agents (for example, NH_4Cl, HCl), hydronephrosis, or sickle cell nephropathy.

Metabolic acidosis with an *increased anion gap* (>14 mEq/liter) occurs with conditions characterized by accumulation of organic acids, sulfates, or phosphates:
• Renal failure
• Ketoacidosis, caused by starvation, diabetes mellitus, or alcohol
• Lactic acidosis
• Toxin ingestion, including salicylates, methanol, ethylene glycol (antifreeze), or paraldehyde.

metabolic acidosis. When acidosis results from loss of bicarbonate in the urine or other body fluids, renal reabsorption of sodium promotes retention of chloride, and the anion gap remains unchanged. Thus, metabolic acidosis caused by excessive chloride levels is called *normal anion gap acidosis.*

When acidosis results from accumulation of metabolic acids—as occurs in lactic acidosis, for example—the anion gap increases (above 14 mEq/liter) with the increase in unmeasured anions. Metabolic acidosis caused by such accumulation is known as a *high anion gap acidosis.* (See *How Anion Gap Results Distinguish Causes of Metabolic Acidosis,* for the possible causes of both normal and high anion gap acidoses.)

Because the anion gap only determines total anion-cation balance, it doesn't necessarily reflect abnormal values for individual electrolytes. Further investigation and diagnostic tests are usually necessary to determine the specific cause of metabolic acidosis.

A decreased anion gap (below 8 mEq/liter) is rare. However, it may occur with hypermagnesemia and with paraproteinemic states, such as multiple myeloma and Waldenström's macroglobulinemia.

Post-test care

• If a hematoma develops at the venipuncture site, apply warm soaks to relieve discomfort.

• As ordered, instruct the patient to resume use of any drugs discontinued before the test.

Interfering factors

• Diuretics, lithium, chlorpropamide, and vasopressin suppress serum sodium levels, possibly decreasing the anion gap; corticosteroids and antihypertensives elevate serum sodium levels and may increase the anion gap.

• Salicylates, paraldehyde, methicillin, dimercaprol, ammonium chloride, acetazolamide, ethylene glycol, and methyl alcohol decrease serum bicarbonate levels, possibly increasing the anion gap; ACTH, cortisone, mercurial or chlorthiazide diuretics, and excessive ingestion of alkalis or licorice elevate serum bicarbonate levels and may decrease the anion gap.

• Ammonium chloride, cholestyramine, boric acid, oxyphenbutazone, phenylbutazone, and excessive I.V. infusion of sodium chloride may elevate serum chloride levels and possibly decrease the anion gap.

• Thiazides, furosemide, ethacrynic acid, bicarbonates, or prolonged I.V. infusion of dextrose 5% in water can lower serum chloride levels and may increase the anion gap.

• Iodine absorption from wounds packed with povidone-iodine, or excessive use of magnesium-containing antacids (especially by patients with renal failure) may cause a spuriously low anion gap.

• Hemolysis due to rough handling of the sample may interfere with accurate determination of test results.

ANNETTE L. HARMON, RN, MSN

Antegrade pyelography

This radiographic procedure allows examination of the upper collecting system when ureteral obstruction rules out retrograde ureteropyelography or when cystoscopy is contraindicated. It depends on percutaneous needle puncture for injection of contrast medium into the renal pelvis or calyces. Antegrade pyelography also is indicated when excretory urography or renal ultrasonography demonstrates hydronephrosis and the need for therapeutic nephrostomy. After completion of radiographic studies, a nephrostomy tube can be inserted to provide temporary drainage or access for other therapeutic or diagnostic procedures.

Renal pressure can be measured during the procedure. Also, urine can be collected for cultures and cytologic studies and for evaluation of renal functional reserve before surgery.

Purpose
• To evaluate obstruction of the upper collecting system by stricture, stone, clot, or tumor
• To evaluate hydronephrosis revealed during excretory urography or ultrasonography and to enable accurate placement of a percutaneous nephrostomy tube
• To evaluate the function of the upper collecting system after ureteral surgery or urinary diversion
• To assess renal functional reserve before surgery.

Patient preparation
Explain to the patient that this test allows radiographic examination of the kidney. Instruct him to fast, if ordered, for 4 hours before the test. However, instruct him to continue to drink fluids (antegrade pyelography is most easily performed in dilated collecting systems). Tell the patient who will perform the test and where, and that it will take approximately 1 hour.

Inform the patient that a needle will be inserted into the kidney after he is given a sedative and a local anesthetic. Explain that urine may be collected from the kidney for testing and that, if necessary, a tube will be left in the kidney for drainage. Tell him that he may feel mild discomfort during injection of the local anesthetic and contrast medium and that he may also feel transient burning and flushing from the contrast medium. Warn him that the X-ray machine makes loud clacking sounds as films are taken.

Check the patient's history for hypersensitivity reactions to contrast media. Report any such sensitivities to the doctor. Also check the history and recent coagulation studies for indications of bleeding disorders.

Make sure that the patient or a responsible family member has signed an appropriate consent form. Just before the procedure, administer a sedative, as ordered.

Equipment
X-ray equipment, including a fluoroscope and possibly ultrasound equipment/percutaneous nephrostomy tray/manometer/preparatory tray/gloves and sterile containers for specimens/syringes and needles/contrast medium/local anesthetic/emergency resuscitation equipment.

Procedure
The patient is placed prone on the X-ray table. The skin over the kidney is cleansed with antiseptic solution, and a local anesthetic is injected.

Previous urographic films or ultrasound recordings are studied to identify critical anatomic landmarks. (It's important to determine if the kidney to be studied is in normal position. If not, the angle of the needle entry must be adjusted during percutaneous puncture.) Under guidance of fluoroscopy or ultrasound, the percutaneous needle is inserted below the 12th rib at the level of the transverse process of the 2nd lumbar vertebra. Aspiration of urine confirms that the needle has reached the dilated collecting system (usually 7 to 8 cm below the skin surface in adults).

Flexible tubing is connected to the needle to prevent displacement during the procedure. If intrarenal pressure is to be measured, the manometer is connected to the tubing as soon as it's in place. Urine specimens are then taken if needed.

An amount of urine equal to the amount of contrast medium to be injected is withdrawn to prevent overdistention of the collecting system. The contrast medium is injected under fluoroscopic guidance. Posteroanterior, oblique, and anteroposterior radiographs are taken. Ureteral peristalsis is observed on the fluoroscope screen to evaluate obstruction. A percutaneous nephrostomy tube is inserted at this time if drainage is needed because of increased renal pressure, dilatation, or intrarenal reflux. If drainage is not needed, the catheter is withdrawn and a sterile dressing is applied.

Precautions
• Antegrade pyelography is contraindicated in patients with bleeding disorders.
• Watch for signs of hypersensitivity to the contrast medium.

Findings
After injection of contrast medium, the upper collecting system should fill uniformly and appear normal in size and course. Normal structures should be outlined clearly.

Implications of results
Enlargements of the upper collecting system and parts of the ureteropelvic junction indicate obstruction. Antegrade pyelography shows the degree of dilatation, clearly defines obstructions, and demonstrates intrarenal reflux. In hydronephrosis, the ureteropelvic junction shows marked distention. Results of recent surgery or urinary diversion will be obvious; for example, a ureteral stent or a dilated stenotic area will be clearly visualized.

Intrarenal pressures that exceed 20 cmH_2O indicate obstruction. Cultures or cytologic studies of urine specimens taken during antegrade pyelography can confirm antegrade pyelonephrosis or malignancy.

Post-test care
• Check vital signs every 15 minutes for the first hour, every 30 minutes for the second hour, and every 2 hours for the next 24 hours.
• Check dressings for bleeding, hematoma, or urine leakage at the puncture site at each check of vital signs. For bleeding, apply pressure. For a hematoma, apply warm soaks to relieve discomfort. Report urine leakage to the doctor.
• Monitor fluid intake and urine output for 24 hours. Notify the doctor if the patient doesn't void within 8 hours. Observe each specimen for hematuria. Report hematuria if it persists after the third voiding.
• Watch for and report signs of sepsis or extravasation of contrast medium (chills, fever, rapid pulse or respirations, and hypotension).
• Also watch for and report signs that adjacent organs have been punctured: pain in the abdomen or flank, or pneumothorax (sudden onset of pleuritic chest pain, dyspnea, tachypnea, decreased breath sounds on the affected side, and tachycardia).
• If a nephrostomy tube is inserted, check to be sure that it is patent and draining well.
• Administer antibiotics for several days after the procedure, as ordered, to prevent infection. Administer analgesics as ordered.

Interfering factors
Recent barium procedures or the presence of feces or gas in the bowel can impair visualization of the kidney, inhibiting accurate results.

ELLEN SHIPES, RN, ET, MN, MEd

Antithrombin III test

This test helps detect the cause of impaired coagulation, especially hypercoagulation. Antithrombin III (AT III) inactivates thrombin and inhibits coagulation. Normally, a balance between AT III and thrombin creates hemostasis, whereas AT III deficiency increases coagulation.

Using a fresh, citrated blood sample, this test measures the ability of AT III to inhibit thrombin's enzymatic cleavage of p-nitroaniline (p-NA) from a small polypeptide chain. Cleavage of colored p-NA is measured spectrophotometrically and compared to control samples.

Normal values exceed 50% of control. Lower AT III levels can indicate disseminated intravascular coagulation, thromboembolic or hypercoagulation disorders, or hepatic diseases, such as cirrhosis. Slightly decreased levels can result from use of heparin or oral contraceptives, so be sure to note their use on the laboratory slip. Elevated levels can result from kidney transplant and use of oral anticoagulants or anabolic steroids.

WILLIAM E. KLINE, MS, MT(ASCP), SBB

Chorionic villi sampling

Chorionic villi sampling, or biopsy, is an experimental prenatal test that may someday replace amniocentesis for quick, safe detection of fetal chromosomal and biochemical disorders. Developed in Europe and now being tested in the United States, the procedure is performed during the first trimester of

Autoantibodies in autoimmune disease

When the immune system produces autoantibodies against the antigenic determinants on and in cells, two types of autoimmune disease can result. *Organ-specific disease,* such as pernicious anemia, occurs when the targeted antigenic determinants are specific to an organ or tissue, or to certain cells or cell types. Lymphocytes invade the target organ, tissue, or cell and destroy targeted cells. *Non-organ-specific disease,* such as myasthenia gravis, occurs when the targeted antigenic determinants are shared with other cells (self-antigens). This causes deposition of immune complexes (Type III hypersensitivity), with subsequent lesions anywhere in the body.

Various diagnostic techniques are used to detect antibodies in autoimmune disease, including radioimmunoassay, hemagglutination, complement fixation, and immunofluorescence. The chart shown here lists common test methods and findings in various autoimmune diseases.

SR. REBECCA FIDLER, MT(ASCP), PhD
BEVERLY ZENK WHEAT, RN, MA

COMMON TESTS FOR AUTOIMMUNE DISEASES

DISEASE	AFFECTED AREA
Hashimoto's thyroiditis	Thyroid gland
Pernicious anemia	Hematopoietic system
Pemphigus vulgaris	Skin
Myasthenia gravis	Neuromuscular system
Autoimmune hemolytic anemia	Hematopoietic system
Primary biliary cirrhosis	Small bile ducts in liver
Rheumatoid arthritis	Joints, blood vessels, skin, muscles, lymph nodes
Goodpasture's syndrome	Lungs and kidneys
Systemic lupus erythematosus	Skin, joints, muscles, lungs, heart, kidneys, brain, eyes

pregnancy. Preliminary results may be available within hours; complete results within a few days. In contrast, amniocentesis cannot be performed before the 16th week of pregnancy, and the results aren't available for at least 2 weeks. Thus, chorionic villi sampling offers the advantage of earlier detection of fetal abnormalities.

The chorionic villi are fingerlike projections that surround the embryonic membrane and give rise to the placenta. Cells obtained from sample are of fetal—not maternal—origin and thus can be analyzed for fetal abnormalities. Samples are best obtained between the 8th and 10th weeks of pregnancy. Before 7 weeks, the villi cover the embryo and make selective sampling difficult. After 10 weeks, maternal cells begin to grow over the villi and the amniotic sac begins to fill the uterine cavity, making sampling difficult and possibly dangerous.

ANTIGEN	ANTIBODY	DIAGNOSTIC TECHNIQUE
Thyroglobulin, second colloid antigen, cytoplasmic microsomes, cell-surface antigens	Antibodies to thyroglobulin and to microsomal antigens	Radioimmunoassay, hemagglutination, complement fixation, immunofluorescence
Intrinsic factor	Antibodies to gastric parietal cells and vitamin B_{12} binding site of intrinsic factor	Immunofluorescence, radioimmunoassay
Desmosomes between prickle cells in the epidermis	Antibodies to intercellular substances of the skin and mucous membranes	Immunofluorescence
Acetylcholine receptors of skeletal and heart muscle	Anti-acetylcholine antibody	Immunoprecipitation radioimmunoassay
Red blood cells (RBCs)	Anti-RBC antibody	Direct and indirect Coombs' test
Mitochondria	Mitochondrial antibody	Immunofluorescence of mitochondrial-rich cells (kidney biopsy)
IgG	Anti–gamma globulin antibody	Sheep RBC agglutination, latex immunoglobulin agglutination, radioimmunoassay, immunofluorescence, immunodiffusion
Glomerular and lung basement membranes	Anti–basement membrane antibody	Immunofluorescence of kidney biopsy sample, radioimmunoassay
Deoxyribonucleic acid (DNA), nucleoprotein, blood cells, clotting factors, IgG, cardiolipin antigen	Antinuclear, anti-DNA, anti–ds-DNA, anti–ss-DNA, anti–ribonucleoprotein, anti–gamma globulin, anti-RBC, anti-lymphocyte, anti-platelet, antineuronal cell, and anti-Sm antibodies	Counterelectrophoresis, hemagglutination, radioimmunoassay, immunofluorescence, Coombs' test

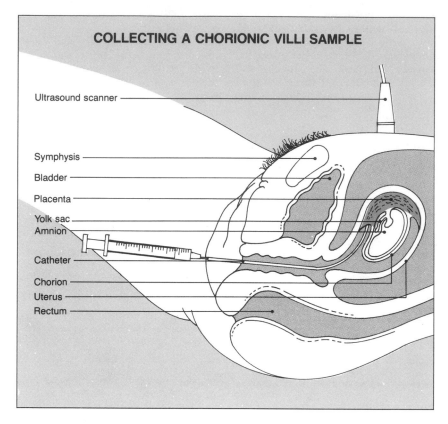

COLLECTING A CHORIONIC VILLI SAMPLE

Ultrasound scanner

Symphysis
Bladder
Placenta
Yolk sac
Amnion
Catheter
Chorion
Uterus
Rectum

To collect a chorionic villi sample, place the patient in the lithotomy position. The doctor checks the placement of the patient's uterus bimanually and then inserts a Graves speculum and swabs the cervix with an antiseptic solution. If necessary, he may use a tenaculum to straighten an acutely flexed uterus, permitting cannula insertion. Guided by ultrasound and possibly endoscopy, he directs the catheter through the cannula to the villi. Suction is applied to the catheter to remove about 30 mg of tissue from the villi. The sample is withdrawn, placed in a Petri dish, and examined with a dissecting microscope. Part of the specimen is then cultured for further testing.

Results of chorionic villi testing can be used to detect about 200 diseases prenatally. For example, direct analysis of rapidly dividing fetal cells can detect chromosomal disorders; DNA analysis can detect hemoglobinopathies; and lysosomal enzyme assays can screen for lysosomal storage disorders, such as Tay-Sachs disease.

The test appears to provide reliable results, except when the sample contains too few cells or the cells fail to grow in culture. Patient risks for this procedure are considered similar to those for amniocentesis—a small chance of spontaneous abortion, cramps, infection, and bleeding.

Unlike amniocentesis, chorionic villi sampling can't detect complications in cases of Rh sensitization, uncover neural tube defects, or determine pulmonary maturity. However, it may prove to be the best way to detect other serious fetal abnormalities early in pregnancy.

FRANK C. RIGGALL, MD

Computed tomography of the spine

Much more versatile than conventional radiography, computed tomography (CT) of the spine provides detailed high-resolution images in the cross-sectional, longitudinal, sagittal, and lateral planes. Multiple X-ray beams from a computerized body scanner are directed at the spine from different angles; these pass through the body and strike radiation detectors, producing electrical impulses. A computer then converts these impulses into digital information, which is displayed as a three-dimensional image on a video monitor. Storage of the digital information allows electronic recreation and manipulation of the image, creating a permanent record of the images to enable reexamination without repeating the procedure.

Two variations of spinal CT further expand the procedure's diagnostic capabilities. Contrast-enhanced CT accentuates spinal vasculature and highlights even subtle differences in tissue density. Air CT, which involves removing a small amount of cerebrospinal fluid (CSF) and injecting air via lumbar puncture, intensifies the contrast between the subarachnoid space and surrounding tissue.

Purpose
• To diagnose spinal lesions and abnormalities
• To monitor the effects of spinal surgery or therapy.

Patient preparation
Explain to the patient that this procedure allows visualization of his spine. Unless contrast enhancement is ordered, tell him that he needn't restrict food or fluids. (If contrast enhancement is ordered, instruct him to fast for 4 hours before the test.) Tell him that a series of X-rays will be taken of his spine. Explain who will perform the procedure and where, and that the test takes 30 to 60 minutes. Reassure him that the procedure is painless.

Explain to the patient that he'll be positioned on an X-ray table inside a CT body scanning unit and asked to lie still; the computer-controlled scanner will revolve around him, taking multiple X-ray exposures. Stress that he should lie as still as possible when asked to do so because movement during the procedure may cause distorted images.

If contrast dye is used, tell him that he may feel flushed and warm and may experience a transient headache, a salty taste, and nausea or vomiting after injection of the contrast dye. Reassure him that this is normal.

Instruct the patient to wear a radiologic examining gown and to remove all metal objects and jewelry that may appear in the X-ray field. Make sure the patient or a responsible family member has signed an appropriate consent form. Check the patient's history for hypersensitivity reactions to iodine, iodine-containing substances such as shellfish, or contrast media. If such reactions have occurred, notify the doctor, who may order prophylactic medications or choose not to use contrast enhancement.

If the patient appears restless or apprehensive about the procedure, notify the doctor, who may prescribe a mild sedative.

Equipment
Computerized body scanner/oscilloscope/recording equipment/contrast medium, as ordered (meglumine iothalamate or diatrizoate sodium)/60-ml syringe/19G to 20G needle/tourniquet.

Procedure
The patient is placed in a supine position on a radiographic table and is told to lie as still as possible. The table is then slid into the circular opening of the body CT scanner. The scanner re-

PRINCIPLES OF COMPUTED TOMOGRAPHY

A computed tomography (CT) scan uses X-rays, radiation detectors, a computer, and a video monitor to create highly accurate pictures of a patient's spine, brain, or other body parts. Here's how it works:

The patient lies motionless on a table surrounded by the scanner unit, which contains X-ray tubes and radiation detectors placed directly opposite each other. As the scanner revolves, a narrow X-ray beam scans the body part while detectors measure the amount of radiation that passes through unabsorbed. Then the detectors send their radiation readings to the computer, which processes them and converts them into an image on the video screen. The images, which appear in different shades of gray, reflect the fact that different densities of tissue absorb radiation at different rates.

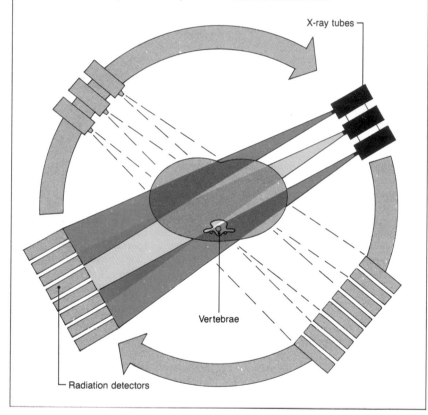

X-ray tubes

Vertebrae

Radiation detectors

volves around the patient, taking radiographs at preselected intervals.

After the first set of radiographs is taken, the patient is removed from the scanner and contrast medium is administered, if ordered. Usually, 50 to 100 ml of contrast dye is injected. Observe the patient for signs and symptoms of a hypersensitivity reaction—pruritus, rash, and respiratory difficulty—for 30 minutes after the contrast dye has been injected.

After dye injection, the patient is moved back into the scanner, and another series of radiographs is taken. The images obtained from the scan are displayed on a video monitor during the procedure and stored on magnetic tape to create a permanent record for subsequent study.

Precautions

● Body CT scanning with contrast enhancement is contraindicated in patients who are hypersensitive to iodine, shellfish, or contrast media.

● Some patients may experience strong feelings of claustrophobia or anxiety when inside the body CT scanner. For such patients, the doctor may order a mild sedative to help reduce anxiety.

Findings

In the CT image, spinal tissue appears black, white, or gray, depending on its density. Vertebrae, the densest tissues, are white; soft tissues appear in shades of gray; CSF is black.

Implications of results

By highlighting areas of altered density and depicting structural malformation, CT scanning can reveal all types of spinal lesions and abnormalities. It's particularly useful in detecting and localizing tumors, which appear as masses varying in density. Measuring this density and noting the configuration and location relative to the spinal cord can often identify the type of tumor. For example, a neurinoma (schwannoma) appears as a spherical mass dorsal to the cord. A darker, wider mass lying more laterally or ventrally to the cord may be a meningioma.

CT also reveals degenerative processes and structural changes in detail. Herniated nucleus pulposus shows as an obvious herniation of disk material with unilateral or bilateral nerve root compression; if the herniation is midline, spinal cord compression will be evident. Cervical spondylosis shows as cervical cord compression due to bony hypertrophy of the cervical spine; lumbar stenosis, as hypertrophy of the lumbar vertebrae, causing cord compression by decreasing space within the spinal column. Facet disorders show as soft-tissue changes, bony overgrowth, and spurring of the vertebrae, which result in nerve root compression. Fluid-filled arachnoidal and other paraspinal cysts show as dark masses displacing the spinal cord. After contrast enhancement, vascular malformations show as masses or clusters, usually on the dorsal aspect of the spinal cord.

Congenital spinal malformations, such as meningocele, myelocele, and spina bifida, show as abnormally large, dark gaps between the white vertebrae.

Post-test care

● If the procedure was done without contrast enhancement, no post-test care is needed.

● After testing with contrast enhancement, observe the patient for residual effects, such as headache, nausea, and vomiting. Also inform the patient that he may resume his usual diet, which was withheld before administration of contrast dye.

Interfering factors

● Excessive movement by the patient during the scanning procedure may distort the images, making them difficult to interpret.

● Radiopaque objects, such as metal objects and jewelry, not removed from the X-ray field may produce unclear images.

ROGER M. MORRELL, MD, PhD, FACP

Digital subtraction angiography

Digital subtraction angiography (DSA) is a sophisticated radiographic technique that uses video equipment and computer-assisted image enhancement to examine the vascular systems. As in conventional angiography, X-ray images are obtained after injection of a contrast medium. However, unlike conventional angiography, in which images of bone and soft tissue often obscure vascular detail, DSA provides a better, high-contrast view of blood vessels, without interfering images or shadows.

This unique view is made possible by digital subtraction, in which fluoroscopic images are taken before and after injection of a contrast medium. A computer converts these images into digital information and then "subtracts" the first image from the second, eliminating most information (mainly bone and soft tissue) common to both images. This technique results in a better image of the contrast-enhanced vasculature.

In addition to superior image quality, DSA has other important advantages over conventional angiography. Because the digital subtraction process allows intravenous rather than intraarterial injection of the contrast medium, DSA avoids one risk of conventional angiography—stroke—and reduces the pain and discomfort of arterial catheterization.

Although DSA has been used to study peripheral and renal vascular disease, it's probably most useful in diagnosing cerebrovascular disorders, such as carotid stenosis and occlusion, arteriovenous malformation, aneurysms, and vascular tumors. It's also useful in visualizing displacement of vasculature by other intracranial pathology or trauma and in detecting lesions often missed by computerized tomography scans, such as thrombosis of the superior sagittal sinus.

Purpose
• To visualize extracranial and intracranial cerebral blood flow
• To detect and evaluate cerebrovascular abnormalities
• To aid postoperative evaluation of cerebrovascular surgery, such as arterial grafts and endarterectomies.

Patient preparation
Explain to the patient that this test visualizes the blood vessels in his head. Instruct him to fast for 4 hours before the test, but inform him that he needn't restrict fluids. Explain that he'll receive an injection of a contrast medium, either by needle or through a venous

catheter inserted in his arm, and that a series of X-rays will be taken of his head. Tell him who will perform the test and where, and that it will take 30 to 45 minutes.

Inform the patient that he'll be positioned on an X-ray table, with his head immobilized, and will be asked to lie still. (Some patients—especially children—may be given a sedative to prevent movement during the procedure.) Instruct him to remove all jewelry, dentures, and other radiopaque objects from the X-ray field. Explain to the patient that he'll probably feel some transient pain from insertion of the needle or catheter and that he may experience mild symptoms from injection of the contrast medium, such as a feeling of warmth, a headache, a metallic taste, and nausea or vomiting. Reassure him that this is normal.

Make sure the patient or a responsible family member has signed a consent form. Check the patient's history for hypersensitivity to iodine, iodine-containing substances such as shellfish, and radiographic contrast media. Report any hypersensitivities to the doctor, who may order prophylactic medications or may choose not to perform the test.

Equipment
I.V. equipment and 250 ml normal saline solution/contrast medium/automatic contrast medium injector/X-ray machine with biplane cassette changer/computer and video monitor/video recorder.

Procedure
The patient is placed in a supine position on an X-ray table and is told to lie still with his arms at his sides. After an initial series of fluoroscopic pictures (mask images) of his head is taken, the injection site—most commonly the antecubital basilic or cephalic vein—is shaved and cleansed with an antiseptic solution.

If catheterization is ordered, a local anesthetic is administered, a venipuncture is performed, and a catheter is inserted and advanced to the superior vena cava. After placement is verified by X-ray, I.V. lines from a bottle of normal saline solution and from an automatic contrast medium injector are connected. While the saline solution is administered, the injector delivers the contrast medium at a rate of about 14 ml/second.

If simple injection of the contrast medium is ordered, a bolus of 40 to 60 ml is administered intravenously by needle.

The patient's vital signs and neurologic status are monitored, and he's observed for signs of a hypersensitivity reaction, such as hives, flushing, and respiratory distress.

After allowing time for the contrast medium to clear the pulmonary circulation and enter the cerebral vasculature, a second series of fluoroscopic images (contrast images) is taken. The computer digitizes the information received from both series and compares mask and contrast images, subtracting the information (images of bone and soft tissue) common to both. A detailed image of the contrast medium–filled vessels is displayed on a video monitor. For many patients, this image may be stored on videotape or a videodisc for future reference.

Precautions

DSA may be contraindicated in patients with iodine or contrast media hypersensitivity or in those who have poor cardiac function; renal, hepatic, or thyroid disease; diabetes; or multiple myeloma.

Findings

The contrast medium should fill and opacify all superficial and deep arteries, arterioles, and veins, allowing visualization of normal cerebral vasculature.

The digital subtraction process may serve to intensify areas that receive only contrast medium. However, conventional angiography provides a more de-

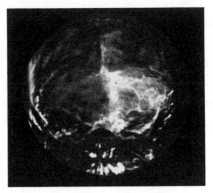

Normal bilateral carotid digital subtraction angiogram (cross-sectional image)

tailed image of the carotids than does DSA.

Implications of results

Vascular filling defects, seen as areas of increased vascular opacity, may indicate arteriovenous occlusion or stenosis, possibly due to vasospasm, vascular malformation or angiomas, arteriosclerosis, or cerebral embolism or thrombosis. Out-pouchings in vessel lumina may reflect cerebral aneurysms; such aneurysms commonly rupture, causing subarachnoid hemorrhage. Vessel displacement or vascular masses may indicate an intracranial tumor. DSA can clearly depict the vascular supply of some tumors, reflecting the tumor's position, size, and nature.

Post-test care

● Because the contrast medium acts as a diuretic, encourage the patient to increase his fluid intake for 24 hours after this test. Advise him that extra fluid intake will also speed excretion of the contrast medium. Monitor intake and output, as ordered.

● Check the venipuncture site for signs of extravasation, such as redness or swelling. If bleeding occurs, apply firm pressure to the puncture site. If a hematoma develops, elevate the arm and apply warm soaks.

● Observe the patient for a delayed hypersensitivity reaction to the contrast

medium. Delayed reaction is rare but can occur up to 18 hours after the procedure.
• Instruct the patient to resume his normal diet.

Interfering factors
• Patient movement during the procedure may cause blurred images that are difficult to interpret.
• Radiopaque objects in the fluoroscopic field may impair image clarity.

ROGER M. MORRELL, MD, PhD, FACP

Extractable nuclear antigen antibodies

[Ribonucleoprotein antibodies; anti-Smith antibodies; Sjögren's antibodies]

Extractable nuclear antigen (ENA) is a complex of at least two and possibly three antigens. One of these—ribonucleoprotein (RNP)—is susceptible to degradation by ribonuclease. The second—Smith (Sm) antigen—is an acidic nuclear protein that resists ribonuclease degradation. The third antigen sometimes included in this group—Sjögren's syndrome B (SS-B) antigen—forms a precipitate when antibody is present. Antibodies to these antigens are associated with certain autoimmune disorders.

Tests to detect ENA antibodies help differentiate autoimmune disorders with similar signs and symptoms. The RNP antibody test detects RNP autoantibodies, which are associated with systemic lupus erythematosus (SLE), progressive systemic sclerosis, and other rheumatic disorders. This test aids in the differential diagnosis of systemic rheumatic disease and is a useful follow-up test for collagen vascular autoimmune disease. The anti-Sm antibody test detects Sm autoantibodies,

which are a specific marker for SLE; positive results are thus highly diagnostic of SLE. This test, too, helps monitor collagen vascular autoimmune disease. The Sjögren's antibody test detects the SS-B autoantibodies produced in Sjögren's syndrome, an immunologic abnormality sometimes associated with rheumatoid arthritis and SLE. However, this test is not diagnostic for Sjögren's syndrome.

To perform these tests, red blood cells from sheep are sensitized with ENA extracted from rabbit thymus and then incubated with serum samples; ENA antibodies present in the serum will agglutinate the cells. If the serum sample shows agglutination, differential double immunoassays are done to determine which antibodies are present. Anti-ENA tests are most useful with anti-DNA, serum complement, and antinuclear antibody tests.

Purpose
• To aid differential diagnosis of autoimmune disease
• To distinguish between anti-RNP and anti-Sm antibodies
• To screen for anti-RNP antibodies (common in mixed connective tissue disease)
• To screen for anti-Sm antibodies (common in SLE)
• To support diagnosis of collagen vascular autoimmune diseases
• To monitor response to therapy.

Patient preparation
Explain to the patient that this test detects certain antibodies and that test results help determine diagnosis and treatment; or, when indicated, explain that the test assesses the effectiveness of treatment.

Advise him he needn't restrict food or fluids. Tell him that the test requires a blood sample; who will perform the venipuncture and when; and that he may experience discomfort from the needle puncture and the tourniquet. Reassure him that the sample collection takes less than 3 minutes.

Procedure

Perform a venipuncture, and collect the sample in a 7-ml *red-top* tube.

Precautions

Send the sample to the laboratory immediately.

Findings

Normally, serum is negative for anti-RNP, anti-Sm, and SS-B antibodies.

Implications of results

The presence of anti-Sm antibodies is highly diagnostic of SLE. A high level of anti-RNP antibodies with a low titer of anti-Sm antibodies suggests mixed connective tissue disease. Although SS-B antibodies are associated with primary Sjögren's syndrome, their presence is not considered diagnostic of this disorder; however, a positive test for SS-B antibodies mandates further testing.

Post-test care

• Check the venipuncture site for infection, and report any change promptly. Keep a clean, dry bandage over the site for at least 24 hours.
• If a hematoma develops at the venipuncture site, apply warm soaks.

Interfering factors

Failure to send the sample to the laboratory immediately may interfere with accurate determination of test results.

SR. REBECCA FIDLER, MT(ASCP), PhD

Endoscopic biopsy of the GI tract

Endoscopy allows direct visualization of the GI tract and any site that requires biopsy of tissue samples for histologic analysis. This relatively painless procedure helps detect, support diagnosis of, or monitor GI tract disorders. Its complications, notably hemorrhage, perforation, and aspiration, are rare.

Patient preparation

Careful patient preparation is vital. Describe the procedure and reassure the patient that he will be able to breathe with the endoscope in place. Tell him to fast for at least 8 hours before the procedure. (For lower GI biopsy, cleanse the bowel, as ordered.) Make sure the patient or a responsible family member has signed a consent form.

Just before the procedure, sedate the patient, as ordered. He should be relaxed but not asleep because his cooperation promotes smooth passage of the endoscope. Spray the back of his throat with a local anesthetic to suppress the gag reflex. Have suction equipment and bipolar cauterizing electrodes available to prevent aspiration and excessive bleeding.

Procedure

After the doctor passes the endoscope into the upper or lower GI tract and visualizes a lesion, node, or other abnormal area, he pushes biopsy forceps through a channel in the endoscope until this, too, can be seen. Then he opens the forceps, positions them at the biopsy site, and closes them on the tissue. The closed forceps and tissue sample are removed from the endoscope, and the tissue is taken from the forceps. The specimen is placed in fixative. After the sample collection, the endoscope is removed. Samples are sent to the laboratory immediately.

Implications of results

Endoscopic biopsy of the GI tract can diagnose cancer, lymphoma, amyloidosis, candidiasis, and gastric ulcers; support diagnosis of Crohn's disease, chronic ulcerative colitis, gastritis, esophagitis, and melanosis coli in laxative abuse; and monitor progression of Barrett's esophagus, multiple gastric polyps, colon cancer and polyps, and chronic ulcerative colitis.

KATHERINE FULTON, RN

RECOGNIZING ENDOSCOPIC LANDMARKS

Certain parts of the upper GI tract act as landmarks during an endoscopic biopsy. Assist the doctor, as ordered, in obtaining specimens at or near these important landmarks.

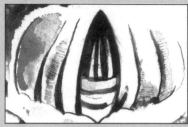

Vocal cords and esophageal orifice

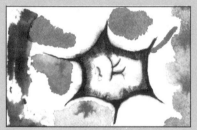

Esophagogastric junction

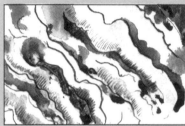

Fundus of stomach

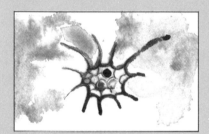

Antrum and pylorus

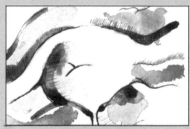

Duodenum and papilla of Vater

Erythrocyte total porphyrins

[Erythropoietic porphyrins]

This test measures total erythrocyte porphyrins—mostly protoporphyrin, but also coproporphyrin and uroporphyrin. Porphyrins are pigments that exist in all protoplasm and are needed for energy storage and use. Protoporphyrin, coproporphyrin, and uroporphyrin are produced during heme biosynthesis. Small amounts of these porphyrins or their precursors normally appear in blood, urine, and feces. Production and excretion of porphyrins or their precursors increase in porphyrias, disorders of porphyrin metabolism, erythropoietic or hepatic. This test detects erythropoietic porphyrias.

After an initial screening test for total porphyrins, quantitative fluorometric analysis can identify specific porphyrins and suggest specific disorders.

Purpose

• To aid diagnosis of congenital or acquired erythropoietic porphyrias
• To help confirm diagnosis of disorders affecting red blood cell (RBC) activity.

Patient preparation

Explain to the patient that this test helps detect RBC disorders. Inform him that he must fast for 12 to 14 hours before the sample is drawn, but that he may drink water. Tell him who will perform the venipuncture and when, and that he may feel some transient discomfort from the needle puncture and the pressure of the tourniquet.

Procedure

Perform a venipuncture and collect the sample in a 5-ml or larger *green-top* tube. Label the sample, place it on ice, and send it to the laboratory promptly.

Precautions

Handle the sample gently to prevent hemolysis.

Values

Total porphyrin levels range from 16 to 60 mg/dl of packed RBCs. Protoporphyrin levels range from 16 to 60 mg/dl; coproporphyrin and uroporphyrin levels are each below 2 mg/dl.

Implications of results

Elevated protoporphyrin levels may indicate erythropoietic protoporphyria, infection, increased erythropoiesis, thalassemia, sideroblastic anemia, iron deficiency anemia, or lead poisoning. Elevated coproporphyrin levels may indicate congenital erythropoietic porphyria, erythropoietic protoporphyria or coproporphyria, and sideroblastic anemia. Elevated uroporphyrin levels typically suggest congenital erythropoietic porphyria or erythropoietic protoporphyria.

Post-test care

If a hematoma develops at the venipuncture site, apply warm soaks.

Interfering factors

Hemolysis or failure to observe dietary restrictions may alter test results.
TOBIE VIRGINIA HITTLE, RN, BSN, CCRN

Evoked potential studies

These tests evaluate the integrity of visual, somatosensory, and auditory nerve pathways by measuring *evoked potentials*—the brain's electrical response to stimulation of the sense organs or peripheral nerves. Evoked potentials are recorded as electronic impulses by surface electrodes attached to the scalp and to the skin over various peripheral sensory nerves. A computer extracts these low-amplitude impulses from background brain-wave activity and averages the signals from repeated stimuli.

Three types of responses are measured. *Visual evoked potentials*, produced by exposing the eye to a rapidly reversing checkerboard pattern, help evaluate demyelinating disease, traumatic injury, and puzzling visual complaints. *Somatosensory evoked potentials*, which are produced by electrically stimulating a peripheral sensory nerve, help diagnose peripheral nerve disease and locate brain and spinal cord lesions. *Auditory brain stem evoked potentials*, produced by delivering clicks to the ear, help locate auditory lesions and evaluate brain stem integrity. Auditory neural activity is recorded as the electric response passes from the peripheral or cochlear end organ through the brain to the cortex.

Evoked potential studies are also useful for monitoring comatose patients and patients under anesthesia, monitoring spinal cord function during spinal cord surgery, and evaluating neurologic function in infants whose sensory systems can't be assessed.

VISUAL AND SOMATOSENSORY EVOKED POTENTIALS

Pattern-shift evoked potentials: In this test, visual neural impulses are recorded as they travel along the pathway from the eye to the occipital cortex. Wave P100 is the most significant component of the resultant waveform—normal P100 latency is approximately 100 msec after the application of visual stimulus, as shown in the top diagram. Increased P100 latency, shown in the bottom diagram, is an abnormal finding indicating a lesion along the visual pathway.

Normal tracing

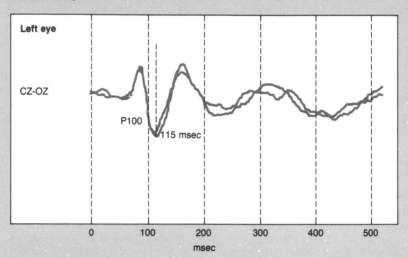

Tracing in multiple sclerosis

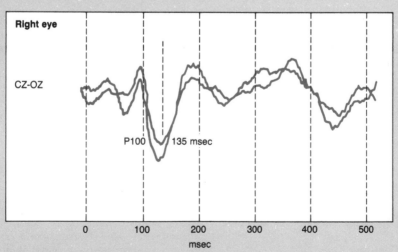

CZ = vertex   OZ = midocciput

Somatosensory evoked potentials: These tests measure the conduction time of an electrical impulse traveling along a somatosensory pathway to the cortex. Interwave latency is the most significant component of the resultant waveform. On the set of upper- and lower-limb tracings shown below, the top tracings represent normal interwave latencies; the bottom tracings, typical abnormal latencies found in a patient with multiple sclerosis. Because of the close correlation between waveforms and the anatomy of somatosensory pathways, such tracings allow precise localization of lesions that produce conduction defects.

Upper limb

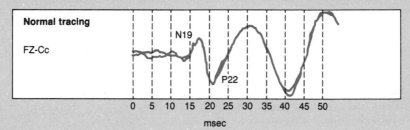

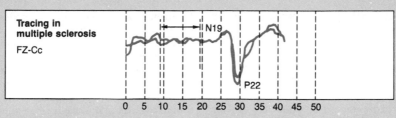

FZ = midfrontal   Cc = sensoparietal cortex contralateral to stimulated limb

Lower limb

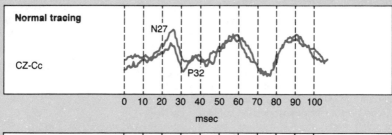

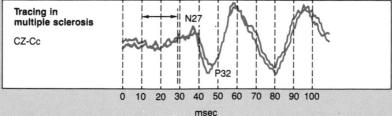

CZ = vertex   Cc = sensoparietal cortex contralateral to stimulated limb

Purpose

• To aid diagnosis of nervous system lesions and abnormalities
• To assess neurologic function.

Patient preparation

Explain to the patient that this group of tests measures the electrical activity of his nervous system. Explain who will perform the procedure and where, and that it takes 45 to 60 minutes.

Tell the patient that he'll be positioned in a reclining chair or on a bed. If visual evoked potentials will be measured, tell him that electrodes will be attached to his scalp; if somatosensory evoked potentials will be measured, that electrodes will be placed on his scalp, neck, lower back, wrist, knee, and ankle.

Assure the patient that the electrodes won't hurt him; encourage him to relax, since tension can affect neurologic function and interfere with test results. Have him remove all jewelry.

Equipment

Evoked potential unit/auditory, visual, or tactile stimuli/amplifier/oscilloscope tube face/magnetic tape.

Procedure

The patient is positioned in a reclining chair or on a bed and is instructed to relax and remain still.

To measure *visual evoked potentials,* electrodes are attached to the patient's scalp at occipital, parietal, and vertex locations; a reference electrode is placed on the midfrontal area or on the ear. The patient is positioned 1 meter from the pattern-shift stimulator—either an electronic stimulator, which displays the pattern on a television screen or uses an array of light-emitting diodes, or a mechanical stimulator, which projects the pattern from a slide projector onto a translucent screen. One eye is occluded, and the patient is instructed to fix his gaze on a dot in the center of the screen. A checkerboard pattern is projected and then rapidly reversed or shifted 100

times, once or twice per second. A computer amplifies and averages the brain's response to each stimulus, and the results are plotted as a waveform. The procedure is repeated for the other eye.

To measure *somatosensory evoked potentials,* electrodes are attached to the patient's skin over somatosensory pathways to stimulate peripheral nerves. Electrode sites usually include the wrist, knee, and ankle. Recording electrodes are placed on the scalp over the sensory cortex of the hemisphere opposite the limb to be stimulated. Additional electrodes may be placed at Erb's point (above the clavicle overlying the brachial plexus) and at the second cervical vertebra for upper-limb stimulation, and over the lower lumbar vertebrae for lower-limb stimulation. Midfrontal or noncephalic electrodes are placed for reference.

A painless electrical shock is delivered to the peripheral nerve through the stimulating electrode. The intensity of the shock is adjusted to produce a minor muscle response, such as a thumb twitch upon median nerve stimulation at the wrist. The shock is delivered at least 500 times, at a rate of five per second. A computer measures and averages the time it takes for the electrical current to reach the cortex; the results, expressed in milliseconds (msec), are recorded as waveforms. The test is repeated once to verify results; then the electrodes are repositioned and the entire procedure is repeated for the other side.

Findings

Visual evoked potentials: On the waveform, the most significant wave is P100, a positive wave appearing about 100 msec after the pattern-shift stimulus is applied. The most clinically significant measurements are absolute P100 latency (the time between stimulus application and peaking of the P100 wave) and the difference between the P100 latencies of each eye. Because many physical and technical factors affect P100 latency, normal results vary greatly between laboratories and patients. The chart on page 34 shows a typical response.

Somatosensory evoked potentials: The waveforms obtained vary, depending on locations of the stimulating and recording electrodes. The positive and negative peaks are labeled in sequence, based on normal time of appearance. For example, N19 is a negative peak normally recorded 19 msec after application of the stimulus. Each wave peak arises from a discrete location: N19 is generated mainly from the thalamus, P22 from the parietal sensory cortex, and so on. Interwave latencies (time between waves), rather than absolute latencies, are used as a basis for clinical interpretation. Latency differences between sides are significant. Normal waveforms for upper and lower limbs appear in the chart on page 35.

Implications of results

Visual evoked potentials: Generally, abnormal (extended) P100 latencies confined to one eye indicate a visual pathway lesion anterior to the optic chiasm. A lesion posterior to the optic chiasm usually doesn't produce abnormal P100 latencies: because each eye projects to both occipital lobes, the unaffected pathway transmits sufficient impulses to produce a normal latency response.

Bilateral abnormal P100 latencies have been found in patients with multiple sclerosis (see the waveform on page 34), optic neuritis, retinopathies, amblyopias (although abnormal latencies don't correlate well with impaired visual acuity), spinocerebellar degeneration, adrenoleukodystrophy, sarcoidosis, Parkinson's disease, and Huntington's chorea.

Somatosensory evoked potentials: Because somatosensory evoked potential components are assumed to be linked in series, an abnormal interwave latency indicates a conduction defect between the generators of the two peaks involved. This often enables precise location of a neurologic lesion.

Abnormal upper-limb interwave latencies may indicate cervical spondylosis, intracerebral lesions, or sensorimotor neuropathies. Abnormalities in the lower limb demonstrate peripheral nerve and root lesions, such as those in Guillain-Barré syndrome, compressive myelopathies, multiple sclerosis (see the chart on pages 34 and 35), transverse myelitis, and traumatic spinal cord injury.

Information from evoked potential studies is useful but insufficient to confirm a specific diagnosis. Test data must be interpreted in light of clinical information.

Post-test care
None.

Interfering factors
• Incorrect placement of electrodes or equipment failure can alter test results.
• Patient tension or failure to cooperate can impair the accuracy of test results.
• Extremely poor visual acuity can hinder accurate determination of visual evoked potentials.

ROGER M. MORRELL, MD, PhD, FACP

External sphincter electromyography

This procedure measures electrical activity of the external urinary sphincter. The electrical activity can be measured in three ways: by needle electrodes inserted in perineal or periurethral tissues, by electrodes in an anal plug, or by skin electrodes. Skin electrodes are used most commonly.

The primary indication for external sphincter electromyography is incontinence. Often, this test is done with cystometry and voiding urethrography as part of a full urodynamic study.

Purpose
• To assess neuromuscular function of

the external urinary sphincter
• To assess the functional balance between bladder and sphincter muscle activity.

Patient preparation

Explain to the patient that this test will determine how well his bladder and sphincter muscles work together. Tell him who will perform the test and where, and that it takes 30 to 60 minutes.

If skin electrodes are to be used, tell the patient where they will be placed. Explain the preparatory procedure, which may include shaving a small area.

If needle electrodes will be used, tell the patient where they will be placed and that the discomfort is equivalent to an intramuscular injection. Assure him that he'll feel discomfort only during insertion. Advise him that the needles are connected to wires leading to the recorder but that there is no danger of electrical shock. Explain to the female patient that she may notice slight bleeding at the first voiding.

If an anal plug will be used, inform the patient that only the tip of the plug will be inserted into the rectum, that he may feel fullness but no discomfort, and that a bowel movement is rare but easily managed.

Check the patient's medications. If he is taking cholinergic or anticholinergic drugs, notify the doctor. Discontinue medications, as ordered.

Equipment

Electromyograph and recorder/skin, needle, or anal plug electrodes/ground plate/electrode paste/tape/antiseptic solution, such as povidone-iodine/preparatory tray, if shaving is necessary.

Procedure

The patient is placed in lithotomy position for electrode placement, then may lie supine. Be sure to record patient position, type of electrode used, measuring equipment used, and any other tests done at the same time. (To obtain comparable results, subsequent studies must be done the same way.)

Electrode paste is applied to the ground plate, which is taped to the thigh and grounded. The electrodes are then placed, as described below, and connected to electrode adaptors.

Placing skin electrodes: The skin is cleansed with antiseptic solution and dried. A small area may be shaved for optimum electrode contact. Electrode paste is applied and the electrodes are taped in place: for females, in the periurethral area; for males, in the perineal area beneath the scrotum.

Placing needle electrodes: With the male patient, a gloved finger is inserted into the rectum. The needles and wires are inserted 1.5″ through the perineal skin toward the apex of the prostate. Needle positions are 3:00 and 9:00. While the needles are withdrawn, the wires are held in place and then taped to the thigh.

With the female patient, the labia are spread, and the needles and wires are inserted periurethrally at 2:00 and 10:00. The needles are withdrawn and the wires taped to the thigh.

Placing anal plug electrodes: The plug is lubricated, and the patient is informed again that only the tip will be inserted into the rectum. The patient is asked to relax by breathing slowly and deeply. He is asked to relax the anal sphincter to accommodate the plug by bearing down as if for a bowel movement.

After the appropriate electrodes are placed and connected to adapters, the adapters are then inserted into the preamplifier and recording is begun. The patient is asked to alternately relax and tighten the sphincter. When sufficient data have been recorded, he is asked to bear down and exhale while the anal plug and needle electrodes are removed. Remove skin electrodes gently to avoid pulling hair and tender skin. Cleanse and dry the area before the patient dresses.

In some urodynamic laboratories, cystometrography is done with electromyography for thorough evaluation of detrusor and sphincter coordination.

Precautions
• Insert needles quickly to minimize discomfort.
• The ground plate should be properly applied and anchored; wires should be taped securely to prevent artifact.

Findings
The electromyogram shows increased muscle activity when the patient tightens the external urinary sphincter and decreased muscle activity when he relaxes it. (The International Continence Society doesn't specify normal findings for sphincter electromyography.)

If electromyography and cystometrography are performed together, a comparison of their results shows that muscle activity of the normal sphincter increases as the bladder fills. During voiding and with bladder contraction, muscle activity decreases as the sphincter relaxes. This comparison is of special significance in assessing external sphincter efficiency and functional balance between bladder and sphincter muscle activity.

Implications of results
Failure of the sphincter to relax or increased muscle activity during voiding demonstrates detrusor–external sphincter dyssynergia. Confirmation of such muscle activity by electromyography may indicate neurogenic bladder, spinal cord injury, multiple sclerosis, Parkinson's disease, or stress incontinence.

Post-test care
• Watch for hematuria after the first voiding in the female patient tested with needle electrodes. If present, report this sign to the doctor.
• Watch for and report symptoms of mild urethral irritation, such as dysuria, hematuria, and urinary frequency.
• Advise the patient to take a warm sitz bath, and encourage fluids (2 to 3 liters/day) unless contraindicated.

Interfering factors
• Patient movement during electromyography may distort recordings.
• Anticholinergic or cholinergic drugs affect detrusor and sphincter activity.
• Improperly placed and anchored electrodes will cause inaccurate recordings.

ELLEN SHIPES, RN, ET, MN, MEd

Gastroesophageal reflux scanning

When results of a barium swallow are inconclusive, gastroesophageal reflux scanning may be done to evaluate esophageal function and detect reflux. This test delivers less radiation than a conventional barium swallow and is a much more sensitive indicator of reflux. It also allows reflux to be measured without insertion of an esophageal tube—an important consideration in testing infants, small children, and other patients for whom intubation is contraindicated.

The patient is instructed to fast after midnight before the test, to clear stomach contents that impede passage of the imaging agent.

As the test begins, the patient is placed in a supine or upright position and is asked to swallow a solution containing a radiopharmaceutical, such as technetium-99m sulfur colloid (^{99m}Tc). A gamma counter placed over the patient's chest records passage of the ^{99m}Tc through the esophagus into the stomach to determine transit time and to evaluate esophageal function. If gastroesophageal reflux is suspected, the patient is repositioned as his stomach distends, and continuous recordings visualize reflux and estimate its quantity. (Depending on hospital policy, manual pressure may be applied to the patient's upper abdomen, and recordings may be taken at specific intervals.)

WHAT HAPPENS IN GASTROESOPHAGEAL REFLUX

Normally, the lower esophageal sphincter (LES)—a high-pressure area just above the stomach—prevents gastric contents from backing up into the esophagus. It does this by closing the lower end of the esophagus to create pressure and then by relaxing after each swallow to allow food into the stomach.
  Gastroesophageal reflux occurs when decreased LES pressure allows stomach contents to regurgitate into the esophagus. These acidic stomach contents can irritate the esophagus, causing hyperemia, friable mucosa, and mucosal ulcers.

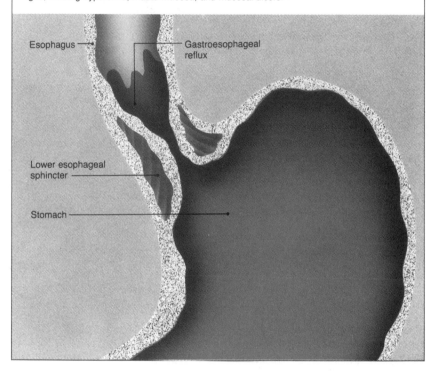

Normally, ^{99m}Tc descends through the esophagus in about 6 seconds; radioactivity is then detected only in the stomach and small bowel. However, diffuse spasm of the esophagus, achalasia, or other esophageal motility disorders may prolong transit time; in gastroesophageal reflux, the gamma counter may detect radioactivity in the esophagus.

Like other radionuclide studies, the gastroesophageal reflux scan is usually contraindicated during pregnancy and lactation. It can be modified for use in infants and children.

FRANCES W. QUINLESS, RN, PhD

Ham test
[Acidified serum lysis test]

The Ham test is performed to determine the cause of undiagnosed hemolytic anemia, hemoglobinuria, and bone marrow aplasia. It helps establish a diagnosis of paroxysmal nocturnal hemoglobinuria (PNH), a rare hematologic disease.

The Ham test relies on the susceptibility of red blood cells (RBCs) to lysis: RBCs from patients with PNH are unusually susceptible to lysis by complement. To perform the test, washed RBCs are mixed with ABO-compatible normal serum and acid. After incubation at 98.6° F. (37° C.), the cells are examined for hemolysis. In the presence of acidified human serum, many PNH cells are lysed, whereas normal RBCs show no hemolysis.

Purpose
To help establish a diagnosis of PNH.

Patient preparation
Explain to the patient that this test helps determine the cause of his anemia or other signs. Advise him he needn't restrict food or fluids. Tell him that the test requires a blood sample, who will perform the venipuncture and when, and that he may experience discomfort from the needle puncture and the tourniquet. Reassure him that the sample collection takes less than 3 minutes.

Procedure
Because the blood sample must be defibrinated immediately, laboratory personnel will perform the venipuncture and collect the sample.

Precautions
None.

Findings
Normally, RBCs undergo no hemolysis.

Implications of results
Hemolysis of RBCs indicates PNH.

Post-test care
If a hematoma develops at the venipuncture site, apply warm soaks.

Interfering factors
• Blood containing large numbers of spherocytes may produce false-positive results.
• Blood from patients with congenital dyserythropoietic anemia or HEMPAS (a rare hematologic disorder) will show false-positive results.
                    BARRY L. TONKONOW, MD

Heparin neutralization assay

This complex, quantitative test is sometimes used to monitor heparin therapy. It can also help determine if prolonged thrombin time results from effective heparin therapy or from the presence of circulating anticoagulants, such as fibrin split products. To perform this test, a specimen is divided into small plasma samples. Thrombin time is determined on one sample; the other samples are added to various dilutions of protamine sulfate. After a brief incubation, equal amounts of thrombin are added to each solution and thrombin time is measured. Because protamine sulfate neutralizes heparin, reduced thrombin time in the protamine samples indicates the presence of heparin.

A fibrometer is used to select the sample with the thrombin time closest to standard. Then a chart or formula is used to convert the sample's protamine concentration to units of heparin/ml, providing an accurate measurement of heparin blood levels. If none of the samples shows a reduced thrombin time, no heparin is present, indicating that the prolonged thrombin time is due to other anticoagulants, such as fibrin split products.
                    WILLIAM E. KLINE, MS, MT(ASCP), SBB

Human leukocyte antigen test

The human leukocyte antigen (HLA) test identifies a group of antigens present on the surfaces of all nucleated cells but most easily detected on lymphocytes. These antigens are essential to

UNDERSTANDING HUMAN LEUKOCYTE ANTIGEN INHERITANCE

Human leukocyte antigen (HLA) plays a major role in the success—or failure—of an organ transplant. Its typical pattern of inheritance appears in the diagram below, where each letter represents an antigen pair, or haplotype. Each child inherits two HLA chromosomal areas: one from the mother and one from the father. Each HLA area contains an antigen pair so that each child shares one antigen pair with each parent. Only four different combinations are possible from one set of parents. Statistically, the chance of each child having the same HLA type is one in four. Siblings who are HLA-identical have the best chance for transplant success.

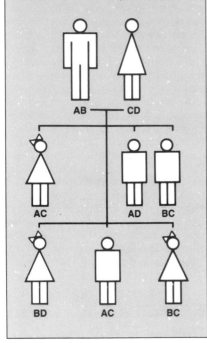

immunity and determine the degree of histocompatibility between transplant recipients and donors. Numerous antigenic determinants (over 60, for instance, at the HLA-B locus) are present for each site; one set of each antigen is inherited from each parent.

Three types of HLA (HLA-A, HLA-B, and HLA-C) are measured with a lymphocyte microcytotoxicity assay. A lymphocyte sample is mixed with known antisera to these antigens and complement. Lymphocytes that react with a specific antiserum lyse and allow a dye to enter; they may then be detected by phase microscopy.

A fourth type of HLA, HLA-D, is measured by a mixed leukocyte reaction. Leukocytes from recipient and donor are combined in a culture to determine HLA-D compatibility. If the leukocytes are incompatible, the culture will demonstrate blast formation, DNA synthesis, and proliferation.

High incidences of specific HLA types have been linked to specific diseases, such as rheumatoid arthritis and multiple sclerosis, but these findings have little diagnostic significance. Thus, HLA testing is best used as an adjunct to diagnosis. In addition, it is useful in genetic counseling and paternity testing.

Purpose
- To provide histocompatibility typing of tissue recipients and donors
- To aid genetic counseling
- To aid paternity testing.

Patient preparation
Explain to the patient that this test detects antigens on white blood cells. Advise him he needn't restrict food or fluids before the test.

Tell the patient that this test requires a blood sample, who will perform the venipuncture and when, and that he may experience transient discomfort from the needle puncture and the pressure of the tourniquet. Reassure him that collecting the blood sample usually takes less than 3 minutes.

Check the patient's history for recent blood transfusions, and report such transfusions to the doctor. He may want to postpone HLA testing.

Procedure
Perform a venipuncture and collect the sample in an ACD collection tube.

Precautions

Handle the sample gently to avoid hemolysis.

Findings

In HLA-A, HLA-B, and HLA-C testing, lymphocytes that react with the test antiserum undergo lysis; they're detected by phase microscopy. In HLA-D testing, leukocyte incompatibility is marked by blast formation, DNA synthesis, and proliferation.

Implications of results

Incompatible HLA-A, HLA-B, HLA-C, or HLA-D groups may cause unsuccessful tissue transplantation.

Many diseases have a strong association with certain types of HLAs. For example, HLA-DR5 is associated with Hashimoto's thyroiditis. B8 and Dw3 are associated with Graves' disease, whereas B8 alone is associated with chronic autoimmune hepatitis, celiac disease, and myasthenia gravis. Dw3 alone is associated with Addison's disease, Sjögren's syndrome, dermatitis herpetiformis, and systemic lupus erythematosus.

In paternity testing, a putative father who has a phenotype (two haplotypes: one from the father and one from the mother) with no haplotype or antigen pair identical to one of the child's is excluded as the father. A putative father with one haplotype identical to one of the child's *may* be the father; the probability varies with the haplotype's incidence in the population.

Post-test care

If a hematoma develops at the venipuncture site, apply warm soaks.

Interfering factors

• Hemolysis caused by rough handling of the sample may interfere with accurate determination of test results.

• HLA from blood transfused within 72 hours before collection of a blood sample may interfere with accurate determination of test results.

BARRY L. TONKONOW, MD

Insulin antibodies test

Using radioimmunoassay, this test detects insulin antibodies in the blood of patients who receive insulin for treatment of diabetes mellitus. Most insulin preparations are derived from beef and pork pancreases and contain insulin-related peptides, impurities that are the major immunogenic components in insulin. IgG antibodies that form in response to these peptides complex with subsequent insulin injections and neutralize the insulin so it cannot regulate glucose metabolism.

Detection of insulin antibodies confirms this process as the cause of insulin resistance and suggests the need for alternate therapy to control hyperglycemia.

Detection of insulin antibodies may also confirm factitious hypoglycemia, an unusual condition that results from insulin injection rather than from a clinical condition, such as insulinoma or chronic pancreatitis.

SR. REBECCA FIDLER, MT(ASCP), PhD
BEVERLY ZENK WHEAT, RN, MA

Insulin tolerance test
[Growth hormone suppression test]

This test measures serum levels of growth hormone (hGH) and adrenocorticotropic hormone (ACTH) after administration of a loading dose of insulin. It's more reliable than direct measurement of hGH and ACTH, because healthy persons often have undetectable fasting levels of these hormones. Insulin-induced hypoglycemia stimulates hGH and ACTH secretion in persons with an intact hypothalamic-pituitary-adrenal axis. Failure of stimulation indicates anterior pituitary or adrenal hypofunction and helps confirm an hGH or ACTH insufficiency.

Because the insulin tolerance test stimulates an adrenergic response, it's not recommended for patients with cardiovascular or cerebrovascular disorders, epilepsy, or low basal plasma cortisol levels.

Purpose
• To aid diagnosis of hGH or ACTH deficiency
• To identify pituitary dysfunction
• To aid differential diagnosis of primary and secondary adrenal hypofunction.

Patient preparation
Explain to the patient or to his family that this test evaluates hormonal secretion. Instruct him to fast and to restrict physical activity for 10 to 12 hours before the test. Explain that the test involves I.V. infusion of insulin and the collection of multiple blood samples. Warn him that he may experience an increased heart rate, diaphoresis, hunger, and anxiety after administration of insulin. Reassure him that these symptoms are transient, but that if they become severe the test will be discontinued. Inform him that the test takes about 2 hours and that results are usually available in 2 days.

Since physical activity and excitement increase hGH and ACTH levels, make sure the patient is relaxed and recumbent for 90 minutes before the test.

Procedure
Between 6 a.m. and 8 a.m., collect three 5-ml samples of venous blood for basal levels—one in a *gray-top* tube (for blood glucose) and two in *green-top* tubes (for hGH and ACTH). Then administer an I.V. bolus of U-100 regular insulin (0.15 U/kg, or as ordered) over a 1- to 2-minute period. Draw additional blood samples 15, 30, 45, 60, 90, and 120 minutes after administration of insulin. Use an indwelling venous catheter to avoid repeated venipunctures. At each interval, collect three samples: one in a *gray-top* tube and two in *green-top* tubes. Label the tubes appropriately and send them to the laboratory immediately.

Precautions
• Have concentrated glucose solution readily available in case of severe hypoglycemic reaction to insulin. To minimize the possibility of such a reaction, use highly purified pork or human insulin.
• Specify the time of collection on the laboratory slip, and send all samples to the laboratory immediately.
• Handle the samples gently to prevent hemolysis.

Values
Normally, blood glucose falls to 50% of the fasting level 20 to 30 minutes after insulin administration. This stimulates a 10 to 20 ng/dl increase over baseline values in both hGH and ACTH, with peak levels occurring 60 to 90 minutes after insulin administration.

Implications of results
Failure of stimulation or a blunted response suggests dysfunction of the hypothalamic-pituitary-adrenal axis. An increase in hGH levels of 10 ng/dl or less above basal suggests hGH deficiency. However, definitive diagnosis of hGH deficiency requires a supplementary stimulation test, such as the arginine test. Additional testing is necessary to determine the site of the abnormality.

An increase in ACTH levels of 10 ng/dl or less above basal suggests adrenal insufficiency. The metyrapone or ACTH stimulation test then confirms the diagnosis and determines whether insufficiency is primary or secondary.

Post-test care
• If a hematoma develops at the I.V. or venipuncture site, ease discomfort by applying warm soaks.
• As ordered, instruct the patient to resume his normal diet, activity, and medications.

Interfering factors
• Failure to follow restrictions of diet, physical activity, and medications can prevent reliable test results.
• Steroids (such as progestogen), estrogen, and pituitary-based drugs elevate hGH levels; glucocorticoids and beta blockers depress hGH levels.
• Glucocorticoids, estrogens, calcium gluconate, amphetamines, methamphetamines, spironolactone, and ethanol depress ACTH levels.
• Hemolysis caused by rough handling of the sample may affect test results.

CAROLYN ROBERTSON, RN, MSN

Leukoagglutinin test
[White cell antibodies]

This test detects leukoagglutinins—antibodies that react with white blood cells and may cause a transfusion reaction. These antibodies usually develop after exposure to foreign white cells through transfusions, pregnancies, or allografts.

If a blood *recipient* has these antibodies, a febrile nonhemolytic reaction may occur 1 to 4 hours after the start of whole blood, red blood cell, platelet, or granulocyte transfusion. (All these blood products contain some granulocytes, which react with the antibodies.) This nonhemolytic reaction (marked by fever and severe chills, sometimes with nausea, headache, and transient hypertension) must be distinguished from a true hemolytic reaction before further transfusion can proceed.

If a blood *donor* has these antibodies, the recipient may develop acute, noncardiogenic pulmonary edema after transfusion of the donor's blood. In this case, the donor's blood must be tested for leukoagglutinins to determine if they have caused the recipient's reaction.

Two methods can detect leukoagglutinins. The older method detects white cell agglutination by microscopic examination of the patient's serum after it's combined with a suspension of granulocytes and lymphocytes. A new method uses a special fluorescence microscope to detect antibodies attached to normal granulocytes that have been incubated with recipient or donor serum. The immunofluorescent method is more sensitive and is now more widely used.

Purpose
• To detect leukoagglutinins in blood recipients who develop transfusion reactions, thus differentiating between hemolytic and febrile nonhemolytic transfusion reactions
• To detect leukoagglutinins in blood donors after transfusion of donor blood causes a reaction.

Patient preparation
If a blood recipient is being tested, explain that this test helps determine the cause of his transfusion reaction. If a blood donor is being tested, explain that this test determines if his blood caused a transfusion reaction in a blood recipient and predicts whether he's likely to have a reaction if he receives blood in the future.

A pretransfusion blood sample taken from the blood bank's cross-match sample is preferred for this test. If such a sample isn't available, tell the patient that the test requires a blood sample. Inform him who will perform the venipuncture and when. Advise him that he may feel some discomfort from the needle puncture and the pressure of the tourniquet. Reassure him that collecting the sample takes only a few minutes.

Be sure to note any recent administration of blood or dextran or testing with I.V. contrast media on the laboratory slip.

Procedure
If a pretransfusion sample isn't avail-

able from the blood bank, perform a venipuncture and collect a blood sample in a 10-ml *red-top* tube. (The laboratory will require 3 to 4 ml of serum for testing.)

Precautions
Label the sample with the patient's name, room number, and hospital or blood bank number. Be sure to include on the laboratory slip the patient's suspected diagnosis and any history of blood transfusions, pregnancies, and drug therapy.

Findings
Normally, test results are negative: agglutination doesn't occur because serum contains no antibodies.

Implications of results
In a recipient's blood, a positive result indicates the presence of leukoagglutinins, identifying his transfusion reaction as a febrile nonhemolytic reaction to these antibodies.

In a donor's blood, a positive result indicates the presence of leukoagglutinins, identifying the cause of a recipient's reaction as an acute, noncardiogenic pulmonary edema.

Post-test care
• If a hematoma develops at the venipuncture site, ease discomfort by applying warm soaks.
• If a transfusion recipient has a positive leukoagglutinin test, continued transfusions require premedication with acetaminophen 1 to 2 hours before the transfusion, specially prepared leukocyte-poor blood, or both to prevent further reactions.
• If a donor has a positive leukoagglutinin test, explain to him the meaning of this result to help prevent future transfusion reactions.

Interfering factors
Previous administration of dextran or I.V. contrast media causes aggregation resembling agglutination.

S. BREANNDAN MOORE, MD, DCH, FACP

Leukocyte alkaline phosphatase stain

Levels of leukocyte alkaline phosphatase (LAP), an enzyme found in neutrophils, may be altered by infection, stress, chronic inflammatory diseases, Hodgkin's disease, and hematologic disorders. Most of these things elevate LAP levels; only a few, notably chronic myelogenous leukemia (CML), depress them. So this test differentiates CML from other disorders that raise the white blood cell count.

To perform this test, a blood sample is obtained by venipuncture or finger stick. The venous blood sample is collected in a 7-ml *green-top* tube and transported immediately to the laboratory, where a blood smear is prepared; the peripheral blood sample is smeared on a 3″ x 1″ glass slide and fixed in cold formalin-methanol. The blood smear is then stained to show the amount of LAP present in the cytoplasm of the neutrophils. One hundred neutrophils are counted and assessed; each is assigned a score of 0 to 4, according to the degree of LAP staining. Normal values for LAP range from 40 to 100, depending on laboratory's standards.

Depressed LAP values typically indicate CML; however, low values may also occur in paroxysmal nocturnal hemoglobinuria, aplastic anemia, and infectious mononucleosis. Elevated values may indicate Hodgkin's disease, polycythemia vera, or a neutrophilic leukemoid reaction—a response to such conditions as infection, chronic inflammation, or pregnancy.

After a diagnosis of CML, the LAP stain may also be used to help detect onset of the blastic phase of the disease, when LAP levels typically rise. However, LAP levels also increase toward normal in response to therapy; because of this, test results must be correlated with the patient's condition.

CLARKE LAMBE, MD

Lymphocyte marker assays

A normal immune response requires a balance between the regulatory activities of several interacting cell types—most notably, T-helper and T-suppressor cells. By using highly specific monoclonal antibodies, levels of lymphocyte differentiation can be defined, and both normal and malignant cell populations can be analyzed. Direct and indirect immunofluorescence, microcytotoxicity, and immunoperoxidase immunoassay techniques are used most frequently: these employ an anticoagulated blood sample combined with monoclonal antibodies that react with specific T- and B-cell markers.

SR. REBECCA FIDLER, MT(ASCP), PhD
BEVERLY ZENK WHEAT, RN, MA

COMMON ASSAYS AND THEIR INDICATIONS

LYMPHOCYTE MARKER ASSAY	PURPOSE
Pan T-cell marker	• To measure mature T cells in immune dysfunction
T-helper/inducer subset marker	• To identify and characterize the proportion of T-helper cells in autoimmune or immunoregulatory disorders • To detect immunodeficiency disorders, such as AIDS • To differentiate T-cell acute lymphoblastic leukemia from T-cell lymphomas and other lymphoproliferative disorders
T-suppressor/cytotoxic subset marker	• To identify and characterize the proportion of T-suppressor cells in autoimmune and immunoregulatory disorders • To characterize lymphoproliferative disorders
T-cell/E-Rosette receptor	• To differentiate lymphoproliferative disorders of T-cell origin, such as T-cell lymphocytic leukemia and lymphoblastic lymphoma, from those of non-T-cell origin
Pan-B (B-1) marker	• To differentiate lymphoproliferative disorders of B-cell origin, such as B-cell chronic lymphocytic leukemia, from those of T-cell origin
Pan-B (BA-1) marker	• To identify B-cell lymphoproliferative disorders, such as B-cell chronic lymphocytic leukemia
CALLA (common acute lymphocytic leukemia antigen) marker	• To identify bone marrow regeneration • To identify non-T-cell acute lymphocytic leukemia
Lymphocyte subset panel (B, pan-T, T-helper/inducer, T-suppressor/cytotoxic, and T-helper/T-suppressor ratio)	• To evaluate immunodeficiencies • To identify immunoregulation associated with autoimmune disorders • To characterize lymphoid malignancies
Lymphocytic leukemia marker panel (T-cell markers [E-Rosette receptor and Leu-9], B-cell markers [B-1 and BA-1], and CALLA)	• To characterize lymphocytic leukemias as T, B, non-T, or non-B, regardless of the stage of differentiation of the malignant cells

Magnetic resonance imaging

Although its full range of clinical applications has yet to be established, magnetic resonance imaging (MRI) is already recognized as a safe, valuable tool for neurologic diagnosis. Like computed tomography (CT), MRI produces cross-sectional images of the brain and spine in multiple planes. However, unlike CT, MRI produces images without use of ionizing radiation or injected contrast solutions.

MRI's greatest advantages are its ability to "see through" bone and to delineate fluid-filled soft tissue in great detail. Thus far, it's proved useful in the diagnosis of cerebral infarction, tumors, abscesses, edema, hemorrhage, nerve fiber demyelination (as in multiple sclerosis), and other disorders that increase the fluid content of affected tissues. It can also show irregularities of the spinal cord with a resolution and detail previously unobtainable. And it holds promise for producing images of organs in motion.

MRI relies on the magnetic properties of the atom. (Hydrogen, the most abundant and magnetically sensitive of the body's atoms, is most commonly selected for MRI studies.) The scanner uses a powerful magnetic field and radiofrequency (RF) energy to produce images based on the hydrogen (primarily water) content of body tissues. Exposed to an external magnetic field, positively charged atomic nuclei and their negatively charged electrons align uniformly in the field. RF energy is then directed at the atoms, knocking them out of this magnetic alignment and causing them to *precess*, or spin. When the RF pulse is discontinued, the atoms realign themselves with the magnetic field, emitting RF energy as a tissue-specific signal based on the relative density of nuclei and the realignment time. These signals are monitored by the MRI computer, which processes them and displays the information on a video monitor as a high-resolution image.

The magnetic fields and RF energy used for MRI are imperceptible by the patient; no harmful effects have been documented. Research is continuing on the optimal magnetic fields and RF waves for each type of tissue.

Purpose
To aid diagnosis of intracranial and spinal lesions and soft-tissue abnormalities.

Patient preparation
Explain to the patient that this test assesses his brain or spinal cord. Tell him who will perform the test and where. Stress that the test is painless and involves no exposure to radiation. Tell him that the procedure may take up to 90 minutes.

Explain to the patient that he'll be positioned on a narrow bed and slid into a large cylinder that houses the MRI magnets. Have him change to a loose-fitting hospital gown (outpatients may wear any comfortable clothing). Since watches and jewelry can be damaged by the strong magnetic field, ask the patient to remove all metal objects before the test begins.

Equipment
MRI scanner and computer/display screen/recorder (film or magnetic tape).

Procedure
The patient is placed in a supine position on a narrow bed and told to lie still. The bed then slides him to the desired position inside the scanner, where RF energy is directed at his head or spine. The resulting images are displayed on a monitor and recorded on film or magnetic tape for permanent storage. The radiologist may vary the RF energy waves and use the computer to manipulate and enhance the magnetic resonance images.

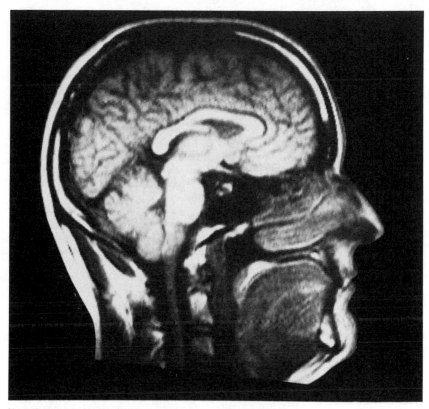

Normal magnetic resonance image of the head (midsagittal view)

Precautions

Because MRI works through a powerful magnetic field, it can't be performed on patients with pacemakers, intracranial aneurysm clips, or other ferrous metal implants.

Findings

MRI can show normal anatomic details of the central nervous system in any plane, without bone interference. Brain and spinal cord structures should appear distinct and sharply defined. Tissue color and shading will vary, depending on the RF energy, magnetic strength, and degree of computer enhancement.

Implications of results

Because the MRI signal represents proton density (water content) of tissue, MRI clearly shows structural changes resulting from disorders that increase tissue water content, such as cerebral edema, demyelinating disease, and pontine and cerebellar tumors. Edematous fluid, for example, generally appears cloudy or gray, whereas blood generally appears dark. Lesions of multiple sclerosis appear as areas of demyelination (curdlike, gray or gray-white areas) around the edges of ventricles. Tumors show as changes in normal anatomy, which computer enhancement may further delineate.

Post-test care

None.

Interfering factors

Excessive movement can blur images.

ROGER M. MORRELL, MD, PhD, FACP

Neonatal thyroid-stimulating hormone
[Neonatal thyrotropin]

This radioimmunoassay confirms congenital hypothyroidism after an initial screening test detects low thyroxine (T_4) levels. Normally, thyroid-stimulating hormone (TSH) levels surge soon after birth, triggering a rise in thyroid hormone, which is essential for neurologic development. However, in primary congenital hypothyroidism, the thyroid gland doesn't respond to TSH stimulation, resulting in diminished thyroid hormone levels and elevated TSH levels. Early detection and treatment of congenital hypothyroidism is critical to prevent mental retardation and cretinism.

Purpose
To confirm diagnosis of congenital hypothyroidism.

Patient preparation
Explain to the infant's parents that this test helps confirm the diagnosis of congenital hypothyroidism. Emphasize the test's importance in detecting the disorder early so that prompt therapy can prevent irreversible brain damage. Tell them further tests will be done if abnormalities are found.

Equipment
For a filter paper sample: Alcohol or povidone-iodine swabs/sterile lancet/specially marked filter paper/2" x 2" sterile gauze pads/adhesive bandage/labels.
For a serum sample: venipuncture equipment.

Procedure
For a filter paper sample: Assemble the necessary equipment and wash your hands thoroughly. Wipe the infant's heel with an alcohol or povidone-io-dine swab, then dry it thoroughly with a gauze pad. Perform a heelstick. Squeezing the infant's heel gently, fill the circles on the filter paper with blood. Make sure the blood saturates the paper. Gently apply pressure with a gauze pad to ensure hemostasis at the puncture site. Allow the filter paper to dry, label it appropriately, and send it to the laboratory.
For a serum sample: Perform a venipuncture and collect the sample in a 5-ml *red-top* tube. Label the sample and send it to the laboratory immediately.

Precautions
If a serum sample is taken, handle it carefully to prevent hemolysis.

Values
At age 1 to 2 days, TSH levels are normally 25 to 30 µIU/ml. Thereafter, levels are normally less than 25 µIU/ml.

Implications of results
Neonatal TSH levels must be interpreted in light of T_4 concentrations. Elevated TSH accompanied by decreased T_4 indicates primary congenital hypothyroidism (thyroid gland dysfunction). Depressed TSH and T_4 may be present in secondary congenital hypothyroidism (pituitary or hypothalamic dysfunction). Normal TSH accompanied by depressed T_4 may indicate hypothyroidism due to a congenital defect in thyroxine-binding globulin or may indicate transient congenital hypothyroidism due to prematurity or prenatal hypoxia. A complete thyroid workup must be done to confirm the cause of hypothyroidism before treatment can begin.

Post-test care
If a hematoma develops at the venipuncture site, apply warm soaks to relieve the patient's discomfort. Heelsticks require no special care.

Interfering factors
• Corticosteroids, T_3, and T_4 lower TSH

levels; potassium iodide, excessive topical resorcinol, and TSH injection raise TSH levels.

• Failure to let a filter paper sample dry completely may alter test results.

• Rough handling of a serum sample may cause hemolysis and may interfere with accurate testing.

WENDY BAKER, RN, MS, CCRN

Neutrophil function tests

Normal neutrophils—the body's primary defense against bacterial invasion—engulf and destroy bacteria and foreign particles by a process known as phagocytosis. In patients who suffer from repeated bacterial infections, neutrophil function tests may reveal the inability of neutrophils to kill target bacteria or to migrate to the bacterial site (chemotaxis).

Neutrophil killing ability can be evaluated by the *nitroblue tetrazolium (NBT) test*, which relies on neutrophil generation of bactericidal enzymes and toxins during killing. This action results in increased oxygen consumption and glucose metabolism, which reduces colorless NBT to blue formazan. The reduced dye is then extracted with pyridine and measured photometrically; the level of reduction indicates phagocytic activity.

Neutrophil killing activity can also be evaluated by noting the *chemiluminescence*—or ability to emit light—of neutrophils. After a neutrophil phagocytizes a microorganism, oxygen-containing substances form within phagocytic vacuoles. As the cell is stimulated, it emits light in proportion to the amount of oxygen-containing substances that are formed, providing an indirect measurement of phagocytosis.

Chemotaxis can be assessed in vitro by placing bacteria in the lower half of a two-part chamber and phagocytic neutrophils in the upper half. After incubation, migrating cells are counted microscopically and compared to standard values.

SR. REBECCA FIDLER, MT(ASCP), PhD
BEVERLY ZENK WHEAT, RN, MA

Nipple discharge cytology

Nipple discharge occurs normally only during lactation. However, when this discharge can't be attributed to lactation or occurs without breast masses or other signs of breast cancer, cytologic study of the discharge can help determine its cause. (The presence of signs of breast cancer necessitates breast biopsy and other tests.) For example, cytologic study of discharge can differentiate between malignant conditions, such as intraductal papillary carcinoma and intracystic infiltrating carcinoma, and benign conditions, such as mastitis and intraductal papilloma.

Before obtaining a discharge specimen, wash the patient's nipple and pat it dry. Then show the patient how to "milk" the breast to express the fluid. Discard the first drop and collect the next drop by moving a labeled glass slide across the nipple. (If a larger specimen is required, you'll need to collect it with a breast pump.)

Fix the specimen immediately with cytology spray, or place it in 95% ethanol solution. Label the specimen and send it to the laboratory immediately for staining. Document which breast was used to obtain the specimen. In addition, be sure to record if the patient is pregnant, perimenopausal, or taking drugs that alter hormonal balance, such as oral contraceptives, phenothiazines, digitalis, diuretics, or steroids.

SHIRLEY GIVEN, HT (ASCP)

Oral lactose tolerance test

This test measures plasma glucose levels after ingestion of a challenge dose of lactose. It's used to screen for lactose intolerance due to lactase deficiency.

Lactose, a disaccharide, is found in milk and other dairy products. The intestinal enzyme lactase splits lactose into the monosaccharides glucose and galactose for absorption by the intestinal epithelium. Absence or deficiency of lactase causes undigested lactose to remain in the intestinal lumen, producing such symptoms as abdominal cramps and watery diarrhea. True congenital lactase deficiency is rare. Usually, lactose intolerance is acquired, as lactase levels generally fall with age.

Purpose
To detect lactose intolerance.

Patient preparation
Explain to the patient that this test determines if his symptoms are due to an inability to digest lactose. Instruct him to fast and to avoid strenuous activity for 8 hours before the test. Tell him this test may require a stool sample. Also tell him that this test requires four blood samples, who will perform the venipunctures and when, and that he may feel transient discomfort from the needle punctures and the pressure of the tourniquet. Reassure him that collecting each blood sample takes less than 3 minutes, but explain that the entire procedure may take as long as 2 hours. As ordered, withhold drugs that may affect plasma glucose levels. If these drugs must be continued, note this on the laboratory slip.

Procedure
After the patient has fasted for 8 hours, perform a venipuncture and collect a blood sample in a 7-ml *gray-top* tube. Then administer the test load of lactose—for an adult, 50 g of lactose dissolved in 400 ml of water; for a child, 50 g per square meter of body surface area. Record the time of ingestion.

Draw a blood sample 30, 60, and 120 minutes after giving the loading dose, using 7-ml *gray-top* tubes. Collect a stool sample 5 hours after the loading dose, if ordered.

Precautions
• Send blood and stool samples to the laboratory immediately, or refrigerate them if transport is delayed. Specify the time of collection on the laboratory slips.
• Watch for symptoms of lactose intolerance—abdominal cramps, nausea, bloating, flatulence, and watery diarrhea—caused by the loading dose.

Values
Normally, plasma glucose levels rise more than 20 mg/dl over fasting levels within 15 to 60 minutes after ingestion of the lactose loading dose. Stool sample analysis shows normal pH (7 to 8) and low glucose content (less than 1 + on a glucose-indicating dipstick).

Implications of results
A rise in plasma glucose levels of less than 20 mg/dl indicates lactose intolerance, as does stool acidity (pH of 5.5 or less) and high glucose content (greater than 1 + on the dipstick). Related signs and symptoms provoked by the test also suggest but do not confirm it because such symptoms may develop for patients with normal lactase activity after a loading dose of lactose. Small-bowel biopsy with lactase assay may be done to confirm the diagnosis.

Post-test care
• If a hematoma develops at the venipuncture site, apply warm soaks.
• As ordered, instruct the patient to resume diet, activity, and medications withheld before the test.

Interfering factors
• Drugs that affect plasma glucose lev-

els—such as thiazide diuretics, oral contraceptives, benzodiazepines, propranolol, and insulin—may alter test results.
• Delayed emptying of stomach contents can cause depressed glucose levels.
• Failure to follow diet and exercise restrictions may alter test results.
• Glycolysis may cause false-negative results.

CLARKE LAMBE, MD
LAUREL LAMBE, MS, RD

Paranasal sinus radiography

The paranasal sinuses—air-filled cavities lined with mucous membrane—lie within the maxillary, ethmoid, sphenoid, and frontal bones. Sinus abnormalities, resulting from inflammation, trauma, cysts, mucoceles, granulomatosis, and other conditions, may include distorted bony sinus walls, altered mucous membranes, and fluid or masses within the cavities.

In paranasal sinus radiography, X-rays or gamma rays penetrate the paranasal sinuses and react on specially sensitized film, forming an image of sinus structures. The air that normally fills the paranasal sinuses appears black on film, but fluid in a sinus appears cloudy to opaque and may reveal an air-fluid level. A bone fracture is visible as a linear, radiolucent defect; cysts, polyps, and tumors are visible as soft-tissue masses projecting into the sinus.

When surrounding facial structures—superimposed on the paranasal sinuses—interfere with visualization of relevant areas, tomography may be done to provide further information. Tomography is especially useful in evaluating facial trauma and neoplastic disease.

PARANASAL SINUS TOMOGRAPHY

Tomography of the paranasal sinuses is performed by moving an X-ray beam and X-ray film simultaneously and in opposite directions around a pivot point during film exposure. The resulting image produces a sharply focused selected section, with blurred areas above and below it. This test supplements radiography when surrounding facial structures obscure relevant areas. Because tomography visualizes the paranasal sinuses in very thin sections, one section at a time, it's especially useful in detecting tumor involvement of bone and locating fractures of bony sinus walls and foreign bodies.

To prepare a patient for paranasal sinus tomography, describe the procedure to him and advise him to remain motionless while the tomograms are being taken; patient movement during filming interferes with test results. A normal paranasal sinus tomogram shows structures equivalent to a normal X-ray film of this area without superimposition of other structures.

Purpose
• To detect unilateral or bilateral abnormalities, possibly indicating trauma or disease
• To confirm diagnosis of neoplastic or inflammatory paranasal sinus disease
• To determine the location and size of a malignant neoplasm.

Patient preparation
Describe the procedure to the patient, and explain that this test helps evaluate abnormalities of the paranasal sinuses. Tell him who will perform the test, where and when it will be performed, and that it usually takes 10 or 15 minutes to complete.

Tell the patient that his head may be immobilized in a foam vise during the test to help him maintain the correct position, but that the vise doesn't hurt. Explain that he'll be asked to sit upright and avoid moving while the X-rays are being taken to prevent blurring of the image and to allow visualization of air-fluid levels, if present. Emphasize the importance of his cooperation. Instruct

IMPLICATIONS OF ABNORMAL RADIOGRAPHIC FINDINGS

DISORDER	ABNORMAL FINDINGS
Paranasal sinus trauma or fracture	• Edema or hemorrhage in mucous membrane lining or sinus cavity • Clouded sinus air cells • Air-fluid level • Radiolucent, linear bone defects • Irregular, overriding bone edges • Depression or displacement of bone fragments • Foreign bodies
Acute sinusitis	• Swollen, inflamed mucous membrane • Inflammatory exudate • Hazy to opaque sinus air cells • Air-fluid level
Chronic sinusitis	• Thickened mucous membrane • Hazy to opaque sinus air cells • Air-fluid level • Thickening or sclerosis of bony wall of affected sinus
Wegener's granulomatosis	• Clouded to opaque sinus air cells • Destruction of bony sinus wall
Malignant neoplasm	• Rounded or lobulated soft-tissue mass, projecting into sinus • Destruction of bony sinus wall
Benign bone tumor	• Distortion of bony sinus wall in specific patterns
Cyst, polyp, or benign tumor	• Rounded or lobulated soft-tissue mass, projecting into sinus
Mucocele	• Clouded sinus air cells • Destruction of bony sinus wall, resulting in various degrees of radiolucency

him to remove dentures, all jewelry, or metal in the X-ray field.

Equipment
Franklin radiographic head unit.

Procedure
The patient sits upright (possibly with his head in a foam vise) between the X-ray tube and a film cassette. During the test, the X-ray tube is positioned at specific angles and the patient's head is placed in various standard positions while his paranasal sinuses are filmed from different angles. If necessary, help position the patient.

Precautions
• Paranasal sinus radiography is usu-ally contraindicated during pregnancy; however, when this test is absolutely necessary, a lead-lined apron placed over the patient's abdomen can shield the fetus.

• To avoid exposure to radiation, leave the room or the immediate area during the test; if you must stay in the area, wear a lead-lined apron.

Findings
Normal paranasal sinuses are radio-lucent and filled with air, which appears black on paranasal sinus films.

Implications of results
See the chart on this page for common implications of abnormal radiographic findings.

Post-test care
None.

Interfering factors
• Failure to remove dentures, jewelry, and metal within the X-ray field, or the presence of numerous metallic foreign bodies in or around the paranasal sinuses may interfere with accurate determination of test results.
• Patient movement during filming may necessitate additional X-ray filming.
• The patient's inability to sit upright during filming may necessitate performing the test on an X-ray table. This impairs visualization and diminishes the diagnostic values of the test.
• The superimposition of surrounding facial structures on the film may impair visualization of paranasal sinuses.
BONNIE L. ANDERSON, MD

Plasma plasminogen

Plasminogen, the precursor molecule of plasmin, is measured to assess fibrinolysis. During fibrinolysis, plasmin dissolves fibrin clots to prevent excessive coagulation and the resultant impairment of blood flow. Plasmin doesn't circulate in active form, so it can't be measured directly. However, its circulating precursor, plasminogen, *can* be measured and provides an estimate of fibrinolysis.

This test assesses plasminogen levels by adding streptokinase, a plasminogen activator, to a plasma sample. Streptokinase converts plasminogen to active plasmin; the plasmin then converts substrate *a*-casein to tyrosine, a colored substance that's measured spectrophotometrically. The amount of color that develops represents the amount of functional plasminogen in the sample.

Purpose
• To assess fibrinolysis

• To detect congenital and acquired fibrinolytic disorders.

Patient preparation
Explain to the patient that this test evaluates blood clotting. Inform him that he needn't restrict food or fluids. Tell him that the test requires a blood sample, who will perform the venipuncture and when, and that he may experience minor discomfort from the needle puncture and the pressure of the tourniquet. Reassure him that collecting the sample takes less than 3 minutes. Check the patient's history for use of streptokinase or other drugs that may cause inaccurate test results. If these drugs must be continued, note this on the laboratory slip.

Procedure
Perform a venipuncture and collect the sample in a 7-ml *blue-top* tube.

Precautions
• Collect the sample as quickly as possible to prevent stasis, which can slow blood flow, causing coagulation and plasminogen activation.
• To prevent hemolysis, avoid excessive probing during venipuncture and rough handling of the specimen.
• Immediately after collection, invert the tube gently several times; then send the sample to the laboratory. If testing is delayed, plasma must be separated and frozen at −94° F. (−70° C.).

Values
Normal plasminogen levels are 65% or greater (expressed as a percentage of normal), or 2.7 to 4.5 μ/ml (expressed as activity units).

Implications of results
Diminished plasminogen levels can result from disseminated intravascular coagulation, tumors, preeclampsia, and eclampsia, which accelerate plasminogen conversion to plasmin and increase fibrinolysis. Some liver diseases prevent formation of sufficient plasminogen, decreasing fibrinolysis.

Post-test care
• If a hematoma develops at the venipuncture site, apply warm soaks.
• Resume medications, as ordered.

Interfering factors
• Failure to use the proper tube, to mix the sample and citrate adequately, to send the sample immediately, or to have it separated and frozen may alter results.
• Hemolysis from excessive probing during venipuncture or rough handling of the sample may alter results. '
• Prolonged tourniquet use before venipuncture may cause stasis, falsely decreasing plasminogen levels.
• Oral contraceptives may slightly increase plasminogen levels. Thrombolytic drugs, such as streptokinase or urokinase, may decrease levels also.
    WILLIAM E. KLINE, MS, MT(ASCP), SBB

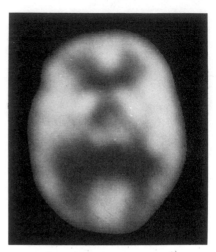

Normal positron emission tomogram of the brain (cross-sectional image)

Positron emission tomography

Like computed tomography (CT) scanning and magnetic resonance imaging (MRI), positron emission tomography (PET) provides images of the brain through sophisticated computer reconstruction algorithms. However, PET images detail brain function as well as structure and thus differ significantly from the images provided by these other advanced techniques.

PET combines elements of both CT scanning and conventional radionuclide imaging. For example, PET measures the emissions of injected radioisotopes and converts these to a tomographic image of the brain. But, unlike conventional radionuclide imaging, PET uses radioisotopes of biologically important elements—oxygen, nitrogen, carbon, and fluorine—that emit particles called *positrons.*

During positron emission, pairs of gamma rays are emitted; the PET scanner detects these and relays the information to a computer for reconstruction as an image. Positron emitters can be chemically "tagged" to biologically active molecules, such as carbon monoxide, neurotransmitters, hormones, and metabolites (particularly glucose), enabling study of their uptake and distribution in brain tissue. For example, blood tagged with ^{11}C-carbon monoxide allows study of hemodynamic patterns in brain tissue, whereas tagged neurotransmitters, hormones, and drugs allow mapping of receptor distribution. Isotope-tagged glucose (which penetrates the blood-brain barrier rapidly) allows dynamic study of brain function, since PET can pinpoint the sites of glucose metabolism in the brain under various conditions. This last application is particularly promising—researchers expect it to prove useful in the diagnosis of psychiatric disorders, transient ischemic attacks, amyotrophic lateral sclerosis, Parkinson's disease, Wilson's disease, multiple sclerosis, seizure disorders, cerebrovascular disease, and Alzheimer's disease. The reason: All of these disorders may alter the location and patterns of cerebral glucose metabolism.

PET is a costly test because the radioisotopes used have very short half-lives and must be produced at an on-site cyclotron and attached quickly to the desired tracer molecules. So far, this prohibitive cost has limited PET's use, except as a research tool. However, PET has already provided significant information about the brain and may someday have widespread clinical applications.

ROGER M. MORRELL, MD, PhD, FACP

Red blood cell survival time

Normally, red blood cells (RBCs) are destroyed only when they reach senility. However, in hemolytic diseases, RBCs of all ages are randomly destroyed, resulting in anemia. This test measures the survival time of circulating RBCs and detects sites of abnormal RBC sequestration and destruction, aiding evaluation of unexplained anemia.

Survival time is measured by labeling a random sample of RBCs with radioactive chromium-51 sodium chromate (^{51}Cr). The ^{51}Cr quickly crosses RBC membranes, reduces to chromium ions, and binds to hemoglobin. This labeled group of RBCs is then injected back into the patient. Serial blood samples measure the percentage of labeled cells per unit volume over 3 to 4 weeks, until 50% of the cells disappear (disappearance rate corresponds to destruction of a random cell population). A normal RBC survives about 120 days (half-life of 60 days); the ^{51}Cr-labeled RBCs have a shorter half-life (25 to 35 days) because about 1% of senescent RBCs are removed from the circulation each day and about 1% of ^{51}Cr is spontaneously eluted from the labeled RBCs each day.

During the test period, a gamma camera scans the body for sites of abnormally high radioactivity, which indicate sites of excessive RBC sequestration and destruction. Other tests performed with the RBC survival time test may include spot checks of the stool to detect GI blood loss; hematocrit tests; blood volume studies; and radionuclide iron uptake and clearance tests to aid differential diagnosis of anemia.

Purpose
● To help evaluate unexplained anemia, particularly hemolytic anemia
● To identify sites of abnormal RBC sequestration and destruction.

Patient preparation
Explain to the patient that this test helps identify the cause of his anemia. Advise him that he needn't restrict food or fluids. Inform him that the test involves labeling a blood sample with a radioactive substance and that it requires regular blood samples at 3-day intervals for 3 to 4 weeks. Tell him who will perform the procedures and when, and that he may experience slight discomfort from the needle punctures. Reassure him that collecting each sample takes less than 3 minutes and that the small amount of radioactive substance used is harmless.

If the doctor orders a stool collection to test for GI bleeding, teach the patient the proper collection technique.

Procedure
A 30-ml blood sample is drawn and mixed with 100 microcuries (μCi) of ^{51}Cr for an adult; less for a child. After an incubation period, the mixture is injected intravenously into the patient. A blood sample is drawn 30 minutes after injection to determine blood and RBC volumes.

A 6-ml sample is collected in a *green-top* tube after 24 hours; follow-up samples are collected at 3-day intervals for 3 to 4 weeks. (The interval between samples may vary, depending on the laboratory.) To avoid error from physical decay of the ^{51}Cr, each sample is measured with a scintillation well counter on the day it's drawn. Radioactivity per ml of RBCs is calculated; these values are then plotted to determine mean RBC survival time. Simultaneous gamma camera scans of the precordium, sacrum, liver, and spleen detect radioactivity at sites of excess RBC sequestration. A hematocrit is done on a small portion of each blood sample to check for blood loss.

At the end of the study, a sample is drawn to compare ending blood and RBC volumes with beginning volumes.

Precautions

• This test is contraindicated during pregnancy, because it exposes the fetus to radiation.

• Because excess blood loss can invalidate test results, this test is usually contraindicated for a patient with active bleeding or poor clotting function. However, if the test is necessary for a patient with poor clotting function, observe the venipuncture sites carefully for signs of hemorrhage.

• The patient should not receive blood transfusions during the test period and should not have blood samples drawn for other tests.

Findings

Normal half-life for RBCs labeled with ^{51}Cr is 25 to 35 days. Normal gamma camera scans reveal slight radioactivity in the spleen, liver, and sometimes the bone marrow.

Implications of results

Decreased RBC survival time indicates a hemolytic disease, such as chronic lymphocytic leukemia, congenital nonspherocytic hemolytic anemia, hemoglobin C disease, hereditary spherocytosis, idiopathic acquired hemolytic anemia, paroxysmal nocturnal hemoglobinuria, elliptocytosis, pernicious anemia, sickle cell anemia, sickle cell hemoglobin C disease, or hemolytic-uremic syndrome. If hemolytic anemia is diagnosed, tests using cross transfusion of labeled RBCs can determine if anemia results from an intrinsic RBC defect or an extrinsic factor.

A gamma camera scan that detects a site of excess RBC sequestration provides direction for treatment. For example, abnormally high RBC sequestration in the spleen may require a splenectomy.

Post-test care

If a hematoma develops at the venipuncture site, apply warm soaks.

Interfering factors

• Dehydration, overhydration, or blood loss (from hemorrhage or blood samples drawn for other tests) can change the circulating RBC volume and invalidate test results.

• Blood transfusions during the test period alter the proportion of labeled RBCs to total RBCs, thus altering results.

BONNIE L. ANDERSON, MD

Renal venography

This relatively simple procedure allows radiographic examination of the main renal veins and their tributaries. In this test, contrast medium is injected by percutaneous catheter passed through the femoral vein and inferior vena cava into the renal vein. Indications for renal venography include renal vein thrombosis, tumor, and venous anomalies. This test helps distinguish renal parenchymal disease and aneurysms from pressure exerted by an adjacent mass. When other diagnostic tests yield ambiguous results, renal venography can definitively differentiate renal agenesis from a small kidney.

Renal venography is also useful in assessing renovascular hypertension. Blood samples can be collected from renal veins during the procedure, and renin assays of the samples can differentiate essential renovascular hypertension from hypertension due to unilateral renal lesions.

Purpose

- To detect renal vein thrombosis
- To evaluate renal vein compression due to extrinsic tumors or retroperitoneal fibrosis
- To assess renal tumors and detect invasion of the renal vein or inferior vena cava
- To detect venous anomalies and defects
- To differentiate renal agenesis from a small kidney
- To collect renal venous blood samples for evaluation of renovascular hypertension.

Patient preparation

Explain to the patient that this test permits radiographic study of the renal veins. If ordered, instruct him to fast for 4 hours before the test. Tell him who will perform the test and where, and that it takes about 1 hour.

Inform the patient that a catheter will be inserted into a vein in the groin area after he is given a sedative and a local anesthetic. Tell him that he may feel mild discomfort during injection of the local anesthetic and contrast medium and that he may feel transient burning and flushing from the contrast medium. Warn him that the X-ray equipment will make loud clacking noises.

Check the patient's history for hypersensitivity to contrast media, iodine, or iodine-containing foods, such as shellfish. Report any sensitivities to the doctor. Check the patient's history and any coagulation studies for indications of bleeding disorders.

If renin assays will be done, review the patient's diet and medications with the doctor. As ordered, restrict the patient's salt intake and discontinue antihypertensive drugs, diuretics, estrogen, and oral contraceptives.

Make sure the patient or a responsible family member has signed a consent form. Just before the procedure, administer a sedative, as ordered.

Equipment

X-ray equipment/renal venography tray with flexible guide wires, polyethylene radiopaque vascular catheters, needle and cannula or 18G Becton Dickinson needle, three-way stopcock, and flexible tubing/preparatory tray/syringes and needles/contrast medium/local anesthetic/emergency resuscitation equipment.

Procedure

The patient is placed in a supine position on the X-ray table, with his abdomen centered over the film. The skin over the right femoral vein near the groin is cleansed with antiseptic solution and draped. A local anesthetic is injected, and the femoral vein is cannulated. Under fluoroscopic guidance, a guide wire is threaded a short distance through the cannula, which is then removed. A catheter is passed over the wire into the inferior vena cava.

When catheterization of the femoral vein is contraindicated, the right antecubital vein is punctured, and the catheter is inserted and advanced through the right atrium of the heart into the inferior vena cava.

A test bolus of contrast medium is injected to determine that the vena cava is patent. If so, the catheter is advanced into the right renal vein and contrast medium is injected. The volume, usually 20 to 40 ml, depends on indications for the procedure. When studies of the right renal vasculature are completed, the catheter is withdrawn into the vena cava, rotated, and guided into the left renal vein.

If visualization of the renal venous tributaries is indicated, epinephrine can be injected into the ipsilateral renal artery by catheter before contrast medium is injected into the renal vein. Epinephrine temporarily blocks arterial flow and allows filling of distal intrarenal veins. Obstructing the artery briefly with a balloon catheter is an alternative method.

After anteroposterior films are made, the patient is placed prone for posteroanterior films. If renin assays are indicated, blood samples are withdrawn under fluoroscopy up to 15 minutes after venography. The catheter is removed and a dressing applied.

Precautions
• Renal venography is contraindicated in severe thrombosis of the inferior vena cava.
• The guide wire and catheter should be advanced carefully if severe renal vein thrombosis is suspected.
• Watch for signs of hypersensitivity to the contrast medium.

Findings
After injection of the contrast medium, opacification of the renal vein and tributaries should occur immediately.

Normally, the renin content of venous blood measured in a supine adult is 1.5 to 1.6 ng/ml/hr.

Implications of results
Occlusion of the renal vein near the inferior vena cava or the kidney indicates renal vein thrombosis. If the clot is outlined by contrast medium, it may look like a filling defect. However, a clot can usually be identified because it is within the lumen and less sharply outlined than a filling defect. Collateral venous channels, which opacify with retrograde filling during contrast injection, often surround the occlusion. Complete occlusion prolongs contrast medium transit through the renal veins.

A filling defect of the renal vein may indicate obstruction or compression by an extrinsic tumor or retroperitoneal fibrosis. A renal tumor that invades the renal vein or inferior vena cava usually produces a filling defect with a sharply defined border.

Venous anomalies are indicated by opacification of abnormally positioned or clustered vessels. Absence of a renal vein differentiates renal agenesis from a small kidney.

Elevated renin content in renal venous blood usually indicates essential renovascular hypertension when assay results correspond for both kidneys. Elevated renin levels in one kidney indicate a unilateral lesion and usually require further evaluation by arteriography.

Post-test care
• Check vital signs and distal pulses every 15 minutes for the first hour, every 30 minutes for the second hour, then every 2 hours for 24 hours.
• Check the puncture site for bleeding or hematoma; if a hematoma develops, apply warm soaks.
• Report signs of vein perforation, embolism, and extravasation of contrast medium. These include chills, fever, rapid pulse and respiration, hypotension, dyspnea, and chest, abdominal, or flank pain. Also report complaints of paresthesias or pain in the catheterized limb—symptoms of nerve irritation or vascular compromise.
• Administer a sedative and antibiotics, as ordered.
• Instruct the patient to resume his usual diet and any medications that were discontinued before the test.

Interfering factors
• Recent contrast studies or the presence of feces or gas in the bowel impairs visualization of the renal veins.
• Failure to restrict salt, antihypertensive drugs, diuretics, estrogen, and oral contraceptives can interfere with renin assay results.

ELLEN SHIPES, RN, ET, MN, MEd

Serum glucagon

Glucagon, a polypeptide hormone secreted by the alpha cells of the islets of Langerhans in the pancreas, acts primarily on the liver to promote glucose production and control glucose storage. Glucagon is secreted in response to hypoglycemia; secretion is inhibited by the other pancreatic hormones, insulin and somatostatin. Normally, the coordinated release of glucagon, insulin, and somatostatin ensures an adequate and constant fuel supply while maintaining blood glucose levels within relatively stable limits.

This test, a quantitative analysis of serum glucagon by radioimmunoassay, evaluates patients suspected of having glucagonoma (alpha cell tumor) or hypoglycemia due to idiopathic glucagon deficiency or pancreatic dysfunction. Glucagon is usually measured concomitantly with serum glucose and insulin, since glucose and insulin levels influence glucagon secretion.

Purpose
To aid diagnosis of glucagonoma and hypoglycemia due to chronic pancreatitis or idiopathic glucagon deficiency.

Patient preparation
Explain to the patient that this test helps evaluate pancreatic function. Instruct him to fast for 10 to 12 hours before the test. Tell him that the test requires a blood sample, who will perform the venipuncture and when, and that he may feel transient discomfort from the needle puncture. Reassure him that collecting the sample takes only a few minutes.

As ordered, withhold insulin, catecholamines, and other drugs that could influence test results. If these drugs must be continued, note this on the laboratory slip.

Since exercise and stress elevate serum glucagon levels, make sure the patient is relaxed and recumbent for 30 minutes before the test.

Procedure
Perform a venipuncture, and collect a blood sample in a chilled 10-ml *lavender-top* tube.

Precautions
• Make sure the patient is relaxed before sample collection since stress may elevate glucagon levels.
• Place the sample on ice and send it to the laboratory immediately.
• Handle the sample gently to prevent hemolysis.

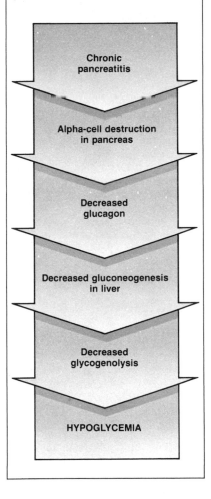

HOW PANCREATIC DYSFUNCTION CAUSES HYPOGLYCEMIA

As you know, alpha cells in the pancreas secrete glucagon—a hormone that promotes glucose production and controls glucose storage. Normally, glucagon works with three other hormones to raise blood glucose levels back to normal after they drop. The hormones do this by assisting in glycogenolysis (conversion of glycogen back to glucose) and gluconeogenesis (creation of new glucose from noncarbohydrates, such as amino acids or fatty acids).

Hypoglycemia can result when chronic pancreatitis destroys alpha cells in the pancreas, as shown below.

Chronic pancreatitis

Alpha-cell destruction in pancreas

Decreased glucagon

Decreased gluconeogenesis in liver

Decreased glycogenolysis

HYPOGLYCEMIA

Values

Fasting glucagon levels are normally less than 250 pg/ml.

Implications of results

Markedly elevated fasting glucagon levels occur in glucagonoma; values may range from 900 to 7,800 pg/ml. Elevated levels also occur in diabetes mellitus, acute pancreatitis, and pheochromocytoma.

Abnormally low glucagon levels are associated with idiopathic glucagon deficiency and hypoglycemia due to chronic pancreatitis. Stimulation or suppression tests may be necessary to confirm diagnosis.

Post-test care

• If a hematoma develops at the venipuncture site, apply warm soaks.
• As ordered, resume diet and administration of drugs.

Interfering factors

• Prolonged fasting, undue stress, or use of catecholamines or insulin before the collection of blood samples may elevate glucagon levels.
• Failure to pack the sample in ice and send it to the laboratory immediately may affect test results.
• Hemolysis caused by rough handling of the sample may interfere with accurate determination of test results.

WENDY BAKER, RN, MS, CCRN

Serum myoglobin

Using radioimmunoassay, this test measures serum levels of myoglobin, an oxygen-binding muscle protein similar to hemoglobin. Myoglobin binds, stores, and transports oxygen to the muscle cells' mitochondria, where oxygen generates energy by converting glucose into carbon dioxide and water. Myoglobin is normally found in skeletal and cardiac muscle but is released into the blood after muscle injury. Thus, serum myoglobin levels help estimate the severity of muscle damage. However, because myoglobin levels don't indicate the site of injury, they're commonly used to confirm other studies, such as total creatine phosphokinase (CPK) or the myocardial-specific isoenzyme, CPK-MB.

Purpose

• To estimate damage caused by myocardial infarction (MI) or skeletal muscle injury
• To predict exacerbation of polymyositis, a degenerative muscle disease.

Patient preparation

Explain to the patient that this test helps determine the severity of muscle damage. Inform him that he needn't restrict food or fluids. Tell him that the test requires a blood sample, who will perform the venipuncture and when, and that he may feel some discomfort from the needle puncture and the pressure of the tourniquet. Reassure him that collecting the sample takes only a few minutes.

Procedure

Perform a venipuncture and collect the sample in a 10-ml *red-top* tube.

Precautions

None.

Values

Normal serum myoglobin levels range from 30 to 90 ng/ml.

Implications of results

Elevated serum myoglobin levels help estimate the severity of damage after MI or skeletal muscle injury. In a patient with polymyositis, elevated levels may signal exacerbation of the disease. However, elevated myoglobin levels are also associated with dermatomyositis, systemic lupus erythematosus, shock, or severe renal failure. Because test results are nonspecific, elevated serum myoglobin levels must be correlated with the patient's signs and symptoms.

Post-test care

If a hematoma develops at the venipuncture site, apply warm soaks.

Interfering factors

• Recent cardioversion or angina attacks may increase myoglobin levels.
• Performing this test immediately after onset of an acute MI produces misleading results, since myoglobin levels don't peak for 4 to 8 hours.
• A radioactive scan performed within 1 week before the test may affect results.

TOBIE VIRGINIA HITTLE, RN, BSN, CCRN

Siderocyte stain

Siderocytes are red blood cells (RBCs) containing particles of nonhemoglobin iron known as siderocytic granules. In newborn infants, siderocytic granules are normally present in normoblasts and reticulocytes during hemoglobin synthesis. However, the spleen removes most of these granules from normal RBCs, and they disappear rapidly with age. In adults, an elevated siderocyte level usually indicates abnormal erythropoiesis, as in congenital spherocytic anemia, chronic hemolytic anemias (such as the thalassemias), pernicious anemia, hemochromatosis, toxicities (such as lead poisoning), infection, or severe burns. Elevated levels may also follow splenectomy since the spleen normally removes siderocytic granules.

Procedure

The siderocyte stain test measures the number of circulating siderocytes. Venous blood is drawn into a 7-ml *lavender-top* tube or, for infants and children, collected in a Microtainer or pipette and smeared directly on a 3″ × 1″ glass slide. When the blood smear is stained, siderocytic granules appear as purple-blue specks clustered around the periphery of mature erythrocytes. Cells containing these granules are

counted as a percentage of total RBCs. The results aid differential diagnosis of the anemias and hemochromatosis, and help detect toxicities.

Implications of results

Normally, newborn infants have a slightly elevated siderocyte level, which reaches the normal adult value of 0.5% of total RBCs in 7 to 10 days. In patients with pernicious anemia, the siderocyte level is 8% to 14%; in chronic hemolytic anemia, 20% to 100%; in lead poisoning, 10% to 30%; and in hemochromatosis, 3% to 7%. A high siderocyte level mandates additional testing—including bone marrow examination—to determine the cause of abnormal erythropoiesis.

WILLIAM M. DOUGHERTY, BS

Small-bowel biopsy

Small-bowel biopsy helps evaluate diseases of the intestinal mucosa, which may cause malabsorption or diarrhea. Using a capsule, it produces larger specimens than does endoscopic biopsy and allows removal of tissue from those areas beyond an endoscope's reach.

Several types of capsules are available, all similar in design and use. The Carey capsule, for example, is a spring-loaded, two-piece capsule, 8 mm in diameter and 2.6 cm long. A mercury-weighted bag is attached to one end of the capsule; a thin polyethylene tube about 150 cm long is attached to the other end. Once the bag, capsule, and tube are in place in the small bowel, suction applied to the tube causes the mucosa to enter the capsule. Continued suction closes the capsule, cutting off the piece of tissue within.

The biopsy sample verifies diagnosis of some diseases, such as Whipple's disease, and may help confirm others, such as tropical sprue. Capsule biopsy is an invasive procedure, but it causes little pain and complications are rare.

Purpose

To help diagnose diseases of the intestinal mucosa.

Patient preparation

Describe the procedure to the patient, and ask if he has any questions. Explain that this test helps identify intestinal disorders. Tell him to restrict food and fluids for at least 8 hours before the test. Also tell him who will perform the biopsy and where, and that the procedure takes 45 to 60 minutes but causes little discomfort.

Make sure the patient or a responsible family member has signed a consent form. Ensure that coagulation tests have been performed and that the results are recorded on the patient's chart.

Withhold aspirin and anticoagulants, as ordered. If they must be continued, note this on the laboratory slip.

Procedure

Check the tubing and the mercury bag for leaks. Lightly lubricate the tube and the capsule with a water-soluble lubricant, and moisten the mercury bag with water. Spray the back of the patient's throat with a local anesthetic, as ordered, to decrease gagging during passage of the tube. Ask the patient to sit upright. The capsule is placed in his pharynx, and he is asked to flex his neck and swallow as the doctor advances the tube about 50 cm. (If a local anesthetic is used to control the gag reflex, the patient must not receive any fluids to help him swallow the capsule.) Place the patient on his right side; the doctor then advances the tube another 50 cm. The tube's position must be checked by fluoroscopy or by instilling air through the tube and listening with a stethoscope for air to enter the stomach.

Next, the tube is advanced 5 to 10 cm at a time to pass the capsule through the pylorus. Talk to the patient about food to stimulate the pylorus and help the capsule pass. When fluoroscopy confirms that the capsule has passed the pylorus, keep the patient on his right side to allow the capsule to move into the second and third portions of the small bowel. Tell the patient that he may hold the tube loosely to one side of his mouth, if it makes him more comfortable. Capsule position is checked again by fluoroscopy.

When the capsule is at or beyond the ligament of Treitz, the biopsy sample can be taken. (The doctor will determine the biopsy site.) Place the patient supine so the capsule's position can be verified fluoroscopically. A 100-ml glass syringe is placed on the end of the tube, and steady suction is applied to close the capsule and cut off a tissue specimen. Suction is maintained on the syringe as the tube and capsule are removed; then the suction is released. This opens the capsule and exposes the specimen, mucosal side down. The specimen is gently removed with forceps, placed mucosal side up on a piece of mesh, and placed in a biopsy bottle with the required fixative. Send the specimen to the laboratory immediately.

Precautions

- Keep suction equipment nearby to prevent aspiration if the patient vomits.
- Do not allow the patient to bite the tubing.
- Handle the tissue carefully and place it correctly on the slide, as ordered.
- Biopsy is contraindicated in uncooperative patients, in those taking aspirin or anticoagulants, and in those with uncontrolled coagulation disorders.

Findings

A normal small-bowel biopsy sample consists of fingerlike villi, crypts, columnar epithelial cells, and round cells.

Implications of results

Small-bowel tissue that reveals histologic changes in cell structure may indicate abetalipoproteinemia, Whipple's disease, eosinophilic enteritis, lymphoma, lymphangiectasia, and such parasitic infections as giardiasis and coccidiosis. Abnormal samples may also suggest celiac sprue, tropical sprue, infectious gastroenteritis, intraluminal bacterial overgrowth, folate and B_{12} deficiency, radiation enteritis, and malnutrition, but such disorders require further studies.

Post-test care
• As ordered, resume diet after confirming return of the gag reflex.
• Complications are rare. However, watch for signs of hemorrhage, bacteremia with transient fever and pain, and bowel perforation. Tell the patient to report abdominal pain or bleeding.

Interfering factors
• Mechanical failure of the biopsy capsule or any hole in the tubing can prevent removal of a tissue sample.
• Incorrect handling or positioning of the specimen may alter test results.
• Failure to fast before the biopsy may yield a poor specimen or cause vomiting and aspiration.
• Failure to place the specimen in fixative or a delay in transport may alter test results.

KATHERINE FULTON, RN

T3 (Cytomel) thyroid suppression test

The T_3 (Cytomel) thyroid suppression test helps determine whether areas of excessive iodine uptake in the thyroid (hot spots) are autonomous (as in some cases of Graves' disease) or reflect pituitary overcompensation (as in iodine-deficient goiter). Autonomous hot spots function independently of pituitary control. However, hot spots caused by iodine deficiency stem from reduced T_4 production, which decreases T_3 production and increases thyroid-stimulating hormone (TSH) production. Increased TSH production, in turn, overstimulates the thyroid and causes excessive iodine uptake.

After a baseline reading of thyroid function is obtained by a radioactive iodine uptake (RAIU) test, a dosage of 100 mcg of synthetic T_3 (Cytomel) is

TESTING THYROID RESPONSE

NORMAL FEEDBACK MECHANISM

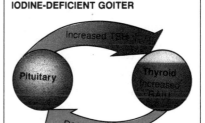

BASELINE TEST IN IODINE-DEFICIENT GOITER

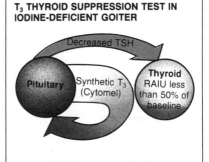

T3 THYROID SUPPRESSION TEST IN IODINE-DEFICIENT GOITER

administered for 7 days. (Normally, T_3 acts through a negative feedback mechanism to suppress pituitary release of TSH; TSH suppression then suppresses thyroid function and iodine uptake.) During the last 2 days of Cytomel administration, RAIU tests are repeated to assess thyroid response. Suppression of RAIU to at least 50% of baseline shows that the hot spot is under pituitary control and suggests iodine deficiency as the cause of increased iodine uptake. Failure to suppress RAIU by 50% suggests autonomous thyroid hyperfunction, possibly caused by Graves' disease or a toxic thyroid nodule.

BONNIE L. ANDERSON, MD

Terminal deoxynucleotidyl transferase test

Using indirect immunofluorescence, this test measures levels of terminal deoxynucleotidyl transferase (TdT), an intranuclear enzyme found in certain primitive lymphocytes in the normal thymus and bone marrow. Since TdT acts as a biochemical marker for these lymphocytes, it can help classify the origin of a particular tissue. Thus, the TdT test is useful in differentiating certain types of leukemias and lymphomas marked by primitive cells that can't be identified by histology alone. Measurement of TdT may also help determine the prognosis for these diseases and may provide early diagnosis of a relapse.

Purpose
• To help differentiate acute lymphocytic leukemia (ALL) from acute non-lymphocytic leukemia
• To help differentiate lymphoblastic lymphomas from non-Hodgkin's lymphomas
• To monitor response to therapy.

Patient preparation
Explain to the patient that this test detects an enzyme that can help classify tissue origin. If the patient is scheduled for a blood test, tell him to fast for 12 to 14 hours before the test. Tell him that the test requires a blood sample, who will perform the venipuncture and when, and that he may experience transient discomfort from the pressure of the tourniquet. Reassure him that collecting the sample takes less than 3 minutes.

If the patient is scheduled for a bone marrow aspiration, describe the procedure to him and answer any questions. Inform the patient that he needn't restrict food or fluids before the test. Tell him who will perform the biopsy and where, and that it usually takes only 5 to 10 minutes to perform. Make sure the patient or a responsible family member has signed a consent form. Check the patient's history for hypersensitivity to the local anesthetic. After checking with the doctor, tell the patient which bone will be the biopsy site. Inform him that he will receive a local anesthetic but will feel pressure on insertion of the biopsy needle and a brief, pulling pain when the marrow is withdrawn. As ordered, administer a mild sedative 1 hour before the test.

Procedure
If a blood test is scheduled, perform a venipuncture and collect the sample in two 7-ml *green-top* tubes. Wrap the tubes in a paper towel, refrigerate them on cold packs or wet ice, and send them to the laboratory immediately.

If assisting with a bone marrow aspiration, inject 1 ml of bone marrow into a 7-ml *green-top* tube and dilute it with 5 ml of sterile saline solution. Wrap the tube in a paper towel and refrigerate it on cold packs or wet ice. Be sure to send it to the laboratory immediately.

Precautions
• Contact the laboratory before performing the venipuncture to ensure that

they are able to process the sample and to find out how much blood to draw.

• Since patients with leukemia are more susceptible to infection, cleanse the skin thoroughly before performing the venipuncture.

• Send the sample to the laboratory immediately.

Values

Normal serum TdT levels range from 0 to 10 IU/10¹³ cells. Normal TdT levels in bone marrow have not been established but are similar to serum TdT levels.

Implications of results

TdT levels are elevated in ALL, the blastic phase of chronic myelogenous leukemia, lymphoblastic lymphoma, acute lymphoblastic leukemia, and a small percentage of acute nonlymphocytic leukemias. TdT-positive cells are absent in patients with ALL who are in remission.

Post-test care

• Since patients with leukemia may bleed excessively, apply pressure to the venipuncture site until bleeding stops. If a hematoma develops at the venipuncture site, apply warm soaks.

• Check the bone marrow aspiration site for bleeding and inflammation, and observe the patient for signs of hemorrhage and infection.

Interfering factors

• Failure to obtain a representative sample may interfere with accurate results of bone marrow aspiration.

• Performing a bone marrow aspiration on a child may produce false-positive results, since TdT is normally present in bone marrow during proliferation of prelymphocytes.

• Bone marrow regeneration, idiopathic thrombocytopenic purpura, and neuroblastoma may produce false-positive bone marrow aspiration results since these conditions cause TdT-positive bone marrow.

BARRY L. TONKONOW, MD

Ultrasonography of the abdominal aorta

In this safe, noninvasive test, a transducer directs high-frequency sound waves into the abdomen over a wide area from the xiphoid process to the umbilical region. The sound waves, echoing to the transducer from interfaces between tissues of different densities (acoustic interfaces), are transmitted as electrical impulses and displayed on an oscilloscope or television screen to reveal internal organs, the vertebral column, and, most importantly, the size and course of the abdominal aorta and other major vessels.

Ultrasonography helps confirm a suspected aortic aneurysm and is the method of choice for determining its diameter. Several scans may be performed to detect expansion of a known aneurysm because the risk of rupture is highest when the aneurysmal diameter is 7 cm or greater. However, angiography is indicated preoperatively to visualize the extent of atherosclerotic changes and to discover anatomic anomalies, such as three renal arteries. It's also indicated when diagnosis is unclear. Once an aneurysm is detected, ultrasonography is used every 6 months to monitor changes in patient status.

Purpose

• To detect and measure a suspected abdominal aortic aneurysm

• To measure and detect expansion of a known abdominal aortic aneurysm.

Patient preparation

Explain to the patient that this test allows examination of the abdominal aorta. Instruct him to fast for 12 hours before the test to minimize bowel gas and motility. Tell him who will perform the test and where, that the room light may be reduced to improve visualization, and that the test takes 30 to 45 minutes.

Tell the patient that mineral oil or a gel will be applied to his abdomen and will feel cool. Explain that a transducer will pass over his skin, from the costal margins to the umbilicus or slightly below, directing inaudible sound waves into the abdominal vessels and organs. Assure him that this is safe and painless but that he will feel slight pressure. If he has a known aneurysm, reassure him that the sound waves will not cause it to rupture. Instruct him to

---

SCANNING THE ABDOMINAL AORTA

Ultrasonography can reveal characteristic pathology of the abdominal aorta. For example, the cross-sectional view of one patient reveals calcification at the aneurysm site. The longitudinal view of another patient reveals a thickened aortic wall, calcification, a blood clot, and a slightly dilated aorta.

CROSS-SECTIONAL VIEW

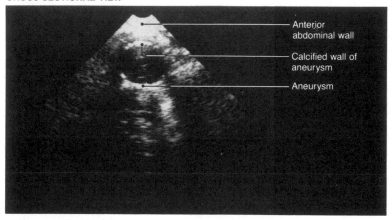

Anterior abdominal wall

Calcified wall of aneurysm

Aneurysm

LONGITUDINAL VIEW

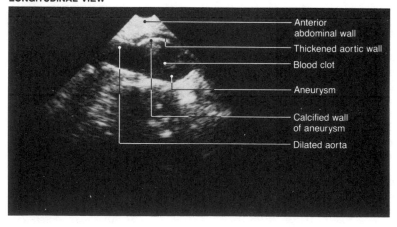

Anterior abdominal wall

Thickened aortic wall

Blood clot

Aneurysm

Calcified wall of aneurysm

Dilated aorta

remain still during scanning and to hold his breath when requested.

If ordered, give simethicone to reduce bowel gas. Just before the test, instruct the patient to put on a hospital gown.

Procedure

The patient is placed in a supine position, and acoustic coupling gel or mineral oil is applied to his abdomen. Longitudinal scans are made at 0.5- to 1-cm intervals left and right of the midline until the entire abdominal aorta is outlined. Transverse scans are made at 1- to 2-cm intervals from the xiphoid to the bifurcation at the common iliac arteries. The patient may be placed in right and left lateral positions. Appropriate views are photographed or videotaped.

Precautions

None.

Findings

In adults, the normal abdominal aorta tapers from about 2.5 to 1.5 cm in diameter along its length from the diaphragm to the bifurcation. It descends through the retroperitoneal space, anterior to the vertebral column and slightly left of the midline. Four of its major branches are usually well visualized: the celiac trunk, the renal arteries, the superior mesenteric artery, and the common iliac arteries.

Implications of results

Luminal diameter of the abdominal aorta greater than 4 cm is aneurysmal; over 7 cm, aneurysmal with high risk of rupture.

Post-test care

• Remove the acoustic coupling gel from the patient's skin.
• Instruct the patient to resume his usual diet and medications.
• Aneurysms may expand and dissect rapidly, so check the patient's vital signs frequently. Remember that sudden onset of constant abdominal or back pain

accompanies rapid expansion of the aneurysm; sudden, excrutiating pain with weakness, sweating, tachycardia, and hypotension signals rupture.

Interfering factors

• Bowel gas and motility, excessive body movement, surgical wounds, and severe dyspnea may prevent adequate imaging.
• Residual barium from gastrointestinal contrast studies within the past 24 hours and air introduced during endoscopy within the past 12 to 24 hours hinder ultrasound transmission.
• In obese patients, mesenteric fat may impair transmission of ultrasound waves during testing.

PATRICIA L. BAUM, RN, BSN

Urinary tract brush biopsy

Retrograde brush biopsy of the urinary tract may be used to obtain a renal tissue specimen when X-rays show a lesion in the renal pelvis or calyx. It can also be used to obtain specimens from other areas of the urinary tract. However, retrograde brush biopsy is contraindicated in patients with acute urinary tract infection or an obstruction at or below the biopsy site.

Patient preparation

To prepare the patient for brush biopsy, describe the procedure and tell him he may feel some discomfort. Inform him who will perform the biopsy and when. Reassure the patient that the procedure will take only 30 to 60 minutes.

Make sure the patient or a responsible family member has signed an appropriate consent form. Because this procedure requires the use of a contrast agent and a general, local, or spinal anesthetic, check the patient's history for hypersensitivity to anesthetics, contrast media, or iodine-containing foods, such as shellfish. Just before the biopsy procedure, administer a sedative to the patient, as ordered.

Procedure

After the patient has received a sedative and an anesthetic, place him in the lithotomy position. Using a cystoscope, the doctor passes a guide wire up the ureter and passes a urethral catheter over the guide wire. Contrast medium is instilled through the catheter, which is positioned next to the lesion under fluoroscopic guidance. The contrast medium is washed out with normal saline solution to prevent cell distortions from the dye. A nylon or steel brush is passed up the catheter and the lesion is brushed. This procedure is repeated at least six times, using a new brush each time.

As each brush is removed from the catheter, a smear is made for Papanicolaou staining and the brush tip is cut off and placed in formalin for 1 hour. The biopsy material is then removed from the brush tip for histologic examination. When the last brush is withdrawn, the catheter is irrigated with normal saline solution to remove additional cells. These cells are also sent for histologic examination.

Implications of results

Results of the urinary tract brush biopsy differentiate between malignant and benign lesions, which may appear the same on X-rays.

Post-test care

Because brush biopsy may cause such complications as perforation, hemorrhage, sepsis, or contrast medium extravasation, carefully monitor the patient's vital signs. Be sure to record the time, color, and amount of voiding, being alert for hematuria and abdominal or flank pain. Report any abnormal findings to the doctor immediately, and administer analgesics and antibiotics, as ordered.

ELLEN SHIPES, RN, ET, MN, MEd

Urine cytology

Epithelial cells line the urinary tract and exfoliate easily into the urine. So a simple cytologic examination of these cells can aid diagnosis of urinary tract disease. Although urine cytology is not done routinely, it's particularly useful for detecting cancer and inflammatory diseases of the renal pelvis, ureters, bladder, and urethra. In fact, it's especially useful for detecting bladder cancer in high-risk groups, such as smokers, people who work with aniline dyes, and patients who have received treatment for bladder cancer. Urine cytology can also determine whether bladder lesions that appear on X-rays are benign or malignant. This test can also detect cytomegalovirus infection and other viral diseases.

Procedure

To perform the test, the patient must collect a 100- to 300-ml clean-catch urine specimen 3 hours after his last voiding. (He should not use the first-voided specimen of the morning.) The urine specimen is sent to the cytology laboratory immediately so that it can be examined before the cells begin to degenerate.

The specimen is prepared in one of the following ways and stained with Papanicolaou's stain:
• *Centrifuge:* After the urine is spun down, the sediment is smeared on a glass slide and stained for examination.
• *Filter:* Urine is poured through a filter, which traps the cells so that they can be stained and examined directly.
• *Cytocentrifuge:* After the urine is centrifuged, the sediment is resuspended and placed on slides, which are spun in a cytocentrifuge and stained for examination.

Implications of results

Normal urine is relatively free of cellular debris but should have some epithelial and squamous cells that appear normal under a microscope. Identification of malignant cells or any other signs of malignancy may indicate cancer of the kidney, renal pelvis, ureters, bladder, or urethra. It could also indicate a metastatic tumor. An overgrowth of epithelial cells, an excess of red blood cells, or the presence of leukocytes or atypical cells may indicate a lower urinary tract inflammation, which can result from prostatic hyperplasia, urinary calculi, bladder diverticula, strictures, or malformations. Large intranuclear inclusions may indicate a cytomegalovirus infection, which usually affects the renal tubular epithelium. This viral infection generally occurs in cancer patients undergoing chemotherapy and transplant patients receiving immunosuppressive drugs. Cytoplasmic inclusion bodies may also indicate measles and may precede the characteristic Koplik's spots.

ELLEN SHIPES, RN, ET, MN, MEd

Urine hydroxyproline

This test measures total urine levels of hydroxyproline, an amino acid found mainly in collagen (a component of skin and bone). Urine hydroxyproline levels are a good index of bone matrix turnover because levels increase when collagen breaks down during bone resorption. Bone matrix turnover and hydroxyproline levels normally rise in children during periods of rapid skeletal growth. However, they also rise in disorders that increase bone resorption, such as Paget's disease, metastatic bone tumors, and certain endocrine disorders. This test helps diagnose these disorders, but it's more commonly used to monitor response to drug therapy in conditions marked by rapid bone resorption.

Hydroxyproline levels are most often determined colorimetrically on a timed urine sample; they may also be determined by ion-exchange or gas-liquid chromatography. A collagen-restricted diet is essential for this test because hydroxyproline levels reflect collagen intake. Free hydroxyproline, a small component of total hydroxyproline and a sensitive indicator of dietary collagen intake, may be measured to validate results.

Purpose
● To monitor treatment for disorders characterized by bone resorption, primarily Paget's disease
● To aid diagnosis of disorders characterized by bone resorption.

Patient preparation
Explain to the patient that this test helps monitor treatment or detect an amino acid disorder related to bone formation. Inform him that he must not eat meat, fish, poultry, jelly, or any foods containing gelatin for 24 hours before the test or during the test. Tell him the test requires a 2-hour or 24-hour urine specimen, as appropriate, and teach him the collection technique.

Note the patient's age and sex on the laboratory slip. Check his history for drugs that may alter test results. Restrict such drugs as ordered.

Procedure
Collect a 2-hour or 24-hour urine specimen, as ordered, in a container that has a preservative to prevent degradation of hydroxyproline.

Precautions
Refrigerate the specimen or keep it on ice during the collection period, and send it to the laboratory immediately.

Values
Normal values for adults are 14 to 45 mg/24 hours. For a 2-hour specimen, normal values are 0.4 to 5 mg for males and 0.4 to 2.9 mg for females. Normal values for children are much higher and peak between ages 11 and 18. Values also rise during the third trimester of

pregnancy, reflecting fetal skeletal growth.

Implications of results
Hydroxyproline levels should decrease slowly during therapy for bone resorption disorders. Elevated levels may indicate bone disease, metastatic bone tumors, or endocrine disorders that stimulate hormonal secretion.

Post-test care
As ordered, resume foods and drugs withheld before the test.

Interfering factors
• Ascorbic acid, vitamin D, aspirin, glucocorticoids, 'and calcitonin and mithramycin (used to treat Paget's disease) can decrease urine hydroxyproline levels.
• Failure to observe restrictions, to collect all urine during the test period, or to store the specimen correctly may alter test results.
• Psoriasis and burns can promote collagen turnover, elevating urine hydroxyproline levels.
TOBIE VIRGINIA HITTLE, RN, BSN, CCRN

Urine potassium

This quantitative test measures urine levels of potassium, a major intracellular cation that helps regulate acid-base balance and neuromuscular function. Potassium imbalance may cause such signs and symptoms as muscle weakness, nausea, diarrhea, confusion, hypotension, EKG changes, and even cardiac arrest.

Most commonly, a serum potassium test is performed to detect hyperkalemia (abnormally high levels) or hypokalemia (abnormally low levels). A urine potassium test may be done to evaluate hypokalemia when a history and physical examination fail to uncover the cause. Since the kidneys regulate potassium balance through potassium excretion in the urine, measuring urine potassium levels can determine if hypokalemia results from a renal disorder, such as renal tubular acidosis, or an extrarenal disorder, such as malabsorption syndrome. If results suggest a renal disorder, further renal function tests may be ordered.

Purpose
To determine whether hypokalemia is caused by renal or extrarenal disorders.

Patient preparation
Explain to the patient that this test evaluates his kidney function. Tell him that the test requires a 24-hour urine specimen. If it's to be collected at home, teach him the correct collection technique. Check his history for drugs that may alter test results. If they must be continued, note this on the laboratory slip.

Procedure
Collect a 24-hour urine specimen.

Precautions
• Tell the patient not to contaminate the specimen with toilet tissue or stool.
• Refrigerate the specimen or place it on ice during the collection period.
• Send the specimen to the laboratory immediately or refrigerate it.

Values
Normal potassium excretion is 25 to 125 mEq/24 hours, with an average potassium concentration of 25 to 100 mEq/liter. In a patient with hypokalemia and normal kidney function, potassium concentration will be less than 10 mEq/liter, indicating that potassium loss is most likely the result of a gastrointestinal disorder, such as malabsorption syndrome.

Implications of results
In a patient with hypokalemia lasting more than 3 days, urine potassium levels above 10 mEq/liter indicate renal losses that may result from such dis-

orders as aldosteronism, renal tubular acidosis, or chronic renal failure. However, extrarenal disorders, such as dehydration, Cushing's disease, or salicylate intoxication, may also elevate urine potassium levels.

Post-test care
• Monitor the hypokalemic patient for diminished reflexes; rapid, weak, irregular pulse; mental confusion; hypotension; anorexia; muscle weakness; and paresthesias. Watch for EKG changes and signs of ventricular fibrillation, respiratory paralysis, and cardiac arrest.
• Administer potassium supplements and monitor serum levels, as ordered.
• Provide dietary supplements and nutritional counseling, as ordered.
• Replace volume loss with I.V. or oral fluids, as ordered.
• Resume drugs, as ordered.

Interfering factors
• Excess dietary potassium raises urine potassium levels.
• When excessive vomiting or stomach suctioning causes alkalosis, urine potassium levels will not reflect actual potassium depletion.
• Potassium-wasting medications, such as ammonium chloride and thiazide diuretics raise potassium levels.
• Failure to collect all urine or incorrect specimen storage may alter results.

CLARKE LAMBE, MD

Uroflowmetry

This simple, noninvasive test uses a uroflowmeter to detect and evaluate dysfunctional voiding patterns. The uroflowmeter, contained in a funnel into which the patient voids, measures flow rate (volume of urine voided per second), continuous flow (time of measurable flow), and intermittent flow (total voiding time, including any interruptions).

Several types of uroflowmeters are available: rotary disk, electromagnetic, spectrophotometric, and gravimetric systems. The gravimetric system, which weighs urine as it's voided and plots the weight against time, is the simplest to use and is widely available.

Purpose
• To evaluate lower urinary tract function
• To show bladder outlet obstruction.

Patient preparation
Explain to the patient that this test evaluates his pattern of urination. Advise him not to urinate for several hours before the test and to increase fluid intake so he'll have a full bladder and a strong urge to void. Tell him who will perform the test and where, and that it will take 10 to 15 minutes. Instruct the patient to remain still while voiding during the test to help ensure accurate results.

Assure the patient that he will have complete privacy during the test. As ordered, discontinue drugs that may affect bladder and sphincter tone.

Equipment
Commode chair with funnel containing a uroflowmeter/beaker to hold urine/transducer/start and flow cables/data recording module.

Procedure
The test procedure is the same with all types of equipment. A male patient is asked to void while standing; a female patient, while sitting. The patient is asked to avoid straining to empty the bladder. Cable connections are checked, and the patient is left alone.

The patient pushes the start button on the commode chair, counts for 5 seconds, and voids. When finished, he counts for 5 seconds and pushes the button again. The volume of urine voided is then recorded and plotted as a curve over the time of voiding. The patient's position and the route of fluid intake (oral or intravenous) are noted.

CHARACTERISTIC UROFLOW CURVES

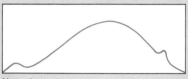

Normal curve.

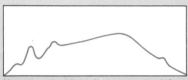

Normal peak with hesitancy may result from the patient's embarrassment or advanced age.

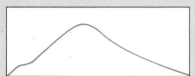

High peak flow over short voiding time may indicate incontinence.

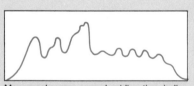

Many peaks over normal voiding time indicate abdominal straining and detrusor muscle weakness.

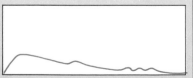

Low peak with long voiding time and urethral dribbling indicates obstruction.

Precautions

• The transducer must be level, and the beaker centered beneath the funnel.
• The beaker must be large enough to hold all urine; overflow can invalidate results and damage the transducer.

Values

Flow rate varies according to the patient's age and sex and the volume of urine voided. Normal values are listed below for minimum volumes.

Age	Minimum volume (ml)	Male (ml/sec)	Female (ml/sec)
4 to 7	100	10	10
8 to 13	100	12	15
14 to 45	200	21	18
46 to 65	200	12	15
66 to 80	200	9	10

Implications of results

Increased flow rate indicates reduced urethral resistance, which may be associated with external sphincter dysfunction. A high peak on the curve plotted over the voiding time indicates decreased outflow resistance, which may be due to stress incontinence. Decreased flow rate indicates outflow obstruction or hypotonia of the detrusor muscle. More than one distinct peak in a normal curve indicates abdominal straining, which may be due to pushing against an obstruction to empty the bladder. (See chart at left.)

Post-test care

Instruct the patient to resume any medications, as ordered.

Interfering factors

• Drugs that affect bladder and sphincter tone, such as spasmolytics and anticholinergics, will alter test results.
• Strong drafts can affect transducer function.
• Patient movement on the commode chair may make the flow recording inaccurate.
• The presence of toilet tissue in the beaker will invalidate test results.

• Straining to void will alter test results.

ELLEN SHIPES, RN, ET, MN, MEd

Uroporphyrinogen I synthase

[Uroporphyrinogen I synthetase, porphobilinogen deaminase]

This test measures blood levels of uroporphyrinogen I synthase, an enzyme that converts porphobilinogen to uroporphyrinogen during heme biosynthesis. This enzyme is normally present in erythrocytes, fibroblasts, lymphocytes, liver cells, and amniotic fluid cells. However, a hereditary deficiency can reduce uroporphyrinogen I synthase levels by 50% or more, resulting in acute intermittent porphyria (AIP). An autosomal-dominant disorder of heme biosynthesis, AIP can be latent until certain factors (some sex hormones and drugs, a low-carbohydrate diet, or an infection) activate it.

Traditional urine tests can only detect AIP during an acute episode. But the uroporphyrinogen I synthase test can detect AIP even during its latent phase. Thus, it can identify affected individuals before their first acute episode. Also, its specificity for AIP allows it to differentiate AIP from other porphyrias.

Enzyme activity is determined by fluorometrically measuring the conversion rate of porphobilinogen to uroporphyrinogen. If levels are indeterminate, urine and stool tests for aminolevulinic acid (ALA) and porphobilinogen may be ordered since excretion of these porphyrin precursors increases substantially during an acute episode of AIP and may increase slightly during the latent phase.

Purpose
To aid diagnosis of AIP.

Patient preparation
Explain to the patient that this test helps detect a red blood cell disorder. Inform him that he must fast for 12 to 14 hours before the test, but that he may drink water. Tell him that the test requires a blood sample, who will perform the venipuncture and when, and that he may experience discomfort from the needle puncture and the tourniquet. Reassure him that sample collection takes less than 3 minutes.

If the patient's hematocrit values are available, record them on the laboratory slip. As ordered, withhold any medications that may decrease enzyme levels. If they must be continued, note this on the laboratory slip.

Procedure
Perform a venipuncture and collect the sample in a 10-ml *green-top* tube.

Precautions
• Handle the sample gently to prevent hemolysis.
• Place the sample on dry ice and send it frozen to the laboratory. (Frozen samples may be stable for up to 1 month.)

Values
Normal values for uroporphyrinogen I synthase are 8.1 to 16.8 nm/sec/liter for females and 7.9 to 14.7 nm/sec/liter for males.

Implications of results
Decreased levels generally indicate latent or active AIP; symptoms differentiate these phases. Levels below 6.0 nm/sec/liter confirm AIP, but levels between 6.0 and 8.0 nm/sec/liter are indeterminate. Indeterminate results may require urine and stool tests for porphyrin precursors ALA and porphobilinogen to support the diagnosis.

Post-test care
• If a hematoma develops at the venipuncture site, apply warm soaks.
• As ordered, instruct the patient to resume diet and medications.

• If the patient has AIP, provide nutritional and genetic counseling. Teach him to avoid low-carbohydrate diets, alcohol, and such drugs as estrogens, steroid hormones, barbiturates, sulfonamides, phenytoin, griseofulvin, and others that may precipitate an acute episode. Remind him to seek care for all infections promptly since these may also precipitate an acute episode.

Interfering factors
• Hemolytic and hepatic diseases may elevate uroporphyrinogen I synthase levels.
• Hemolysis due to rough handling of the sample may cause inaccurate results.
• Failure to freeze the sample will cause false-positive results.
• Failure to fast before the test may increase enzyme levels.
• A low-carbohydrate diet, alcohol, infection, and certain drugs may decrease enzyme levels.

WENDY BAKER, RN, MS, CCRN

Whitaker test
[Pressure/flow study]

This study of the upper urinary tract correlates radiographic findings with measurements of pressure and flow in the kidneys and ureters. It assesses the upper tract's efficiency in emptying. Radiographs are taken after urethral catheterization, I.V. administration of a contrast medium, percutaneous cannulation of the kidney, and renal perfusion of the contrast medium. Intrarenal and bladder pressures are then measured.

The Whitaker test may be performed as a primary study to detect intrarenal obstruction and to help determine if surgery is needed. It may also follow other procedures, such as percutaneous nephrostomy, for further evaluation of obstruction.

Purpose
To identify and evaluate renal obstruction.

Patient preparation
Explain to the patient that the test evaluates kidney function. Instruct him to avoid food and fluids for at least 4 hours before the test. Tell him who will perform the test and where, and that it will take about 1 hour.

Describe the procedure to the patient. Inform him that he will receive a mild sedative, that he may feel some discomfort during catheter insertion and anesthetic injection, and that he may sense transient burning and flushing after contrast medium injection. Warn him that the X-ray machine makes loud clacking sounds.

Make sure the patient or a responsible family member has signed a consent form. Check the patient's history and recent coagulation studies for bleeding disorders. Also check his history for hypersensitivity reactions to iodine, iodine-containing foods, such as shellfish, and contrast media. Tell the doctor of any sensitivities.

Just before the procedure, instruct the patient to void, and administer a sedative, as ordered. Give prophylactic antibiotics, as ordered, to prevent infection from instrumentation.

Equipment
X-ray equipment/perfusion pump with 50 ml Luer-Lok syringe/transducer and recorder/manometer/three-way and four-way stopcocks/I.V. extension set/manometer lines/one double-male connector to connect urethral catheter and stopcock/sterile water and normal saline solution/contrast medium/local anesthetic/percutaneous puncture tray with 4″ to 6″ 18G Longdwel cannula/gloves/preparatory tray/emergency resuscitation equipment.

Procedure
The patient is placed in a supine position on the X-ray table. The table is horizontal and must remain at the same

height throughout the test. To prepare to measure bladder pressure, a urethral catheter is placed in the bladder, which may or may not be emptied. (If obstruction is suspected, the patient will be asked to void before the test. If a condition such as bladder hypertonia is suspected, he should not void.) A plain film of the urinary tract is taken to obtain anatomic landmarks. The catheter is connected to a three-way stopcock on a manometer line linked to the transducer and recorder. The line is filled with sterile water.

The contrast medium is injected intravenously, and the patient is placed prone and made comfortable. The side to be examined is closest to the doctor. When urography shows the contrast medium in the kidney, the skin is cleansed with antiseptic solution and draped. Pressure recording equipment is calibrated. The renal perfusion tubing is filled with sterile water or saline solution and held at kidney level.

A local anesthetic is injected, and an incision is made through the flank for kidney cannulation. The patient holds his breath while the needle is inserted into the renal pelvis. Aspiration of urine confirms that the needle is in place. The cannula is then connected by a four-way stopcock to the perfusion tubing and the manometer line.

Perfusion of the contrast medium is begun, serial X-rays are taken, and intrarenal pressure is measured. Bladder pressure is then measured. Perfusion continues steadily at 10 ml/minute until bladder pressure is constant. When pressure holds steady for a few minutes and adequate films have been taken, perfusion ends. Residual fluid is aspirated from the kidney, the cannula is removed, and the wound is dressed.

Precautions

Contraindications include bleeding disorders and severe infection.

Findings

Visualization of the kidney after gradual perfusion of the contrast medium shows normal outlines of the renal pelvis and calyces. The ureter should fill uniformly and appear normal.

Normal intrarenal pressure is 15 cmH$_2$O; normal bladder pressure, 5 to 10 cmH$_2$O.

Implications of results

Enlargement of the renal pelvis, calyces, or ureteropelvic junction may indicate obstruction. Subtraction of bladder pressure from intrarenal pressure results in a differential that aids diagnosis. A differential of 12 to 15 cmH$_2$O indicates obstruction. A differential of less than 10 cmH$_2$O indicates a bladder abnormality, such as hypertonia or neurogenic bladder.

Post-test care

● Keep the patient in a supine position for 12 hours after the test.
● Check vital signs every 15 minutes for the first hour, every 30 minutes for the next hour, and then every 2 hours for 24 hours.
● Check the puncture site for bleeding, hematoma, or urine leakage each time vital signs are checked. If bleeding occurs, apply pressure. If a hematoma develops, apply warm soaks. If urine leaks, report it to the doctor.
● Monitor fluid intake and urine output for 24 hours. If hematuria persists after the third voiding, notify the doctor.
● Watch for signs of sepsis (fever, tachycardia, tachypnea, or hypotension) or similar signs of contrast medium extravasation.
● Tell the patient that colicky pains will pass. Administer analgesics, as ordered.
● Give antibiotics after the test, as ordered, to prevent infection.

Interfering factors

● Recent barium studies or the presence of feces or gas in the bowel hinders accurate needle placement and visualization of the upper urinary tract.
● Patient movement interferes with accurate needle placement.

ELLEN SHIPES, RN, ET, MN, MEd

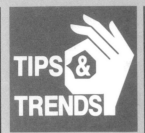

TIPS & TRENDS

Lixi™ Imaging Scope

The first completely portable X-ray machine, called the Lixi™ Imaging Scope, can provide X-rays on the spot. It's hand-held, emits less than one millirad (mrad) of radiation per second, and can X-ray a 2″ area of the body. It helps diagnose athletic injuries, such as a fractured wrist or ankle, right on the field. It can also help surgeons insert catheters and position pins, and screen auto accident victims, helping ensure they're safely removed from their vehicles. A camera can be attached to permanently record each X-ray.

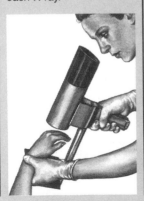

CLONED CELLS DETECT EARLY CANCER

Monoclonal antibodies

When tagged with radioactive isotopes and injected into the body, biochemicals called monoclonal antibodies help detect cancer by attaching to tumor cells. They're produced in the laboratory, based upon the immune response, and may detect a tumor's location and extent earlier and more accurately than traditional methods. Typically, a selected antigen is injected into a mouse, stimulating B lymphocyte antibody production. After a few days, the mouse's spleen cells—rich in B lymphocytes—are removed and fused with rapidly dividing mouse myeloma cells that secrete no antibodies. These fused cells, or hybridomas, are grown in culture, tested for the desired antibody, and cloned. Hybridomas with the desired antibody are either grown in a culture or injected into a mouse's peritoneum, so the monoclonal antibodies can proliferate for later retrieval and purification.

Purified monoclonal antibodies attach themselves to specific antigenic determinants on cell surfaces. This specificity allows radiolabelled monoclonal antibodies for colon cancer, for example, to seek out colon cancer cells in a tumor and elsewhere. In the future, monoclonal antibodies may be linked with toxins to destroy specific cancer cells without harming nearby healthy cells.

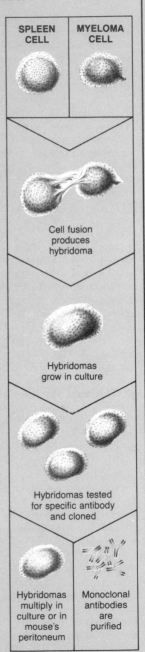

SPLEEN CELL	MYELOMA CELL

Cell fusion produces hybridoma

Hybridomas grow in culture

Hybridomas tested for specific antibody and cloned

Hybridomas multiply in culture or in mouse's peritoneum	Monoclonal antibodies are purified

E.L.I.S.A. TEST DETECTS HTLV-III ANTIBODIES IN DONATED BLOOD

Tests screen blood for AIDS antibodies

Tests that measure serum antibodies for human T-cell lymphotropic virus Type III (HTLV-III), the AIDS virus, have been licensed by the Food and Drug Administration and are now commercially available. The tests are used to screen donated blood for AIDS antibodies, preventing contamination of the blood supply. Based on an enzyme-linked immunosorbent assay (ELISA), the tests detect antibodies to the AIDS virus, not the virus itself.

Limitations
The ELISA test sometimes gives false results. For instance, a false-negative result may be caused by a variance in test sensitivity between laboratories. A positive result in an asymptomatic person may be due to immunity, subclinical infection, or cross-reactivity with other viral antigens. False-positives may result from laboratory error. Therefore, any positive result must be confirmed using the accurate but technically difficult Western blot test.

Clinical implications of a positive test for an asymptomatic patient are currently unknown.

Your role
When caring for a seropositive patient, encourage him to seek medical follow-up. If he's asymptomatic, tell him to watch for—and report—any early signs of AIDS, such as fever, weight loss, swollen glands, rash, and persistent cough.

Until further data is available, assume that the seropositive patient can transmit the disease to others. To reduce the risk of transmission, instruct him not to share razors, toothbrushes, or utensils (which may be contaminated with blood). Teach him to clean anything that becomes contaminated with blood, using household bleach diluted 1:10 in water. Advise the patient not to donate blood, tissue, or organs. If you suspect I.V. drug abuse, warn him not to share needles. Tell him to alert his doctor and dentist to his condition, so they can take precautions.

D.N.A. PROBES IDENTIFY GENETIC DEFECT

Prenatal test for Duchenne's MD

A new test can diagnose Duchenne's muscular dystrophy (MD) in the fetus. In fact, prenatal detection of this most common form of MD can occur as early as the eighth week of pregnancy.

The test uses DNA probes to identify genetic variations called restriction fragment length polymorphisms (RFLPs) on the short arm of the X chromosome. It can detect Duchenne's MD with 96% to 99% accuracy and can also identify female carriers of the disease, making genetic counseling

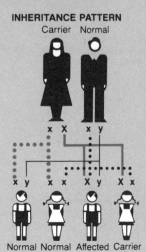

INHERITANCE PATTERN
Carrier Normal

x X   x y

x y   x x   X y   X x

Normal Normal Affected Carrier

and planning now possible. (Previously, only the serum creatine phosphokinase test could detect carriers—and it was unreliable.)

Duchenne's MD, an X-linked recessive disorder, affects boys almost exclusively. This progressive degenerative muscular disorder typically begins between ages 3 and 5, immobilizes the boys by ages 9 to 12, and results in death—usually from sudden heart or respiratory failure—by early adulthood. Females carry it on the X chromosome.

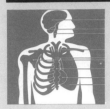

Diseases

IMMUNE DISORDERS

Acquired immunodeficiency syndrome (AIDS)

Currently a widely publicized disease, AIDS is characterized by progressively weakened cell-mediated (T cell) immunity, which makes the patient susceptible to opportunistic infections and unusual cancers. AIDS was first defined by the Centers for Disease Control (CDC) in 1981. Recent studies point overwhelmingly to a retrovirus—the human T cell leukemia/lymphoma virus (HTLV-III)—as its cause.

The population most at risk for contracting AIDS consists of homosexual and bisexual men who are sexually active with many partners. Other risk groups include intravenous drug abusers and hemophiliacs. Most recently, heterosexual partners and children of patients with AIDS or of those in high-risk groups and persons receiving multiple blood transfusions have been added to the high-risk category. More than 75% of AIDS victims die within 2 years of diagnosis. To date, no effective therapy has been found to stop the growth of the virus or to correct the immune defect.

The CDC has also defined an AIDS-related complex (ARC), in which the patient develops some of the nonspecific symptoms of AIDS but not the typical opportunistic infections. Occasionally, this complex is mistakenly labeled pre-AIDS; some, but not all, cases progress to AIDS.

Causes

AIDS results from infection with the HTLV-III virus, which selectively

COMMON INFECTIOUS ORGANISMS IN A.I.D.S.

PROTOZOA

Pneumocystis carinii
Cryptosporidium
Toxoplasma gondii
Entamoeba histolytica
Giardia lamblia

FUNGI

Candida species
Cryptococcus neoformans

MYCOBACTERIA

Mycobacterium avium-intracellularis

VIRUSES

Cytomegalovirus
Epstein-Barr virus
Herpes simplex virus
Herpes zoster
Poxvirus
Polyomavirus

strikes T_4 helper lymphocytes, gradually depleting their number and impairing their function. The resultant decrease in the T_4:T_8 (helper:suppressor) lymphocyte ratio profoundly impairs cell-mediated immunity. Natural killer cells and cytotoxic T cells also display limited activity. Although B cell production of immunoglobulin increases, these cells respond poorly to new antigens. (T_4 helper lymphocytes normally enhance B cell recognition of antigen.) The HTLV-III virus appears to be transmitted by direct inoculation alone via intimate sexual contact, especially associated with rectal mucosal trauma; by administration of blood or blood products such as cryoprecipitate, Factor VIII, or Factor IX; by contaminated needles; or by maternal-fetal transplacental contact. The time between probable exposure to the virus and diagnosis averages 1 to 3 years.

Signs and symptoms

Some patients with AIDS are asymptomatic until they abruptly develop an opportunistic infection or the purple

KAPOSI'S SARCOMA

Kaposi's sarcoma is a vascular tumor that was rare in the U.S. and Europe until the recent outbreak of AIDS. This rare tumor formerly affected elderly Jewish and Italian men, young black Africans, and patients with depressed immune function. It commonly produced purple and brown plaques or nodules on the lower legs. The Kaposi's sarcoma associated with AIDS, although histologically identical to the rarer form, is more rapidly progressive and often involves many body sites (instead of just the lower extremities), including the oral cavity, hard palate, gastrointestinal tract, lymph nodes, and lungs.

skin nodules that typify Kaposi's sarcoma. More often, though, patients have a recent history of mild to severe nonspecific symptoms, such as fatigue, afternoon fevers, night sweats, weight loss, diarrhea, or cough. Soon after these appear, the patient often develops several infections concurrently.

This clinical course varies slightly in children with AIDS. First, incubation time appears to be shorter, with a mean of 8 months. Signs and symptoms in children resemble those in adults with AIDS, except for those findings related to venereal disease. Finally, in children, the most common effect—and cause of death—is diffuse interstitial pneumonitis, not *Pneumocystis carinii* pneumonia as in adults.

Patients with ARC display some of the nonspecific symptoms of AIDS, but not the typical opportunistic infections. Most of these patients have a history of unexplained fever, lymphadenopathy, weight loss, diarrhea, sore throat, fatigue, and night sweats.

Diagnosis
The CDC defines AIDS as the presence of an opportunistic infection or unusual cancer (such as Kaposi's sarcoma) in a person with no known cause of immunodeficiency. Diagnosis rests on careful correlation of the patient's history and clinical features with

this definition. To date, the presence of the HTLV-III virus or antibody is not considered diagnostic of AIDS.

Several blood tests help evaluate immunity and support the diagnosis, including complete blood count with differential, fluorescent activated cell sorter (FACS) analysis of total T cell and B cell number, and the T_4:T_8 ratio. A decreased T_4:T_8 ratio associated with a severely depleted T_4 lymphocyte population is characteristic. Skin testing with common antigens confirms impaired cell-mediated immunity.

Treatment
Currently, no cure exists for the immunodeficiency of AIDS. However, researchers continue to explore methods to arrest growth of the HTLV-III virus or to restore lost immune function. Although bone marrow transplantation has failed to improve immune function, intravenous infusion of interleukin-2 and interferon has shown limited effectiveness. New antiviral drugs also offer some hope.

Supportive measures in AIDS aim to reduce the risk of infection, to treat existing infections and malignancies, to maintain adequate nutrition, and to provide emotional and psychological support.

Drug treatment for AIDS varies. Although many of the causative infectious organisms are responsive to drugs, infection tends to recur when treatment is discontinued. The drug of choice for *P. carinii* pneumonia is an oral or I.V. preparation of co-trimoxazole (Bactrim or Septra). If treatment fails or if toxicity occurs, pentamidine (Pentam 300) may be substituted; however, this drug may cause side effects such as azotemia, liver dysfunction, tachycardia, hypotension, hypoglycemia, and skin rashes.

Antineoplastic drugs, such as vincristine and etoposide (VP-16), may be used to treat Kaposi's sarcoma; however, aggressive treatment increases the likelihood of infection. Alpha-interferon is also being used to treat Kaposi's

HOW THE A.I.D.S. VIRUS AFFECTS IMMUNITY

NORMAL IMMUNE FUNCTION

1. When viruses enter a healthy body, they are detected and identified as antigens by macrophages. Macrophages process the antigens and present them to T cells and B cells.

2. The antigen-activated T cells proliferate and form several kinds of T cells. Helper T cells stimulate B cells. Suppressor T cells control the amount of T cell help for B cells. Lymphokine-producing T cells are involved in delayed hypersensitivity and other immune reactions. Cytotoxic (killer) T cells directly destroy antigenic agents. Memory T cells are stored to recognize and attack the same antigen on subsequent invasions.

3. The B cells proliferate, forming memory cells and plasma cells that produce antigen-specific antibodies, which then attack and kill the invading virus.

ALTERED IMMUNE FUNCTION

1. The AIDS virus infects helper T cells, first blocking their ability to recognize antigens, then allowing the AIDS virus to proliferate within the T cells.

2. Cell-mediated immunity is weakened, making the patient vulnerable to bacterial, viral, and fungal infections and certain malignancies, all of which can be fatal in the immunocompromised patient. Meanwhile, the damaged T cells produce more AIDS virus, which invades other T cells, compounding the problem.

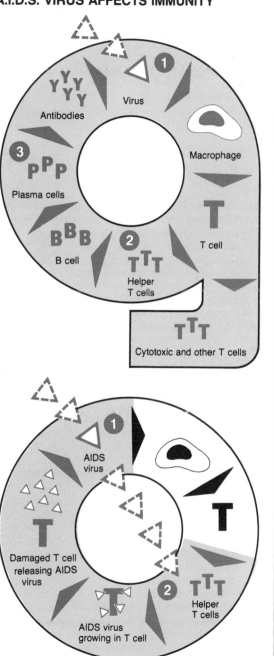

sarcoma. Radiation and laser therapy are palliative measures for local lesions.

To reduce the risk of contracting AIDS, the U.S. Public Health Service recommends avoiding sexual contact with persons known to have or suspected of having AIDS. It also advises that members of high-risk groups refrain from donating blood.

Nursing intervention

Although AIDS is not thought to be transmitted by casual contact, you should observe special precautions when caring for an AIDS patient. Wear gloves and a gown when handling blood, other body fluids, excretions, or potentially contaminated objects or surfaces. If such contact occurs, wash your hands immediately with soap and water. Of course, thorough hand washing is necessary before and after any contact with suspected or diagnosed AIDS patients. Generally, follow precautions appropriate for hepatitis B: properly label all specimens collected from the patient; place soiled linen from the patient in a labeled, impervious bag; and dispose of needles (unsheathed) in a puncture-resistant container.

• Monitor the patient for fever, noting its pattern. Also assess for tender, swollen lymph nodes and check laboratory values regularly. Be alert for signs of infection, such as skin breakdown, cough, sore throat, and diarrhea.

• Encourage daily oral rinsing with normal saline solution or bicarbonate. To relieve oral *Candida* infection or stomatitis, offer hydrogen peroxide or a mixture of Benadryl and Kaopectate (swish and spit). Avoid glycerin swabs, which dry mucous membranes.

• Record the patient's caloric intake. Intravenous hyperalimentation may be necessary to maintain adequate caloric intake, although it provides a potential route for infection.

• If the patient develops Kaposi's sarcoma, monitor the progression of lesions. Provide meticulous skin care, es-

pecially in the debilitated patient.

• Recognize that diagnosis of AIDS is typically emotionally charged because of the disease's social impact and discouraging prognosis. The patient may face the loss of his job and financial security as well as the support of his family. Coping with an altered body image and the emotional burden of untimely death may also overwhelm the patient. Be as supportive as possible.

ELIZABETH JOHNSTONE, RNC, BS

Ataxia-telangiectasia

Inherited as an autosomal recessive disorder, ataxia-telangiectasia is characterized by progressively severe ataxia; telangiectasia, particularly of the face, earlobes, and conjunctivae; and chronic sinopulmonary infections that may reflect both antibody-mediated (B cell) and cell-mediated (T cell) immune deficiencies. Ataxia usually appears within 2 years after birth, but may develop as late as age 9. The degree of immunodeficiency determines the prognosis. Some patients die within several years; others survive until their 30s. Severe abnormalities cause rapid deterioration and premature death from overwhelming sinopulmonary infection or malignancy.

Causes

In this autosomal recessive disorder, immunodeficiency may result from defective embryonic development of the mesoderm, hormone deficiency, or defective DNA repair.

Signs and symptoms

The earliest and most dominant signs of cerebellar ataxia usually develop by the time the infant begins to use his motor skills. They typically include continual and involuntary jerky (choreoathetoid) movements, nystagmus, extrapyramidal symptoms (pseudoparkinsonism, motor restlessness, and dystonias), and posterior column signs (unsteady gait, with forward leaning to maintain balance; decreased arm movements; and purposeless tremors). The associated telangiectasia usually appears later and may not develop until age 9, appearing first as a vascular lesion on the sclera and later on the bridge or side of the nose, the ear, or the antecubital or popliteal areas. Approximately 80% of affected children develop recurrent or chronic respiratory infections because of IgA deficiency early in life, but some may be symptom-free for 10 years or more. These children are unusually vulnerable to lymphomas, particularly lymphosarcomas and lymphoreticular malignancies, and they may also develop leukemia, adenocarcinoma, dysgerminoma, or medulloblastoma. They may fail to develop secondary sex characteristics during puberty and eventually may become mentally retarded. Rarely, a patient shows signs of progeria: premature graying, senile keratoses, and vitiligo.

Diagnosis

If a patient has the complete syndrome (ataxia, telangiectasia, and recurrent sinopulmonary infection), the diagnosis can be made on these clinical facts alone. However, the complete syndrome may not be apparent, and ataxia may be the only symptom for 6 years or longer. If this is the case, early diagnosis usually depends on immunologic tests. A patient with ataxia-telangiectasia usually shows:

• selective absence of IgA (in 60% to 80% of patients) or deficient IgA and IgE

• normal B cell count but diminished antibody responses

• absence of Hassall's corpuscles on examination of thymic tissue

• high serum levels of oncofetal proteins

• decreased number of T cells.

   Physical examination reveals degenerative neurologic changes; these can also be demonstrated by computed to-mography scan, magnetic resonance imaging, and pneumoencephalography.

Treatment and nursing intervention

No treatment is yet available to stop progression of this disease. However, prophylactic or early and aggressive use of broad-spectrum antibiotics is essential to prevent or control recurrent infections.

   To help parents protect their child from infections, advise them to keep the affected child away from crowds and from persons who have active infections, and teach them to recognize early signs of infection. Also teach physical therapy and postural drainage techniques if their child has chronic bronchial infections. As always, stress the importance of proper nutrition and adequate hydration.

   Immune globulin infusion or injection can passively replace missing antibodies in an IgG-deficient patient, and may also help prevent infection. The effectiveness of other forms of immunotherapy—fetal thymus transplant, repeated doses of thymosin, or histocompatible bone marrow transplant—is unproven.

   Parents of a child with ataxia-telangiectasia may have questions about the vulnerability of future offspring and may need genetic counseling. Some parents may also require psychological therapy to help them cope with the child's long-term illness and inevitable early death.

   NORA LYNN BOLLINGER, RN, MSN
   CHRISTINE GRADY, RN, MSN, CNS

Blood transfusion reaction

Mediated by immune or nonimmune factors, a transfusion reaction accompanies or follows I.V. administration of blood components. Its severity varies from mild (fever and chills) to severe (acute renal failure or complete vascular collapse and death), depending on the amount of blood transfused, the type of reaction, and the patient's general health.

Types and causes

Hemolytic reactions follow transfusion of mismatched blood. Transfusion with serologically incompatible blood triggers the most serious reaction, marked by intravascular agglutination of red blood cells (RBCs). The recipient's antibodies (IgG or IgM) attach themselves to the donated RBCs, leading to the clumping and destruction of large numbers of the recipient's RBCs.

Transfusion with Rh-incompatible blood triggers a less serious reaction within several days to 2 weeks. Rh reactions are most likely in women sensitized to RBC antigens by prior pregnancy or by unknown factors such as bacterial or viral infection, and in those who have received more than five transfusions.

Allergic reactions are fairly common but only occasionally serious. Here, transfused soluble antigens react with surface IgE molecules on mast cells and basophils, causing degranulation and release of allergic mediators. Antibodies against IgA in a recipient who is IgA-deficient can also trigger a severe allergic reaction (anaphylaxis).

Febrile nonhemolytic reactions, the most common type of reaction, apparently develop when cytotoxic or agglutinating antibodies in the recipient's plasma attack antigens on transfused lymphocytes, granulocytes, or plasma cell membranes.

Although fairly uncommon, *bacterial contamination* of donor blood can occur during donor phlebotomy. Offending organisms are usually gram-negative, especially *Pseudomonas* species, *Citrobacter freundii,* and *Escherichia coli.*

Also possible is contamination of donor blood with viruses, such as hep-atitis, cytomegalovirus, and malaria.

Signs and symptoms

Immediate signs and symptoms of hemolytic transfusion reaction develop within a few minutes or hours after the start of transfusion and may include chills, fever, urticaria, tachycardia, dyspnea, nausea, vomiting, tightness in the chest, chest and back pain, hypotension, bronchospasm, angioedema, anaphylaxis, shock, pulmonary edema, and congestive heart failure. In a surgical patient under anesthesia, these symptoms are masked, but blood oozes from mucous membranes or the incision site.

Delayed hemolytic reactions can occur up to several weeks after transfusion, causing fever, an unexpected fall in the patient's serum hemoglobin level, and jaundice.

Allergic reactions are afebrile and characterized by urticaria and angioedema, possibly progressing to cough, respiratory distress, nausea and vomiting, diarrhea, abdominal cramps, vascular instability, shock, and coma.

The hallmark of febrile nonhemolytic reactions is mild to severe fever, which may begin at the start of transfusion or within 2 hours after it's completed.

Bacterial contamination causes high fever, nausea and vomiting, diarrhea, abdominal cramps, shock, and hemoglobinuria, possibly leading to disseminated intravascular coagulation (DIC) and renal failure.

Diagnosis

Confirming a hemolytic transfusion reaction requires proof of blood incompatibility and evidence of hemolysis, such as hemoglobinuria, anti-A or anti-B antibodies in the serum, low serum hemoglobin levels, and elevated bilirubin levels. When you suspect such a reaction, draw blood; have the patient's blood retyped and cross-matched with the donor's blood. After a hemolytic transfusion reaction, laboratory tests will show increased indirect bilirubin, decreased haptoglobin, and increased serum hemoglobin levels, and hemoglobin in urine. Later, as the reaction progresses, tests may show signs of DIC (thrombocytopenia, increased prothrombin time, and decreased fibrinogen level) and acute tubular necrosis (increased serum BUN and creatinine levels).

Blood cultures to isolate the causative organism should be done when bacterial contamination is suspected.

Treatment and nursing intervention

At the first sign of a hemolytic reaction, *stop the transfusion immediately,* maintain a patent I.V. line, and notify the doctor.

Subsequent procedures may include the following:

• Monitor the patient's vital signs every 15 to 30 minutes, watching for signs of shock.

• As ordered, insert an indwelling catheter and monitor intake and output, observing carefully for hematuria, oliguria, and anuria.

• Cover the patient with blankets to ease chills, and explain what is happening to allay his fears.

• Administer, as ordered, an I.V. antihypotensive drug and normal saline solution to combat shock, oxygen (by nasal cannula or Venturi mask at low flow rates), epinephrine to treat dyspnea and wheezing, diphenhydramine to combat cellular histamine released from mast cells, corticosteroids to reduce inflammation, and mannitol or furosemide to maintain urinary function. Administer parenteral antihistamines and corticosteroids for allergic reactions. Severe reactions—anaphylaxis—may require epinephrine. Administer antipyretics for febrile nonhemolytic reactions and appropriate intravenous antibiotics for bacterial contamination.

• Remember to fully document the transfusion reaction on the patient's chart, noting duration of transfusion, amount of blood absorbed, and a com-

---

Rh SYSTEM

The Rh system contains more than 30 antibodies and antigens. Eighty-five percent of the world's population are Rh-positive, which means their red blood cells carry the D or Rh antigen. The remaining 15% of the population, who are Rh-negative, do not carry this antigen.

When Rh-negative persons receive Rh-positive blood for the first time, they become sensitized to the D antigen but show no immediate reaction to it. If they receive Rh-positive blood a second time, they then develop a massive hemolytic reaction. For example, an Rh-negative mother who delivers an Rh-positive baby is sensitized by the baby's Rh-positive blood. During her next Rh-positive pregnancy, her sensitized blood would cause a hemolytic reaction in fetal circulation. Thus, the Rh-negative mother should receive Rh$_o$ (D) immune globulin (human) I.M. within 72 hours after delivering an Rh-positive baby to prevent formation of antibodies against Rh-positive blood.

---

plete description of the reaction.

• To prevent hemolytic transfusion reaction: Before giving a blood transfusion, be sure you know your hospital policy about giving blood. Then make sure you have the right blood and the right patient. Check and double-check with another nurse the patient's name, hospital number, ABO group, and Rh status. If you find the smallest discrepancy, don't give the blood. Notify the blood bank immediately and return the unopened unit.

BASIA BELZA TACK, RN, MSN, ANP

Chédiak-Higashi syndrome (CHS)

CHS is characterized by morphologic changes in granulocytes that impair their ability to respond to chemotaxis and to digest or "kill" invading organisms. This rare syndrome has been documented in about 100 cases worldwide. It also affects certain animals, including cows, mice, whales, tigers, and mink. Partial albinism is typically associated with CHS.

Causes

CHS is transmitted as an autosomal recessive trait. In many cases, it seems linked to consanguinity. The genetic defect is expressed by morphologic changes in the granulocytes, which contain giant granules with abnormal lysosomal enzymes. These abnormal granulocytes display delayed chemotaxis and impaired intracellular digestion of organisms, both of which diminish the inflammatory response.

Signs and symptoms

The child with CHS has recurrent bacterial infections, most commonly caused by *Staphylococcus aureus* but also by streptococci and pneumococci. These infections occur primarily in the skin, subcutaneous tissue, and lungs and may be accompanied by fever, thrombocytopenia, neutropenia, and hepatosplenomegaly.

Partial albinism in CHS involves the ocular fundi, skin, and hair, which has a characteristic silvery sheen. Most patients also have significant photophobia. Progressive motor and sensory neuropathy may eventually cause debilitation and inability to walk or perform activities of daily living. Patients who survive recurrent bouts of infection commonly develop marked proliferation of granulocytes or lymphocytes resembling lymphoreticular malignancy. These cells infiltrate the liver, spleen, and bone marrow, causing progressively severe and ultimately fatal hepatosplenomegaly, thrombocytopenia, neutropenia, and anemia.

Diagnosis

Diagnosis rests on detection of characteristic morphologic changes in granulocytes on a peripheral smear. Function studies confirm delayed chemotaxis of granulocytes and impaired intracellular digestion of organisms.

Treatment

When prevention of infection fails, the next best step is early detection and vigorous treatment of infection with antimicrobials and surgical drainage, if indicated. In a few patients, large doses of vitamin C (ascorbic acid) have helped enhance chemotaxis of abnormal granulocytes, although without associated clinical improvement.

Nursing intervention

● Provide meticulous skin care to maintain skin integrity and prevent infection.

● Teach the patient and his family how to prevent and recognize infection, especially in areas of decreased sensation.

● After surgical drainage of infection, provide diligent wound care. Irrigate draining or open wounds and change sterile dressings frequently.

● Administer antimicrobials, as ordered, and monitor the patient for drug side effects. Also check the I.V. site frequently.

● Suggest sunglasses and/or a visor to minimize discomfort associated with photophobia. Also teach the patient how to avoid injury associated with decreased sensation or motor coordination.

● Offer emotional support to help the patient and his family cope with this difficult disorder and maintain as normal a life-style as possible.

CHRISTINE GRADY, RN, MSN, CNS

Chronic granulomatous disease (CGD)

In CGD, abnormal neutrophil metabolism impairs phagocytosis—one of the body's chief defense mechanisms—resulting in increased susceptibility to low-virulent or nonpathogenic organisms, such as *Staphylococcus epidermidis, Serratia marcescens, E. coli, Aspergillus,* and *Nocardia.* Phagocytes attracted to sites of infection can engulf these invading organisms but are unable to digest or "kill" them. Patients with CGD may develop granulomatous inflammation, which leads to ischemic tissue damage.

Causes
CGD is usually inherited as an X-linked trait, although a variant form—probably autosomal recessive—also exists. The genetic defect may be linked to deficiency of the enzymes NADH, NADPH oxidase, or NADH reductase.

Signs and symptoms
Usually, the patient with CGD displays signs and symptoms by age 2, associated with infections of the skin, lymph nodes, lung, liver, and bone. Skin infection is characterized by small, well-localized areas of tenderness. Seborrheic dermatitis of the scalp and axilla is also common. Lymph node infection typically causes marked lymphadenopathy with draining lymph nodes and hepatosplenomegaly. Many patients develop liver abscess, which may be recurrent and multiple; abdominal tenderness, fever, anorexia, and nausea point to abscess formation. Other common infections include osteomyelitis, which causes localized pain and fever; pneumonia; and gingivitis with severe periodontal disease.

Diagnosis
Clinical features of osteomyelitis, pneumonia, liver abscess, or chronic lymphadenopathy in a young child provide the first clues to diagnosis of CGD. An important tool for confirming this diagnosis is the nitroblue tetrazolium (NBT) test. A clear yellow dye, NBT is normally reduced by neutrophil metabolism, resulting in a color change from yellow to blue. Quantifying this color change estimates the degree of neutrophil metabolism. Patients with CGD show impaired or absent reduc-

tion of NBT, indicating abnormal neutrophil metabolism. Another test can measure the rate of intracellular killing by neutrophils; in CGD, killing is delayed or absent.

Other laboratory values may support the diagnosis or help monitor disease activity. Osteomyelitis typically causes an elevated white blood cell count and erythrocyte sedimentation rate; bone scans help locate and size such infections. Recurrent liver or lung infection may eventually cause abnormal function studies. Cell-mediated and humoral immunity are usually normal in CGD, although some patients have hypergammaglobulinemia.

Treatment and nursing intervention
Early, aggresssive treatment of infection is the chief goal in CGD. Areas of suspected infection should be biopsied or cultured, and broad-spectrum antibiotics usually started immediately, without waiting for results of cultures. Confirmed abscesses may be drained or surgically removed. Provide meticulous wound care after such treatment, including irrigation or packing.

Many patients with CGD receive a combination of intravenous antibiotics, often extended beyond the usual 10- to 14-day course. However, for fungal infections with *Aspergillus* or *Nocardia,* treatment involves amphotericin B in progressively higher doses to achieve a maximum cumulative dose. During I.V. drug therapy, monitor the patient's vital signs frequently. Rotate the I.V. site every 48 to 72 hours.

To help treat life-threatening or antibiotic-resistant infection or to help localize infection, the patient may receive granulocyte transfusions—usually once daily until the crisis has passed. During such transfusions, watch for fever and chills (these effects can sometimes be prevented by premedication with acetaminophen). Transfusions should not be given within 6 hours before or after administration of amphotericin B to avoid severe pulmonary edema and, possibly, respiratory arrest.

If prophylactic antibiotics are ordered, teach the patient and his family how to administer them properly and how to recognize side effects. Advise them to promptly report any signs or symptoms of infection. Stress the importance of good nutrition and hygiene, especially meticulous skin and mouth care.

During hospitalizations, encourage the patient to continue his activities of daily living as much as possible. Try to arrange for a tutor to help the child keep up with his school work.

CHRISTINE GRADY, RN, MSN, CNS

Common variable immunodeficiency
(Acquired hypogammaglobulinemia, agammaglobulinemia with Ig-bearing B cells)

Common variable immunodeficiency is characterized by progressive deterioration of B cell (humoral) immunity, resulting in increased susceptibility to infection. Unlike X-linked hypogammaglobulinemia, this disorder usually causes symptoms after infancy and childhood, between ages 25 and 40. It affects males and females equally and usually doesn't interfere with normal life span or with normal pregnancy and offspring.

Causes
The cause of common variable immunodeficiency is unknown. Most patients have a normal circulating B cell count but defective synthesis or release of immunoglobulins. Many also exhibit progressive deterioration of T cell (cell-mediated) immunity, revealed by delayed hypersensitivity skin testing.

Signs and symptoms
In common variable immunodeficiency, pyogenic bacterial infections are characteristic but tend to be chronic rather than acute (as in X-linked hypogammaglobulinemia). Recurrent sinopulmonary infections, chronic bacterial conjunctivitis, and malabsorption (often associated with infestation by *Giardia lamblia*) are usually the first clues to immunodeficiency.

Common variable immunodeficiency may be associated with autoimmune diseases, such as systemic lupus erythematosus, rheumatoid arthritis, hemolytic anemia, and pernicious anemia, and with malignancies, such as leukemia and lymphoma.

Diagnosis
Characteristic diagnostic markers in this disorder are decreased serum IgM, IgA, and IgG levels, detected by immunoelectrophoresis, along with a normal circulating B cell count. Antigenic stimulation confirms an inability to produce specific antibodies; cell-mediated immunity may be intact or delayed. X-rays usually show signs of chronic lung disease or sinusitis.

Treatment and nursing intervention
Treatment and nursing care for common variable immunodeficiency are essentially the same as for X-linked hypogammaglobulinemia.

Intramuscular or intravenous injection of immune globulin (usually weekly to monthly) helps maintain immune response. Since these injections are very painful, give them deep into large muscle mass, such as the gluteal or thigh muscles, and massage well. If the doctor orders more than 1.5 ml, divide the dose and inject it into more than one site; for frequent injections, rotate the injection sites. Because immune globulin is composed primarily of IgG, the patient may also need fresh frozen plasma infusions to provide IgA and IgM.

Antibiotics are the mainstay for combatting infection. Regular X-rays and pulmonary function studies help monitor infection in the lungs; chest physiotherapy may be ordered to forestall or help clear such infection.

To help prevent severe infection, teach the patient and his family how to recognize its early signs. Warn them to avoid crowds and persons who have active infections. Also stress the importance of good nutrition and regular follow-up care.

ELIZABETH JOHNSTONE, RNC, BS

Complement deficiencies

Complement is a series of circulating enzymatic serum proteins with nine functional components, labeled C1 through C9. (Historically, the first four complement components are numbered out of sequence—C1, C4, C2, and C3—but the remaining five are numbered sequentially.) When the immunoglobulins IgG or IgM react with antigens as part of an immune response, they activate C1, which then combines with C4, initiating the classic complement pathway, or cascade. (An alternative complement pathway involves the direct activation of C3 by the serum protein properdin, bypassing the initial components [C1, C4, C2] of the classic pathway.) Complement then combines with the antigen-antibody complex and undergoes a sequence of complicated reactions that amplify the immune response against the antigen. This complex process is called complement fixation.

Complement deficiency or dysfunction may cause increased susceptibility to infection and also seems related to certain autoimmune disorders. Theoretically, any complement component may be deficient or dysfunctional, and many such disorders are under investigation. Primary complement deficiencies are rare. The most common ones are C2, C6, and C8 deficiencies and C5 familial dysfunction. More common secondary complement abnormalities have been confirmed in patients with lupus erythematosus, in some with dermatomyositis, in one with scleroderma (and in his family), and in a few with gonococcal and meningococcal infections. Prognosis varies with the abnormality and the severity of associated diseases.

Causes
Primary complement deficiencies are inherited as autosomal recessive traits, except for deficiency of C1 esterase inhibitor, which is autosomal dominant. Secondary deficiencies may follow complement-fixing (complement-consuming) immunologic reactions, such as drug-induced serum sickness, acute streptococcal glomerulonephritis, and active systemic lupus erythematosus.

Signs and symptoms
Clinical effects vary with the specific deficiency. C2 and C3 deficiencies and C5 familial dysfunction increase susceptibility to bacterial infection (which may involve several body systems simultaneously). C2 deficiency is also related to collagen vascular disease, such as lupus erythematosus, and chronic renal failure. C5 dysfunction, a familial defect in infants, causes failure to thrive, diarrhea, and seborrheic dermatitis. C1 esterase inhibitor deficiency (hereditary angioedema) may cause periodic swelling in the face, hands, abdomen, or throat, with potentially fatal laryngeal edema.

Diagnosis
Diagnosis of a complement deficiency is difficult and requires careful interpretation of both clinical features and laboratory results. Total serum complement level (CH50) is low in various complement deficiencies. In addition, specific assays may be done to confirm deficiency of specific complement components. For example, detection of

complement components and IgG by immunofluorescent examination of glomerular tissues in glomerulonephritis strongly suggests complement deficiency.

Treatment

Primary complement deficiencies have no known cure. Associated infection, collagen vascular disease, or renal disease requires prompt, appropriate treatment. Transfusion of fresh frozen plasma to provide replacement of complement components is controversial, because replacement therapy doesn't cure complement deficiencies and any beneficial effects are transient. Bone marrow transplant may be helpful, but can cause a potentially fatal graft-versus-host (GVH) reaction. Anabolic steroids and antifibrinolytic agents are often used to reduce acute swelling in

---

COMPLEMENT CASCADE

The complement system plays an indispensable role in the humoral immune response. Activation of this system, the complement cascade, follows one of two pathways: the *classical pathway*, initiated by antigen-antibody complexes, or the *alternative pathway*, triggered by IgA; some IgG molecules; and certain polysaccharides, lipopolysaccharides, and trypsin-like enzymes. The diagram below shows how these pathways work.

CLASSICAL PATHWAY

Initiated by antigen-antibody complexes (IgG, IgM)

▼

C1qrs generates an enzyme that cleaves C4 and C2

▼

C1$\overline{42}$ is formed, which cleaves C3

▼

C3a (anaphylatoxin) and C3b are formed; C3a is released and functions in inflammation; C3b is an opsonin and is active in the enzyme C1423b

▼

C1$\overline{423}$b induces cleavage of C5

ALTERNATIVE PATHWAY

Initiated by IgA, some IgG, and certain polysaccharides, lipopolysaccharides, and trypsin-like enzymes

▼

Factor B combines with C3b in the presence of Factor D

▼

C3bBb (stablilized by properdin) is formed, which acts on C3

▼

C3bBbC3b (stabilized by properdin) is formed, which induces cleavage of C5

Forms C5a (anaphylatoxin) and C5b; C5a is released and functions in inflammation; C5b binds to C6,7

▼

C5b,6,7 binds to C8

▼

C5b,6,7,8 binds to C9

▼

C5b,6,7,8,9 causes cell lysis

patients with C1 esterase inhibitor deficiency.

Nursing intervention

• Teach the patient (or his family, if he's a child) the importance of avoiding infection, how to recognize its early signs and symptoms, and the need for prompt treatment if it occurs.
• After bone marrow transplant, monitor the patient closely for signs of transfusion reaction and GVH reaction.
• Meticulous patient care can speed recovery and prevent complications. For example, a patient with renal infection needs careful monitoring of intake and output, tests for serum electrolytes and acid-base balance, and observation for signs of renal failure.
• When caring for a patient with hereditary angioedema, be prepared for emergency management of laryngeal edema; keep airway equipment on hand.

NORA LYNN BOLLINGER, RN, MSN
CHRISTINE GRADY, RN, MSN, CNS

DiGeorge's syndrome

(Congenital thymic hypoplasia or aplasia)

DiGeorge's syndrome is a disorder known typically by the partial or total absence of cell-mediated immunity that results from a deficiency of T cells. It characteristically produces life-threatening hypocalcemia, which may be associated with cardiovascular and facial anomalies. Patients rarely live beyond age 2 without fetal thymic transplant; however, prognosis improves when fetal thymic transplant, correction of hypocalcemia, and repair of cardiac anomalies are possible.

Causes

DiGeorge's syndrome is probably caused by abnormal fetal development of the third and fourth pharyngeal pouches (12th week of gestation),

---

ROLE OF THE THYMUS IN IMMUNE RESPONSE

Although the exact relationship between the thymus and the immune system remains unclear, possible thymic functions include:
• destruction of T cells that would have "mistaken" components of the human organism as foreign during the fetal stage. This establishes immunologic differentiation between self and nonself.
• maturation of T cells in the thymic epithelium or mesenchymal cells. These mature cells help regulate the humoral immune response.

---

which interferes with the formation of the thymus. As a result, the thymus is completely or partially absent and abnormally located, causing deficient cell-mediated immunity. This syndrome has been associated with maternal alcoholism and resultant fetal alcohol syndrome.

Signs and symptoms

Symptoms are usually obvious at birth or shortly thereafter. An infant with DiGeorge's syndrome may have low-set ears, notched ear pinnae, a fish-shaped mouth, an undersized jaw, and abnormally wide-set eyes (hypertelorism) with antimongoloid eyelid formation (downward slant).

Cardiovascular abnormalities include great blood vessel anomalies (these may also develop soon after birth) and tetralogy of Fallot. The thymus may be absent or underdeveloped, and abnormally located. An infant with thymic hypoplasia (rather than aplasia) may experience a spontaneous return of cell-mediated immunity but can develop severe T cell deficiencies later in life, causing exaggerated susceptibility to viral, fungal, or bacterial infections, which may be overwhelming. Hypoparathyroidism, usually associated with DiGeorge's syndrome, typically produces tetany, hyperphosphoremia, and hypocalcemia. Hypocalcemia develops early and is

SHEEP CELL TEST

When human red blood cells are mixed with sheep red blood cells, the sheep cells aggregate peripherally around human T cells to form characteristic rosettes. An electron microscope scan showing decreased or absent rosettes confirms deficient or absent T cells.

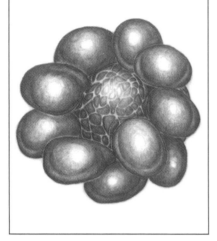

both life-threatening and unusually resistant to treatment. It can lead to seizures, central nervous system damage, and early congestive heart failure.

Diagnosis

Immediate diagnosis is difficult unless the infant shows typical facial anomalies—normally the first clues to the disorder. Definitive diagnosis depends on successful treatment of hypocalcemia and other life-threatening birth defects during the first few weeks of life. Such diagnosis rests on proof of decreased or absent T cells (sheep cell test showing lymphopenia) and of an absent thymus (chest X-ray). Immunoglobulin assays are useless, because the antibodies present are usually from maternal circulation.

Additional laboratory tests showing low serum calcium levels, elevated serum phosphorus levels, and an absence of parathyroid hormone confirm hypoparathyroidism.

Treatment and nursing intervention

Life-threatening hypocalcemia must be treated immediately, but it's unusually resistant and requires aggressive treatment—for example, with a rapid I.V. infusion of 10% calcium gluconate solution. During such an infusion, monitor heart rate and watch carefully to avoid infiltration. Remember that calcium supplements *must* be given with vitamin D, or sometimes also with parathyroid hormone, to ensure effective calcium utilization. After hypocalcemia is under control, fetal thymic transplant may restore normal cell-mediated immunity. Cardiac anomalies require surgical repair when possible.

An infant with DiGeorge's syndrome also needs a low-phosphorus diet and careful preventive measures for infection. Teach the infant's parents to watch for signs of infection and get immediate treatment; to keep the infant away from crowds and other sources of infection; and to provide good hygiene, nutrition, and hydration.

NORA LYNN BOLLINGER, RN, MSN

IgA deficiency
(Janeway Type 3 dysgammaglobulinemia)

Selective deficiency of IgA is the most common immunoglobulin deficiency, appearing in as many as 1 in 800 persons. IgA—the major immunoglobulin in human saliva, nasal and bronchial fluids and intestinal secretions—guards against bacterial and viral reinfections. Consequently, IgA deficiency leads to chronic sinopulmonary infections, gastrointestinal diseases, and other disorders. Prognosis is good for patients who receive correct treatment, especially if they are free of associated disorders. Such patients have been known to survive to age 70.

Causes

IgA deficiency seems to be linked to autosomal dominant or recessive inheritance. The presence of normal numbers of peripheral blood lymphocytes carrying IgA receptors and of normal amounts of other immunoglobulins suggests that B cells may not be secreting IgA. In an occasional patient, suppressor T cells appear to inhibit IgA secretion. IgA deficiency also seems related to autoimmune disorders, since many patients with rheumatoid arthritis or systemic lupus erythematosus are also IgA-deficient. Some drugs, such as anticonvulsants, may cause transient IgA deficiency.

Signs and symptoms

Some IgA-deficient patients have no symptoms, possibly because they have extra amounts of low-molecular-weight IgM (7s), which takes over IgA function and helps maintain adequate immunologic defenses.

Among those patients who do develop symptoms, chronic sinopulmonary infection is most common. Other effects are respiratory allergy, often triggered by infection; gastrointestinal tract diseases, such as celiac disease, ulcerative colitis, and regional enteritis; autoimmune diseases, such as rheumatoid arthritis, systemic lupus erythematosus, immunohemolytic anemia, and chronic hepatitis; and malignant tumors, such as squamous cell carcinoma of the lungs, reticulum cell sarcoma, and thymoma. The age of onset varies. Some IgA-deficient children with recurrent respiratory disease and middle-ear inflammation may begin to synthesize IgA spontaneously as recurrent infections subside and their condition improves.

Diagnosis

Immunologic analyses of IgA-deficient patients show serum IgA levels below 5 mg/dl. While IgA is usually absent from secretions in IgA-deficient patients, levels may be normal in rare cases. IgE levels are normal, while IgM levels may be normal or elevated in serum and secretions. Normally absent low-molecular-weight IgM (7S) may be present.

Tests may also indicate autoantibodies and antibodies against IgG (rheumatoid factor), IgM, and bovine milk. Cell-mediated immunity and secretory piece (the glycopeptide that transports IgA) are usually normal, and most circulating B cells appear normal.

Treatment and nursing intervention

Selective IgA deficiency has no known cure. Treatment aims to control symptoms of associated diseases, such as respiratory and gastrointestinal infections, and is generally the same as for a patient with normal IgA, with one exception: *don't* give an IgA-deficient patient immune globulin, because sensitization may lead to anaphylaxis during future administration of blood products. If transfusion with blood products is necessary, minimize the risk of adverse reaction by using washed red blood cells, or avoid the reaction completely by cross-matching the patient's blood with that of an IgA-deficient donor. Since this is a lifelong disorder, teach the patient to prevent infection, to recognize its early signs, and to seek treatment promptly.

NORA LYNN BOLLINGER, RN, MSN

Immunodeficiency with eczema and thrombocytopenia
(Wiskott-Aldrich syndrome)

Wiskott-Aldrich syndrome is an X-linked recessive immunodeficiency disorder in which both B cell and T cell functions are defective. Its clinical features include thrombocytopenia with severe bleeding, eczema, recurrent infection, and an increased risk of lym-

NURSING MANAGEMENT OF BONE MARROW TRANSPLANT

The patient who undergoes bone marrow transplant needs special nursing care before, during, and after this difficult procedure.

Before transplant
• Assist, as needed, as the patient receives various blood tests for baseline hematologic studies, histocompatibility (human leukocyte antigen typing, and mixed leukocyte culture).
• Monitor the patient during pharmacologic or radiologic treatment to suppress the immune system.
• Impose the use of sterile clothing, sheets, and food equipment; implement reverse isolation or use of laminar flow. Help the patient adjust to the sterile environment, which will protect him from his own flora during extreme immunosuppression.
• During decontamination, provide regular baths with Hibiclens liquid or Betadine, as ordered; administer oral nonabsorbable antibiotics to sterilize the patient's GI tract.
• Monitor vital signs, EKGs, intake and output, and blood chemistries.
• Teach the patient and his family what they need to know about the transplant procedure and the preparations for it. Offer them reassurance and support.

During bone marrow infusion
• Monitor for possible allergic reactions and pulmonary overload.
• Provide meticulous care of the I.V. line and the infusion site.

After the transplant
• Provide meticulous supportive care to avoid complications and to promote successful engraftment.
• During the early weeks of posttransplant pancytopenia, carefully administer ordered transfusions of red blood cells, platelets, or granulocytes.
• Maintain a sterile environment to prevent infection. Assess carefully for signs of infection, and monitor vital signs. Take weekly samples for cultures of stool, urine, throat, and catheter sites.
• Take special care to protect venous access devices, such as a Hickman or Broviac catheter.
• Watch for signs of graft-versus-host disease; administer immunosuppressive drugs as ordered.
• Provide good skin care; as needed, administer topical corticosteroids.
• Ensure adequate nutrition and fluid balance; provide I.V. fluid replacement and hyperalimentation as ordered.
• Watch for opportunistic infections. Monitor closely for signs of respiratory infection. Check respirations and temperature regularly. At the first sign of a fever, obtain chest X-rays and cultures. Commonly, treatment for suspected bacterial infection begins with administration of broad-spectrum antibiotics without delay for the results of culture tests. Treatment for fungal infection usually includes I.V. amphotericin B for *Pneumocystis carinii* pneumonia, with co-trimoxazole (Bactrim, Septra). No effective therapy is available for cytomegalovirus infection.
• Provide continuing emotional support and reassurance for the patient and his family.
CHRISTINE GRADY, RN, MSN, CNS

phoid malignancy. Prognosis is poor. This syndrome causes early death (average life span is 4 years), usually from massive bleeding during infancy or from malignancy or severe infection in early childhood.

Causes
Because Wiskott-Aldrich syndrome results from an X-linked recessive trait, it affects only males. Infants with this genetic defect are born with a normal thymus gland and normal plasma cells and lymphoid tissues. But an inherited defect in both B cell and T cell function compromises immune system re-

sponse, and increases the patient's vulnerability to infection. These patients also have a metabolic defect in platelet synthesis and produce only small, short-lived platelets, resulting in thrombocytopenia.

Signs and symptoms
Characteristically, newborns with Wiskott-Aldrich syndrome develop bloody stools, bleeding from a circumcision site, petechiae, and purpura, resulting from thrombocytopenia. As these infants get older, thrombocytopenia subsides. But beginning at about 6 months, they typically develop re-

current systemic infections, such as chronic pneumonia, sinusitis, otitis media, and herpes simplex of the skin and eyes (which may cause keratitis and vision loss), with hepatosplenomegaly. Usually, *Streptococcus pneumoniae*, meningococci, and *Hemophilus influenzae* are the infecting organisms. At about 1 year, eczema occurs, becoming progressively more severe. Their skin is easily infected because of scratching. These infants are also highly vulnerable to malignancy, especially leukemia and lymphoma.

Diagnosis

The most important clues to diagnosis of Wiskott-Aldrich syndrome are thrombocytopenia (with a platelet count below 100,000/mm³ and prolonged bleeding time) and bleeding disorders at birth. Laboratory tests may show normal or elevated IgE and IgA levels, decreased IgM levels, normal IgG levels, and low to absent isohemagglutinins. Cell-mediated immunity may be normal in newborns but gradually declines with age.

Treatment

Treatment aims to limit bleeding through the use of fresh, cross-matched platelet transfusions; to prevent or control infection with prophylactic or early and aggressive antibiotic therapy; to supply passive immunity with immune globulin injections or infusions; and to control eczema with topical corticosteroids. (Systemic corticosteroids are contraindicated, since they further compromise immunity.) An antipruritic may relieve itching.

Treatment with transfer factor has had limited success. However, bone marrow transplant has been remarkably successful in some patients.

Nursing intervention

Physical and psychological support and patient teaching can help these patients and their families cope with this disorder.

• Teach parents to watch for signs of

bleeding, such as easy bruising, bloody stools, swollen joints, and tenderness in the trunk. Help them plan their child's activity levels to ensure normal development. While the child must avoid contact sports, he can ride a bike (wearing protective football gear) and swim.

• Before giving platelet transfusions, establish a baseline platelet count, and check the count often during therapy. Each platelet unit transfused should raise the count by 10,000/mm³.

• Instruct parents to observe the child for signs of infection, such as fever, coldlike symptoms, or drainage and redness around any superficial wound, and to cleanse all skin wounds carefully. Emphasize the importance of meticulous mouth and skin care, good nutrition, and adequate hydration. Parents should avoid exposing the child to crowds or to persons with active infections.

• As soon as the child is old enough, begin teaching him about his disease and his limitations.

• The parents of children with Wiskott-Aldrich syndrome may need genetic counseling on the vulnerability of future offspring.

NORA LYNN BOLLINGER, RN, MSN
CHRISTINE GRADY, RN, MSN, CNS

Nezelof's syndrome

Nezelof's syndrome is a primary immunodeficiency disease characterized by absent T cell function and variable B cell function, with fairly normal immunoglobulin levels and little or no specific antibody production. The degree of B cell deficiency varies. Nezelof's syndrome causes early onset of recurrent, progressively severe, and eventually fatal infections.

Causes

The cause of Nezelof's syndrome is unknown. It may be a genetic disorder transmitted as an autosomal recessive trait because it affects both male and female siblings. However, not all patients with Nezelof's syndrome have a positive family history, so alternative explanations are possible. For example, the syndrome could result from a stem cell deficiency that causes T cell and B cell deficiencies; from an underdeveloped thymus gland that inhibits T cell development; or from failure to produce or secrete thymic humoral factors, particularly thymosin.

Signs and symptoms

Clinical signs of Nezelof's syndrome may appear in children up to age 4 and usually include recurrent pneumonia, otitis media, chronic fungal infections, upper respiratory tract infections, hepatosplenomegaly, diarrhea, and failure to thrive. Lymph nodes and tonsils may be absent or enlarged; a tendency toward malignancy is common. Eventually, infection may cause sepsis, the usual cause of death in patients with this disorder.

Diagnosis

Failure to thrive, poor eating habits, weight loss, and recurrent infections in children may all suggest Nezelof's syndrome. But definite diagnosis requires the following: evidence of defective cell-mediated immunity and moderate to marked decrease in T cell count. B cell count and function vary; 50% of patients have normal B cells. Immunoglobulin levels also vary. Isohemagglutinins are absent or normal and eosinophilia may be present.

Treatment

Initial treatment is primarily supportive and includes use of antibiotics to fight infection and monthly immune globulin or fresh frozen plasma infusions, especially if the patient can't produce specific antibodies.

Fetal thymus transplant can fully restore cell-mediated immunity within weeks, but its effect is transient, necessitating repeated transplants. Both transfer factor therapy and repeated injections of thymosin are only partially effective in restoring cell-mediated immunity. Histocompatible bone marrow transplants may restore immunity.

Nursing intervention

● When caring for a patient with Nezelof's syndrome, continuously monitor for signs of infection.

● To prevent tissue damage from immune globulin injections, rotate and record injection sites, and inject immune globulin deeply into a large muscle mass. If the child receives more than 1.5 ml of immune globulin, divide the dose and use more than one injection site.

● Since immune globulin injections are very painful, you may find it helpful to prepare the child with "needle play." Let him inject a doll or pretend to inject you.

● Teach the parents of a child with Nezelof's syndrome to recognize signs of infection, and warn them that their child must avoid crowds and persons who have active infections.

NORA LYNN BOLLINGER, RN, MSN
CHRISTINE GRADY, RN, MSN, CNS

Severe combined immunodeficiency disease (SCID)

In SCID, both cell-mediated (T cell) and antibody-mediated (B cell) immunity are deficient or absent, resulting in susceptibility to infection during infancy. At least three types of SCID exist: reticular dysgenesis, the most severe type, in which the hematopoietic stem cell fails to differentiate into lymphocytes and granulocytes; Swiss-type agammaglobulinemia, in which the hematopoietic stem cell fails to differentiate into lymphocytes alone; and enzyme deficiency, such as adenosine deaminase (ADA) deficiency, in which the buildup of toxic products in the lymphoid tissue causes damage and subsequent dysfunction. SCID affects more males than females, with an estimated incidence of 1 in 100,000 to 500,000 births. Most untreated patients die from infection within a year of birth.

Causes
SCID is usually transmitted as an autosomal recessive trait, although it may be X-linked. In most cases, the genetic defect seems associated with failure of the stem cell to differentiate into T and B cells. Less commonly, it results from enzyme deficiency.

Signs and symptoms
An extreme susceptibility to infection becomes obvious in the infant with SCID in the first few months of life. Commonly, such an infant fails to thrive and develops chronic otitis; sepsis; watery diarrhea (associated with *Salmonella* or *Escherichia coli*); recurrent pulmonary infections (usually caused by *Pseudomonas*, cytomegalovirus, or *Pneumocystis carinii*); persistent oral candidiasis, sometimes with esophageal erosions and hoarseness; and common viral infections (such as chicken pox) that are often fatal.

Pneumocystis carinii pneumonia usually strikes a severely immunodeficient infant in the first 3 to 5 weeks of life. Onset is typically insidious, with gradually worsening cough, low-grade fever, tachypnea, and respiratory distress. Chest X-ray characteristically shows bilateral pulmonary infiltrates.

Because of protection by maternal IgG, gram-negative infections don't usually appear until the infant is about 6 months old.

Diagnosis
Diagnosis is generally made clinically, since most SCID infants suffer recurrent, overwhelming infections within a year after birth. Before age 5 months, even normal infants have very small amounts of serum immunoglobulins

IgM and IgA, and normal IgG levels merely reflect maternal IgG. However, severely diminished or absent T cell number (less than 10% T cell rosettes) and function, and lymph node biopsy showing absence of lymphocytes can confirm diagnosis of SCID.

Treatment
Treatment aims to restore immune response and prevent infection. Histocompatible bone marrow transplant is the only satisfactory treatment available to correct immunodeficiency. Since bone marrow cells must be HLA- (human leukocyte antigen) and MLC- (mixed leukocyte culture) matched, the most common donors are histocompatible siblings. However, bone marrow transplant may cause a graft-versus-host (GVH) reaction, which increases vulnerability to infection and may be fatal. Newer methods of bone marrow transplant that eliminate the problem of GVH reaction, such as lectin separation and the use of monoclonal antibodies, are currently being evaluated.

Fetal thymus and liver transplants have achieved limited success. Administration of immune globulin may also play a role in treatment. Some SCID infants have received long-term protection by being isolated in a completely sterile environment. However, this treatment isn't effective if the infant already has had recurring infections.

Nursing intervention
Nursing care is primarily preventive and supportive. Monitor the infant for early signs of infection; if infection develops, provide prompt and aggressive drug therapy, as ordered. Although SCID infants must remain in strict protective isolation, try to provide a stimulating atmosphere to promote growth and development. Encourage parents to visit their child often, to hold him, and to bring him toys that can be easily sterilized. Explain all procedures to them. Maintain a normal day/night

Continued on page 103

T AND B LYMPHOCYTES:
THEIR ORIGIN AND ROLE IN THE IMMUNE RESPONSE

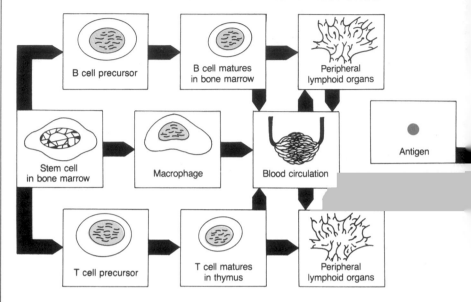

Although both derive from bone marrow stem cells, B and T cells mature differently. *B cell ontogeny* was first detected in the chicken's central lymphoid organ, the bursa of Fabricius. In humans, the bone marrow presumably serves as the bursa equivalent; here, pre-B cells are believed to mature to B cells. These B cells then migrate to peripheral lymphoid organs, such as the lymph nodes and spleen, for storage. When an antigen-presenting cell (APC) presents an antigen to a B cell, with T cell help, the B cell is activated and proliferates. Many of these cells then differentiate into antibody-secreting plasma cells. Others remain in the lymphatic tissue as memory B cells and, upon reexposure to the same antigen, quickly differentiate into antibody-secreting plasma cells for an accelerated immune response.

In *T cell ontogeny*, T cell precursors (pre-T cells) travel to the thymus, where they mature to T cells. These T cells then leave the thymus to circulate in the blood or become constituents of the peripheral lymphoid organs.

When an APC presents an antigen in the presence of the major histocompatibility complex antigen, the T cell activates and differentiates into various subsets with overlapping functions. Helper T cells interact with B cells to stimulate B cell proliferation and differentiation into antibody-secreting cells. Suppressor T cells appear to control the amount of T cell help available to stimulate antibody production. Other T cells produce lymphokines, soluble mediators involved in delayed hypersensitivity and other immune reactions.

Cytotoxic (or killer) T cells and natural killer cells directly destroy the antigenic agent, whereas memory T cells remain in circulation and in lymphatic tissue to recognize and promptly attack that same antigen in any subsequent appearance.

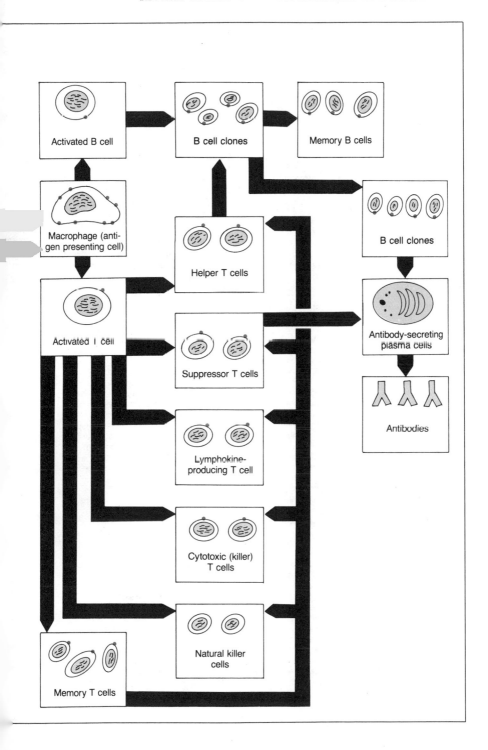

IATROGENIC IMMUNODEFICIENCY

Iatrogenic immunodeficiency may be a complicating side effect of drug or radiation therapy or splenectomy. At times, though, it's the very goal of therapy; for example, to suppress immune-mediated tissue damage in autoimmune disorders or to prevent rejection of an organ transplant.

IMMUNOSUPPRESSIVE DRUG THERAPY

Immunosuppressive drugs fall into several categories:

• **Cytotoxic drugs.** These drugs kill immunocompetent cells while they're replicating. However, because most cytotoxic drugs aren't selective, they interfere with all rapidly proliferating cells, reducing the number of lymphocytes and phagocytes and interfering with lymphocyte synthesis and release of immunoglobulins and lymphokines.

Cyclophosphamide, a potent immunosuppressant frequently used in systemic lupus erythematosus, Wegener's granulomatosis, and other systemic vasculitides and in certain autoimmune disorders, initially depletes the number of B cells, suppressing humoral immunity. Chronic therapy also depletes T cells, suppressing cell-mediated immunity as well. Because it nonselectively destroys rapidly dividing cells, this drug can cause severe bone marrow suppression with neutropenia, anemia, and thrombocytopenia; gonadal suppression with sterility; alopecia; hemorrhagic cystitis; and nausea, vomiting, and stomatitis. It may also increase the risk of lymphoproliferative malignancy.

Among other cytotoxic drugs used for immunosuppression are azathioprine, which is frequently used in kidney transplantation; and methotrexate, which is occasionally used in rheumatoid arthritis and other autoimmune disorders.

When caring for a patient who's receiving cytotoxic drugs, carefully monitor his white blood cell count; if it falls too low, the drug dosage may need to be adjusted. Also monitor urine output and watch for signs of cystitis, especially if the patient's taking cyclophosphamide. Ensure adequate fluid intake (approximately 3 liters/day). Provide antiemetics to relieve nausea and vomiting, as ordered. Provide meticulous oral hygiene and promptly report signs of stomatitis. Warn the patient about his increased risk of infection; be sure he recognizes its early signs and symptoms. Suggest a scarf and/or wig to hide

temporary alopecia; assure the patient that his hair will grow back. Make sure the male patient understands the risk of sterility; advise sperm banking, if appropriate. Generally, young women are advised to take oral contraceptives to minimize ovarian dysfunction and to prevent pregnancy during administration of these potentially teratogenic drugs.

• **Corticosteroids.** These adrenocortical hormones are widely used to treat immune-mediated disorders because of their potent anti-inflammatory and immunosuppressive effects. Corticosteroids stabilize the vascular membrane, blocking migration of neutrophils and monocytes into tissues and thus inhibiting inflammation. They also "kidnap" T cells in the bone marrow, causing transient lymphopenia that resolves itself within 24 hours after the drugs are withdrawn. Corticosteroids also appear to inhibit immunoglobulin synthesis and to interfere with the binding of immunoglobulin to antigen or to cells with Fc receptors.

The most commonly used oral corticosteroid is prednisone. For long-term therapy, it's best given early in the morning to minimize exogenous suppression of cortisol production and with food or milk to minimize gastric irritation. After the acute phase, prednisone is usually reduced to an alternate-day schedule and then gradually withdrawn to minimize potentially harmful side effects. Other corticosteroids used for immunosuppression include hydrocortisone, methylprednisolone, and dexamethasone.

Long-term corticosteroid therapy can cause numerous side effects, which are sometimes more harmful than the disease itself. Neurologic side effects include euphoria, insomnia, or psychosis; cardiovascular effects include hypertension and edema; and GI effects include gastric irritation, ulcers, and increased appetite with weight gain. Other possible effects are cataracts, hyperglycemia, glucose intolerance, muscle weakness, osteoporosis, delayed wound healing, and increased susceptibility to infection.

During corticosteroid therapy, monitor the patient's blood pressure, weight, and intake and output. Instruct him to eat a well-balanced, low-salt diet or to follow the specially prescribed diet to prevent excessive weight gain. Remember that even though the patient is more susceptible to infection, he'll show fewer or less dramatic signs of inflammation.

• **Cyclosporine.** A relatively new immunosuppressant, cyclosporine selectively suppresses proliferation and development of helper T cells, resulting in depressed cell-mediated immunity. This drug is used primarily to prevent rejection of kidney, liver, and heart transplants but is also being investigated for use in several other disorders. Significant toxic effects of cyclosporine primarily involve the liver and kidney, so treatment with this drug requires regular evaluation of renal and hepatic function. Some studies also link cyclosporine with increased risk of lymphoma. Adjusting the dose or duration of therapy helps minimize certain side effects.

• **Antilymphocyte serum or antithymocyte globulin (ATG).** This anti–T cell antibody reduces T cell number and function, thus suppressing cell-mediated immunity. It's been used effectively to prevent cell-mediated rejection of tissue grafts, or transplants. Usually, it's administered immediately before the transplant and continued afterward. Potential side effects include anaphylaxis and serum sickness. Occurring 1 to 2 weeks after injection of ATG, serum sickness is characterized by fever, malaise, rash, arthralgias, and, occasionally, glomerulonephritis or vasculitis.

RADIATION THERAPY

Irradiation is cytotoxic to proliferating and intermitotic cells, including most lymphocytes. As a result, it may induce profound lymphopenia, resulting in immunosuppression. Irradiation of all major lymph node areas— total nodal irradiation—is used to treat certain disorders, such as Hodgkin's lymphoma. Its effectiveness in severe rheumatoid arthritis, lupus nephritis, and prevention of kidney transplant rejection is still under investigation.

SPLENECTOMY

After splenectomy, the patient has increased susceptibility to infection, especially with pyogenic bacteria such as *Streptococcus pneumoniae*. This risk of infection is even greater when the patient is very young or has an underlying reticuloendothelial disorder. The incidence of fulminant, rapidly fatal bacteremia is especially high in splenectomized patients and often follows trauma. These patients should receive Pneumovax immunization for prophylaxis and should be warned to avoid exposure to infection and trauma.

CHRISTINE GRADY, RN, MSN, CNS

routine, and talk to the child as much as possible. If parents cannot visit, call them often to report on the infant's condition.

Since parents will have questions about the vulnerability of future offspring, refer them for genetic counseling. Parents and siblings need psychological and spiritual support to help them cope with the child's inevitable long-term illness and early death. They may also need a social service referral for assistance in coping with the financial burden of the child's long-term hospitalization.

NORA LYNN BOLLINGER, RN, MSN
CHRISTINE GRADY, RN, MSN, CNS

Vasculitis

Vasculitis includes a broad spectrum of disorders characterized by inflammation and necrosis of blood vessels— either the large muscular arteries, medium- to small-sized arteries, arterioles, capillaries, postcapillary venules, or veins. Its clinical effects depend on the vessels involved and reflect tissue ischemia caused by blood flow obstruction. Prognosis is also variable. For example, hypersensitivity vasculitis is usually a benign disorder limited to the skin, whereas more extensive polyarteritis nodosa can be rapidly fatal. Vasculitis can occur at any age, except for mucocutaneous lymph node syndrome, which occurs only during childhood. It may be a primary disorder or occur secondarily to other disorders, such as rheumatoid arthritis or systemic lupus erythematosus.

Causes

Exactly how vascular damage develops in vasculitis is not well understood. Current theory holds that it's initiated by excessive antigen in the circulation, which triggers the formation of soluble antigen-antibody complexes. These complexes cannot be effectively cleared by the reticuloendothelial system and so are deposited in blood vessel walls (Type III hypersensitivity). Increased vascular permeability associated with release of vasoactive amines by platelets and basophils enhances such deposition. The deposited complexes activate the complement cascade, resulting in chemotaxis of neutrophils, which release lysosomal enzymes. In turn, these enzymes cause vessel damage and necrosis, which may precipitate thrombosis, occlusion, hemorrhage, and tissue ischemia.

Another mechanism that may contribute to vascular damage is the cell-mediated immune response. In this response, circulating antigen triggers the release of soluble mediators by sensitized lymphocytes, thus attracting macrophages. The macrophages release intracellular enzymes that cause vascular damage. They can also be transformed into the epithelioid and multinucleated giant cells that typify the granulomatous vasculitides. Phagocytosis of immune complexes by macrophages enhances granuloma formation.

Treatment
Treament of vasculitis aims to minimize irreversible tissue damage associated with ischemia. In primary vasculitis, treatment may involve removal of an offending antigen or use of anti-inflammatory or immunosuppressive drugs. Drug therapy frequently involves low-dose cyclophosphamide (2 mg/kg P.O. daily) with daily corticosteroids. In rapidly fulminant vasculitis, cyclophosphamide dosage may be increased to 4 mg/kg daily for the first 2 to 3 days, followed by the regular dose. Prednisone should be given in a dose of 1 mg/kg daily, in divided doses, for 7 to 10 days, with consolidation to a single morning dose by 2 to 3 weeks. When the vasculitis seems to be in remission, or when prescribed cytotoxic drugs take full effect, corticosteroids are tapered down to a single daily dose and then to an alternate-day schedule.

TYPES OF VASCULITIS

TYPE AND VESSELS INVOLVED

Polyarteritis nodosa
Small- to medium-sized arteries throughout the body. Lesions tend to be segmental, occurring at bifurcations and branchings of arteries and spreading distally to arterioles. In severe cases, lesions circumferentially involve adjacent veins.

Allergic angiitis and granulomatosis
(Churg-Strauss syndrome)
Small- to medium-sized arteries and small vessels, mainly of the lung but also of other organs

Polyangiitis overlap syndrome
Small- to medium-sized arteries and small vessels of the lung and other organs

Wegener's granulomatosis
Small- to medium-sized vessels of the respiratory tract and kidney

Temporal arteritis
Medium- to large-sized arteries, most commonly branches of the carotid artery

Takayasu's arteritis (aortic arch syndrome)
Medium- to large-sized arteries, particularly the aortic arch and its branches and, possibly, the pulmonary artery

Hypersensitivity vasculitis
Small vessels, especially of the skin

Mucocutaneous lymph node syndrome
(Kawasaki disease)
Small- to medium-sized vessels, primarily of the lymph nodes; may progress to involve coronary arteries

Behçet's disease
Small vessels, primarily of the mouth and genitalia but also of the eyes, skin, joints, GI tract, and central nervous system

SIGNS & SYMPTOMS	DIAGNOSIS
Hypertension, abdominal pain, myalgias, headache, joint pain, weakness	History of symptoms; elevated erythrocyte sedimentation rate (ESR); leukocytosis; anemia; thrombocytosis; depressed C3 complement; rheumatoid factor >1:60; circulating immune complexes; tissue biopsy showing necrotizing vasculitis.
Resembles polyarteritis nodosa with severe pulmonary involvement	History of asthma; eosinophilia; tissue biopsy showing granulomatous inflammation with eosinophilic infiltration.
Combines symptoms of polyarteritis nodosa and allergic angiitis and granulomatosis	Possible history of allergy; eosinophilia. Tissue biopsy showing granulomatous inflammation with eosinophilic infiltration.
Fever, pulmonary congestion, cough, malaise, anorexia, weight loss, mild to severe hematuria	Tissue biopsy showing necrotizing vasculitis with granulomatous inflammation; leukocytosis; elevated ESR, IgA, and IgG; low titer rheumatoid factor; circulating immune complexes.
Fever, myalgia, jaw claudication, visual changes, headache (associated with polymyalgia rheumatica syndrome)	Decreased hemoglobin; elevated ESR; tissue biopsy showing panarteritis with infiltration of mononuclear cells, giant cells within vessel wall, fragmentation of internal elastic lamina, and proliferation of intima.
Malaise, pallor, nausea, night sweats, arthralgias, anorexia, weight loss, pain and/or paresthesia distal to affected area, bruits, loss of distal pulses, syncope, and, if carotid artery is involved, diplopia and transient blindness. May progress to congestive heart failure or cerebrovascular accident.	Decreased hemoglobin; leukocytosis; positive lupus erythematosus cell preparation and elevated ESR; arteriography showing calcification and obstruction of affected vessels; tissue biopsy showing inflammation of adventitia and intima of vessels, and thickening of vessel walls.
Palpable purpura, papules, nodules, vesicles, bullae, ulcers, or chronic or recurrent urticaria	History of exposure to an antigen, such as a microorganism or drug; tissue biopsy showing leukocytoclastic venulitis, usually in post-capillary venules, with infiltration of polymorphonuclear leukocytes, fibrinoid necrosis, and extravasation of erythrocytes.
Fever; nonsuppurative cervical adenitis; edema; congested conjunctivae; erythema of oral cavity, lips, and palms; and desquamation of fingertips. May progress to myocarditis, pericarditis, myocardial infarction, and cardiomegaly.	History of symptoms; tissue biopsy showing intimal proliferation and infiltration of vessel walls with mononuclear cells.
Recurrent oral ulcers, eye lesions, genital lesions, and cutaneous lesions	History of symptoms

This alternate-day dosage may continue for 3 to 6 months before steroids are slowly tapered off and discontinued.

In secondary vasculitis, treatment focuses on the underlying disorder, such as rheumatoid arthritis or systemic lupus erythematosus.

Nursing intervention
• Assess for dry nasal mucosa in patients with Wegener's granulomatosis. Instill nose drops or irrigate nasal passages with warm normal saline solution.
• Monitor vital signs. Use a Doppler flowmeter to auscultate blood pressure in patients with Takayasu's arteritis, whose peripheral pulses are frequently difficult to palpate.
• Monitor intake and output. Check daily for edema. Keep the patient well hydrated (3 liters/day) to reduce the risk of hemorrhagic cystitis associated with cyclophosphamide therapy.
• Provide emotional support to help the patient and his family cope with an altered body imaging resulting from the disorder or its therapy. (For example, Wegener's granulomatosis may be associated with saddle noses, steroids may cause weight gain, and cyclophosphamide may cause alopecia.)
• Teach the patient how to recognize drug side effects. Monitor his WBC count during cyclophosphamide therapy to prevent severe leukopenia.

DAWN FLOWERS, RN, BSN

MENTAL AND EMOTIONAL DISORDERS

Anorexia nervosa

Anorexia nervosa, probably a mental disturbance, is characterized by self-imposed starvation and consequent emaciation, nutritional deficiency disorders, and atrophic changes. Gorging and purging by vomiting may occur during starvation, or after normal weight is restored as a means of weight control instead of starvation. This disorder primarily affects adolescent females and young adults but is not uncommon among older women; occasionally, it also affects males. Prognosis varies but is improved if the diagnosis is made early or if the patient voluntarily seeks help and wants to overcome the disorder. Nevertheless, mortality ranges from 5% to 15%, the highest mortality associated with a psychiatric disturbance.

Causes and incidence
No one knows exactly what causes anorexia nervosa. Researchers in neuroendocrinology are seeking a physiologic cause but have found nothing definite yet. Clearly, however, social attitudes that equate slimness with beauty play some role in provoking this disorder; family factors are also clearly implicated.

Anorexia nervosa most often strikes girls from achievement-oriented, upwardly mobile families, but it can occur among those of lower socioeconomic status. It may have a higher incidence in families that stress the importance of certain foods or who have rituals involving them.

Signs and symptoms
Anorexia nervosa usually develops in a patient who is of normal weight or only slightly overweight. One of its cardinal symptoms is a 25% *or greater* weight loss for no organic reason, coupled with a morbid dread of being fat and a compulsion to be thin. Commonly, such a patient tends to be angry and excessively devoted to ritualistic behavior.

The anorectic shows multiple and severe sequelae of chronic undernourishment: skeletal muscle atrophy, loss of fatty tissue, hypotension, constipation, dental caries, susceptibility to infection, blotchy or sallow skin, intolerance to cold, lanugo on the face and body, dryness or loss of scalp hair, and amenorrhea. Oddly, the patient usually demonstrates restless activity and vigor (despite undernourishment), and may exercise avidly without apparent fatigue. Paradoxically, even though she may be obsessed with food or cooking, she refuses to eat and is convinced she's too fat, despite all evidence to the contrary. Gorging, followed by spontaneous or self-induced vomiting or self-administration of laxatives or diuretics, may lead to dehydration or metabolic alkalosis or acidosis; induction of vomiting with ipecac may lead to cardiotoxicity. Circulatory collapse (signaled by a drop in systolic pressure below 50 mm Hg) may prove fatal. Cardiac dysrhythmias due to electrolyte imbalance may cause cardiac arrest.

While anorexia nervosa is not necessarily an expression of a death wish, feelings of despair, hopelessness, and worthlessness produce a higher rate of attempted suicides in these patients.

Diagnosis

Diagnosis requires careful interpretation of clinical status to rule out endocrine, metabolic, and central nervous system abnormalities; malignancy; malabsorption syndrome; and other disorders that cause physical wasting. The patient's obvious physical vigor (despite her emaciated appearance) simplifies this task, and a history of compulsive dieting and bulimic episodes helps confirm the diagnosis.

Initial laboratory analysis should probably include a complete blood count (CBC); measurement of serum levels of creatinine, blood urea nitrogen, uric acid, cholesterol, total protein, albumin, sodium, potassium, chloride, CO_2 content, calcium, SGOT, and SGPT; determination of fasting blood glucose levels; a urinalysis; and an electrocardiogram (EKG). The necessity for periodic repetition of these studies depends on the severity of malnutrition, emesis, and laxative or di-

uretic abuse, as well as on the degree of abnormality of the test results. Laboratory data are usually normal, unless weight loss exceeds 30%.

Treatment

Treatment aims to promote weight gain or control the patient's compulsive gorging and purging, and to correct the underlying dysfunction. Hospitalization in a medical or a psychiatric unit may be required to improve the patient's precarious physical state. The required hospitalization may be as brief as 2 weeks or may stretch from a few months to 2 years or longer. Treatment is difficult and results are often discouraging. Fortunately, many clinical centers are now developing programs for managing eating disorders in both inpatients and outpatients.

Specific approaches to treatment may include behavior modification (privileges are dependent on weight gain); curtailing activity for physical reasons (such as cardiac dysrhythmias); vitamin and mineral supplements; a reasonable diet, with or without liquid supplements; hyperalimentation (subclavian, peripheral, or enteral [enteral and peripheral routes carry less risk of infection]); and group, family, or individual psychotherapy.

All forms of psychotherapy, from psychoanalysis to hypnotherapy, have been used in treating anorexia nervosa, with varying success. To be successful, such therapy should address the patient's underlying problems of low self-esteem, guilt, and anxiety; feelings of hopelessness and helplessness; and depression. Most therapists consider task-centered approaches and therapeutic flexibility important requirements for success in treating anorexia nervosa.

Nursing intervention

• During hospitalization, regularly monitor vital signs and intake and output. Weigh the patient daily—before breakfast, if possible. However, since such a patient often fears being weighed, the routine for this may differ greatly.

• Frequently offer small portions of food or drinks, if the patient wants them. Nutritionally complete liquid feedings are often more acceptable since they eliminate choices between foods—something the anorectic commonly finds difficult.

• If tube feedings or other special feeding measures become necessary, explain these fully to the patient, and be ready to discuss her fears or reluctance; however, limit the discussion about food itself.

• Discuss the patient's need for food with her matter-of-factly; point out how improved nutrition can correct abnormal laboratory findings.

• If edema or bloating occurs after the patient has returned to normal eating behavior, reassure her that this phenomenon is temporary. She will probably find this condition frightening.

• Encourage the patient to recognize and assert her feelings freely. If she understands that she can be assertive, she may gradually learn that expressing her true feelings will not result in her losing control or love.

• Remember: The anorectic uses exercise, preoccupation with food, ritualism, manipulation, and prevarication as mechanisms that preserve the only control she feels she has in her life.

• The patient's family may need therapy to uncover and correct faulty interactions. Advise family members to avoid discussing food. The patient's weight may be monitored by someone who is acceptable to the patient, her family, and her therapist.

You or the doctor may refer the patient and her family to Anorexia Nervosa and Associated Disorders (ANAD), a national information and support organization. This organization may help them understand what anorexia is, convince them they need help, and find a psychotherapist or medical doctor who is experienced in treating this disorder.

VIVIAN MEEHAN, RN

Anxiety states
(Anxiety neuroses)

Anxiety is a feeling of apprehension caused by a threat to a person or his values. Some describe it as an exaggerated feeling of impending doom, dread, or uneasiness. Unlike fear—a reaction to danger from a specific external source—anxiety is a reaction to an internal threat, such as an unacceptable impulse or a repressed thought that's straining to reach a conscious level. Occasional anxiety is a normal part of life as a rational response to a real threat. However, overwhelming anxiety can cause an anxiety state—uncontrollable, unreasonable anxiety that narrows perceptions and interferes with normal functions.

Anxiety states can be acute or chronic. An acute state, or *panic disorder*, often begins between ages 15 and 35. Chronic anxiety that lasts for more than a month is called a *generalized anxiety disorder* and has an uncertain prognosis.

Causes and incidence
Many theorists, such as Freud, Horney, and Rank, describe the cause of anxiety states in different ways. But they all share a common premise: that conflict—whether intrapsychic, sociopersonal, or interpersonal—promotes an anxiety state.

Panic and generalized anxiety disorders are more widespread than previously thought. They affect twice as many women as men, and their symptoms are even more common than depressive symptoms.

Research has proven that anxiety states run in families, suggesting genetic predisposition. Studies also show that families of patients with panic disorders have a high incidence of alcoholism and that these patients have increased mortality caused by suicide and heart disease, especially mitral valve prolapse. Some investigators link physiologic symptoms of anxiety to high serum lactate levels.

Signs and symptoms

The patient with an anxiety state experiences psychological or physiologic symptoms that vary with the degree of anxiety. A mild anxiety causes mainly psychological symptoms with unusual self-awareness and alertness to the environment. Moderate anxiety causes selective inattention, yet with ability to concentrate on a single task. Severe anxiety causes inability to concentrate on more than scattered details of a task. Panic state with acute anxiety causes the patient to lose concentration completely, and his speech is often unintelligible.

In a patient with a *generalized anxiety disorder,* mild to moderate signs and symptoms last for a month or more, but no panic attacks occur. Psychological effects vary in severity but may include restlessness, sleeplessness, appetite changes, irritability, repeated questioning, and constant attention- or reassurance-seeking behavior. The patient feels fatigue on awakening and worries about possible misfortunes. Because he has difficulty concentrating, he is unaware of his surroundings. Typically, he's oriented to the past, not the present or future. He may say that he feels apprehensive, helpless, fearful, "keyed up," angry, tearful, withdrawn, or afraid of losing self-confidence or control. In addition, the patient shows lack of initiative, criticizes himself and others, and is self-deprecating.

Physical effects of a generalized anxiety disorder may include diaphoresis, dilated pupils, dry mouth, a lump in the throat, frequent urination, dysuria, rapid respirations, flushing or pallor, diarrhea, constipation, nausea, vomiting, belching, sexual dysfunction, and cold, clammy hands. The patient's blood pressure and heart rate rise and he feels palpitations and weakness. He displays motor tension by trembling, headaches, muscle aches and spasms,

---

RECOGNIZING A PANIC ATTACK

A panic attack is a brief period of intense apprehension or fear; it may last from minutes to hours. A history of three or more panic attacks within 3 weeks that are unrelated to extreme physical exertion, life-threatening situations, or phobias confirm panic disorder.

During a panic attack, the patient will display four or more of these signs and symptoms:
- chest pains
- palpitations
- dyspnea
- choking or smothering feeling
- vertigo, dizziness, or unsteadiness
- feelings of faintness
- depersonalization or feelings of unreality
- tingling in the hands and feet
- shaking or trembling
- hot and cold flashes
- diaphoresis
- fear of going crazy, dying, or being out of control during a panic attack.

---

inability to relax, twitching eyelids, a strained face, hyperventilation, and easy startle responses.

In a panic disorder, acute anxiety causes a panic attack with severe signs and symptoms. (See *Recognizing a Panic Attack.*) After a panic attack, the patient may not remember what precipitated it and may feel depersonalized. Usually, chronic anxiety persists between attacks.

Diagnosis

A thorough history confirms an anxiety state when it shows a pattern of failure to cope with past or current stress. However, careful evaluation must rule out organic causes of the patient's symptoms, such as hyperthyroidism, pheochromocytoma, coronary artery disease, paroxysmal tachycardia, and Ménière's disease. For instance, if a patient complains of chest pain or other cardiopulmonary symptoms, he should have an EKG to rule out myocardial ischemia. Because anxiety is also the central feature of other psychiatric disorders, additional tests must rule out phobias, obsessive compulsive disorders, depression, and acute schizophrenia. Other tests should include complete blood count, differential, and serum lactate and calcium levels to rule out hypocalcemia.

Treatment
A combination of organic and psychotherapeutic treatments may help a patient with an anxiety disorder. The benzodiazepine antianxiety drugs may relieve mild anxiety and improve ability to cope with stress. Tricyclic antidepressants or higher doses of benzodiazepines may relieve severe anxiety and panic attacks. These drugs can ease distress and facilitate psychotherapy or psychoanalysis.

Nursing intervention
When caring for an anxious patient, your role is primarily supportive and protective. Your goal will be to help the patient develop effective coping mechanisms to manage his anxiety. If the patient must take antianxiety drugs or tricyclic antidepressants, you should:
• administer psychotropic medications and evaluate the patient's response.
• stress the importance of taking the medications exactly as prescribed for maximum effectiveness.
• warn the patient and his family that these drugs may cause side effects, such as drowsiness, fatigue, ataxia, blurred vision, slurred speech, tremors, and hypotension.
• tell the patient to avoid simultaneous use of alcohol or any central nervous system depressants. He should also avoid driving and other hazardous tasks until he develops a tolerance for the drug's sedative effects.
• advise him to discontinue medications only with the doctor's approval because abrupt withdrawal could cause severe symptoms.

If the patient has a panic attack, protect him during the attack. Show him how to take slow, deep breaths if he's hyperventilating. Explain the physio-

logic reasons for these symptoms. Avoid making judgments or critical comments.

When panic subsides, encourage the patient to face his anxiety, because avoidance increases it. Help him recognize his anxiety and his coping mechanisms, such as depression, withdrawal, demanding or violent behavior, denial, and manipulation. Explore alternative behaviors. Encourage him to take up activities that will distract him from anxiety. Make referrals for psychiatric treatment, as needed, for chronic anxiety and disturbed coping mechanisms. Provide telephone numbers for hot lines, psychiatric emergency help, and other emergency interventions.

MARY LOU L. HAMILTON, RN, MS

Bipolar affective disorder

Bipolar affective disorder is marked by severe pathologic mood swings from euphoria to sadness, by spontaneous recoveries, and by a tendency to recur. The cyclic (bipolar) form consists of separate episodes of mania (elation) and depression; however, either the manic or the depressive episodes can be predominant, producing few, if any, mood swings; or the two moods can be mixed. When depression is the predominant mood, the patient has the unipolar form of the disease. The overall incidence of unipolar affective disorder is 3 to 4 per 1,000.

Bipolar affective disorder is 1.5 to 2 times more common among women than men; it is more common in higher socioeconomic groups and is associated with high levels of creativity. It can begin any time after adolescence, but first attacks usually occur between ages 20 and 35; approximately 35% of patients experience onset between ages 35 and 60. The manic form is more prevalent in young patients and the depressive form in older ones. Bipolar disorder recurs in 80% of patients; as they grow older, the attacks of illness recur more frequently and last longer. This illness is associated with a significant mortality; 20% of these patients die as a result of suicide, many just as the depression lifts.

Causes
The causes of bipolar affective disorder are not clearly understood, but hereditary, biologic, and psychological factors may play a part. The incidence of this illness in siblings is 20% to 25%; in identical twins, 66% to 96%. The higher incidence in females suggests a socially learned or sex-linked genetic

---

PRECAUTIONS FOR DRUG THERAPY IN BIPOLAR AFFECTIVE DISORDER AND MAJOR DEPRESSION

Tricyclic antidepressants (TCAs)
• Warn the patient that the TCA may cause drowsiness and fatigue. Tell him to take the drug only as prescribed and to avoid hazardous tasks until he can tolerate its sedative effects. If drowsiness persists, he may take a single daily dose at bedtime.
• Warn him against using alcohol and to use other central nervous system depressants only as prescribed.
• If he's been taking large doses for a long time, advise him not to discontinue the drug without the doctor's guidance, since abrupt withdrawal may cause severe nausea and headache.
• Tell the patient to expect a lag time of 10 to 14 days, or even a month, before the antidepressant effects begin, but that side effects may occur within 24 hours. Side effects include dry mouth (tell the patient to chew gum or use hard candies), urinary retention or constipation (increase fluid intake or administer a stool softener), blurred vision, tachycardia, dysrhythmias, sweating, dizziness, and hallucinations.
• TCAs are contraindicated in males with prostatic hypertrophy.
• TCAs are seldom used with MAO inhibitors because of possible drug interactions.

Monoamine oxidase (MAO) inhibitors
• Emphatically warn the patient on an MAO inhibitor against eating foods containing tryptophan, tyramine, or caffeine (such as cheese; sour cream; beer, chianti, or sherry; pickled herring; liver; canned figs; raisins, bananas, or avocados; chocolate; soy sauce; fava beans; yeast extracts; meat tenderizers; coffee; or colas); severe hypertensive symptoms may occur.
• Carefully monitor blood pressure throughout MAO inhibitor therapy, and keep phentolamine available for possible hypertensive crisis.
• Warn the patient to sit up for at least a

minute before attempting to get out of bed, and then to rise slowly to avoid dizziness. Advise him to lie down or squat if he feels dizzy or faint.
• Warn the patient not to discontinue medication without a doctor's guidance, since abrupt withdrawal may cause severe symptoms; also warn against taking other medications, especially over-the-counter cold, hay fever, or weight-reducing medications for 2 to 3 weeks after discontinuing MAO inhibitor therapy.
• Tell the patient to expect a lag time of 1 to 3 weeks before antidepressant effects begin.
• MAO inhibitors are rarely given with TCAs because of possible drug interactions.
• All patients on antidepressants should be supervised for suicidal ideations as the depression lifts.

Lithium carbonate
• Use with extreme caution with haloperidol (monitor carefully for early signs of encephalopathy, such as lethargy or fever), diuretics, sodium bicarbonate, and I.V. solutions containing sodium chloride.
• Keep daily salt intake constant. Monitor for excessive perspiration, vomiting, or diarrhea.
• Monitor intake and output and serum electrolyte levels closely, since lithium interferes with antidiuretic hormone and is contraindicated in fluid or electrolyte imbalance.
• Watch for side effects (fine tremor, orthostatic hypotension, polyuria, nausea, and diarrhea) and early signs of toxicity (coarse tremor, slurred speech, nystagmus, drowsiness, and ataxia).
• Warn the patient to avoid hazardous tasks until drug response is determined and to carry a Medic Alert card that identifies him as a lithium carbonate user.
• Warn the patient not to stop the drug abruptly without the doctor's supervision.

cause. Other familial influences, especially the early loss of a parent, parental depression, incest, or abuse, may predispose a person to depressive illness. Emotional or physical trauma, such as bereavement, disruption of an important relationship, or severe accidental injury, may precede the onset of bipolar illness, but the disorder often appears without identifiable predisposing factors. Before the onset of overt symptoms, many patients with this illness have an energetic and outgoing personality type with a history of wide mood swings.

Although certain biochemical changes accompany mood swings, it's not clear whether these changes cause the mood swings or result from them. In both mania and depression, intracellular sodium concentration increases during illness and returns to normal with recovery. Biochemical research also reports changes in brain catecholamines that accompany adrenal steroid and other metabolic changes. In depression, brain catecholamine levels decrease; in mania, they increase. These changes can accompany abnormal adrenal steroid levels and other metabolic anomalies.

Signs and symptoms

The manic and depressive phases of bipolar affective disorder produce characteristic mood swings and other behavioral and physical changes. In the depressive phase, the patient experiences loss of self-esteem, overwhelming inertia, hopelessness, despondency, withdrawal, apathy, sadness, and helplessness. He has increased fatigue and difficulty sleeping (falling asleep, staying asleep, or early morning awakening), and awakes feeling tired. He usually feels worse in the morning. He may also have anorexia, causing significant weight loss without dieting, and may become constipated.

The depressed patient also may show psychomotor retardation, with slowed speech, movement, and thoughts, and may complain of difficulty in concentrating. He is usually not disoriented or intellectually impaired but may offer only slow, one-word answers in a monotone. The depressed patient also may express excessive and hypochondriacal concern about body changes and may have multiple somatic complaints, such as constipation, fatigue, headache, and chest pain. He may worry excessively about having cancer or some other severe illness. In an elderly patient, such physical symptoms may be the only clue to depression.

The depressed patient may feel guilt and self-reproach over past events and, as depression deepens, may feel worthless. He may believe he is wicked and deserves to be punished. His deepening sadness, guilt, negativity, and fatigue place extraordinary burdens on his family. Suicide is an ever-present risk, especially when the depression begins to lift. Then a rising energy level may give the patient the strength to carry out suicidal ideas. The suicidal patient may also have homicidal ideas, thinking, for example, of killing his family, either in anger or to spare them pain and disgrace.

The manic phase of bipolar affective disorder is marked by recurrent, distinct episodes of a persistently euphoric, expansive, or irritable mood. It must be associated with four of the following symptoms that persist for at least 1 week:
• increase in social, occupational, or sexual activity with physical restlessness
• unusual talkativeness or pressure to keep talking
• flight of ideas or the subjective experience that thoughts are racing
• inflated self-esteem, grandiosity
• decreased need for sleep
• distractability, attention too easily drawn to trivial stimuli
• excessive involvement in activities that have a high potential for painful but unrecognized consequences (shopping sprees, reckless driving).

The manic patient has little control over incessant pressure of ideas, speech, and activity; he ignores the need to eat, sleep, or relax. Such a patient's constant demands for attention, his high energy level, and his need to test limits and rules can tire even the most energetic nursing staff and frequently causes a major nursing care problem.

Hypomania, more common than acute mania, is marked by a classic triad of symptoms: elated but unstable mood, pressure of speech, and increased motor activity. It too causes patients to be elated, overactive, easily distracted, talkative, irritable, impatient, impulsive, and full of energy but doesn't induce flight of ideas, delusions, or absence of discretion and self-control.

Diagnosis
Diagnosis rests primarily on observation and psychiatric history of pathologic mood swings from elation to sadness. However, rating scales of increased or decreased activity, speech, or sleep and other psychological tests may support the diagnosis of bipolar affective disorder. A manic patient's dramatic improvement in response to treatment with lithium carbonate further validates this diagnosis. A careful history may identify previous mood swings or a family history of manic-depressive illness. Nevertheless, the patient needs careful physical evaluation to rule out possible medical causes (including intraabdominal neoplasm, hypothyroidism, cardiac failure, cerebral arteriosclerosis, parkinsonism, brain tumor, and uremia); amphetamine, alcohol, or phencyclidine (PCP) intoxication; and drug-induced depression.

Treatment
Treatment for an acute manic or depressive episode may require brief hospitalization to provide:
• drug therapy with MAO inhibitors, such as phenelzine (Nardil) and the tricyclic antidepressant imipramine (Tofranil), which relieves depression without causing the amnesia or confusion that commonly follow electroconvulsive therapy (ECT).
• ECT, in which an electric current is passed through the temporal lobe to produce a controlled grand mal seizure. ECT is a well known and effective treatment for persistent depression, though it's less effective in the manic phase. It's the treatment of choice for middle-aged, agitated, and suicidal patients.
• lithium therapy, which can dramatically relieve symptoms of mania and hypomania and may prevent recurrence of depression. In some patients, maintenance therapy with lithium has prevented recurrence of symptoms for decades. Lithium has a narrow therapeutic range, so treatment must include close monitoring of blood levels to avoid dehydration, salt imbalance, and other adverse effects. Because therapeutic doses of lithium produce adverse effects in many patients, compliance may be a problem. In those who fail to respond to lithium and to treat acute symptoms before onset of lithium effect, haloperidol (Haldol) may be effective. (Onset of lithium effect takes 7 to 10 days.)

Nursing intervention
For the depressed patient:
• Provide continual positive reinforcement to help improve his self-esteem.
• Encourage him to talk or to write down his feelings if he's having trouble expressing them. Listen attentively and respectfully, and allow him time to formulate his thoughts if he seems sluggish.
• Provide a structured routine, including activities to boost confidence and promote interaction with others (for instance, group therapy), and keep reassuring him that depression will lift.
• To prevent possible suicide, remove harmful objects from the patient's environment, observe him closely but unobtrusively, and strictly supervise his medications.
• Record all observations and appropriate conversations with the patient,

since these are valuable for evaluating his condition.

• Don't forget the patient's physical needs. If he's too depressed to take care of himself, help him with personal hygiene. Encourage him to eat, or feed him if necessary. If he's constipated, add high-fiber foods to his diet, offer frequent small meals, and encourage physical activity. To help him sleep, give back rubs or warm milk at bedtime.

For the manic patient:

• Remember his physical needs. Encourage him to eat; he may jump up and walk around the room after every mouthful but will sit down again if you remind him.

• Encourage short naps during the day, and assist with personal hygiene.

• Provide emotional support, maintain a calm environment, and set realistic goals for behavior.

• Provide diversionary activities suited to a short attention span; firmly discourage the patient if he tries to overextend himself.

• When necessary, reorient the patient to reality, and tactfully divert conversations when they become intimately involved with other patients or staff members.

• Set limits in a calm, clear, and self-confident manner for the manic patient's demanding, hyperactive, manipulative and acting-out behaviors. Setting limits tells the patient you'll provide security and protection by refusing inappropriate and possibly harmful requests. Avoid leaving an opening for the patient to test or argue.

• Listen to requests attentively and with a neutral attitude, but avoid power struggles if a patient tries to put you on the spot for an immediate answer. Explain that you'll consider the request seriously and will respond later.

• Collaborate with other staff members to provide consistent responses to the patient's manipulations or acting out.

• Watch for early signs of frustration (when the patient's anger escalates from verbal threats to hitting an ob-

ject). Tell the patient firmly that threats and hitting are unacceptable and that these actions show he needs help to control his behavior. Then tell him that staff will help him move to a quiet area and will help him control his behavior so he won't hurt himself or others. Staff who have practiced as a team can work effectively to prevent acting-out behavior or to remove and confine a patient.

• Alert the staff team promptly when acting-out behavior escalates. It's wiser and safer to have help available before you need it than to try controlling an anxious or frightened patient by yourself.

• Once the incident is over and the patient is calm and in control, discuss his feelings with him and offer suggestions to prevent recurrence.

• Treatment sometimes includes ECT, but this is less effective for mania than for depression; the results are better with frequent treatments.

SHARON MCBRIDE VALENTE, RN, MN, CS, FAAN

Bulimia
(Eating disorder)

Bulimia is characterized by recurring episodes of binge-purge behavior. This disorder, of growing concern to health care professionals, primarily affects females of young adult or adolescent age (slightly older than those with anorexia nervosa). Bulimia is much less common, but tends to be more severe, in males.

Causes
The exact cause is unknown, but various psychosocial factors are thought to contribute to its development. Such factors include family disturbance or conflict; maladaptive learned behavior; struggle for control or self-identity; and cultural overemphasis on physical appearance. Recent psychiatric theory

leans strongly toward considering bulimia a syndrome of depression.

Signs and symptoms

Bulimia is marked by episodic binge eating that may occur as often as several times a day. Induced vomiting (purging) allows eating to continue until abdominal pain, sleep, or the presence of another person interrupts it. The preferred food is usually sweet, soft, and high in calories and carbohydrate content. Actually, although the bulimic person's weight fluctuates frequently, it usually stays within the normal range—through the use of diuretics, laxatives, vomiting, and exercise. So, unlike the anorexic, a bulimic person can usually keep her eating disorder hidden. A bulimic person is commonly perceived by others as a "perfect" student, mother, or career woman; an adolescent may be distinguished for participation in competitive activities, such as sports.

Overt clues to this disorder may include hyperactivity, peculiar eating habits or rituals, frequent weighing, and a distorted body image. Repetitive vomiting may cause dental caries, erosions of tooth enamel, and gingival infections.

Diagnosis

Eating disturbances may accompany various neurologic abnormalities, such as central nervous system tumors, or endocrine or metabolic diseases. However, the typical bulimic eating pattern is rarely confused with any physical disorder. Bulimic patients may develop electrolyte imbalance or dehydration and so may require laboratory tests to rule out hypokalemia and alkalosis.

Treatment

The bulimic patient knows her eating pattern is abnormal but can't control it. Therefore, treatment focuses on breaking the binge-purge cycle and helping the patient regain control over eating behavior. Treatment usually occurs in an outpatient setting. It includes

behavior modification therapy, possibly in highly structured psychoeducational group meetings. Individual psychotherapy and family therapy, which address the eating disorder as a symptom of unresolved conflict, may also be used. Antidepressant drugs, such as imipramine, may be helpful because bulimia is often associated with depression. The patient may also benefit from participation in self-help groups such as Overeaters Anonymous.

Nursing intervention

• Help the patient regain control over eating behavior by encouraging her to keep a daily record of everything she has eaten; to eat only at mealtimes and only at the table; and to reduce her access to food by limiting choice or quantity.

• Help the patient develop more adaptive coping skills by encouraging her to recognize and verbalize feelings; by reinforcing realistic perceptions about body weight and appearance; and by encouraging participation in the prescribed therapy program.

Suggest to the patient and her family the American Anorexia/Bulimia Association, Inc. and Anorexia Nervosa and Associated Disorders (ANAD) as sources of additional information and community support.

BARBARA GROSS BRAVERMAN, RN, MSN, CS

Drug abuse and dependence

The National Institute of Drug Abuse defines this condition as the use of a legal or illegal drug that causes physical, mental, emotional, or social harm. Drug abuse is a major health problem today and commonly involves the use of cocaine; however, many drugs are being abused by many groups. The age groups range from adolescents who ex-

PATHOLOGIC SUBSTANCE USE: ABUSE OR DEPENDENCE?

For most classes of substances, pathologic use of substances is divided into abuse and dependence, as defined below according to the *Diagnostic and Statistical Manual of Mental Disorders*, 3rd ed. (DSM-III).

ABUSE	DEPENDENCE
A pattern of pathologic use lasting for at least 1 month, as manifested by the inability to reduce or control intake despite: • a physical disorder that the user knows is made worse by using the substance • the need to use the substance daily for adequate function • episodes of intoxication complication (alcoholic blackouts, opioid overdose); and • impairment in social or occupational function due to substance use.	A severe form of substance use with physiologic dependence demonstrated by tolerance and withdrawal symptoms: • Tolerance means markedly increased amounts of the addicting substance are needed to achieve the desired effect; or regular use of the same dose produces a markedly diminished effect. • Withdrawal is a substance-specific syndrome provoked by stopping or reducing substance intake.

periment with hallucinogens and marijuana to adults who overuse tranquilizers and other prescription drugs. The most dangerous form of drug abuse is that in which users mix several drugs—sometimes with alcohol or other chemicals. Prognosis varies with the drug and the extent of abuse.

Causes

Persons predisposed to drug abuse tend to have an unusually low tolerance for frustration. They demand immediate relief of tension or distress, which they receive from taking the abused drug. Taking the drug gives them pleasure by relieving tension, abolishing loneliness, achieving a temporarily peaceful or euphoric state, or simply relieving boredom.

Drug dependence may follow the use of drugs for relief of physical pain. In young people, it often follows experimentation with drugs that commonly results from peer pressure. Medical professionals are at special risk for drug abuse because of easy access.

Signs and symptoms

Clinical effects vary according to the substance used, duration, and dosage.

(See *Signs and Symptoms of Drug Abuse.*)

Chronic abuse of drugs, especially by intravenous use, can lead to life-threatening complications that may include bacterial endocarditis, hepatitis, thrombophlebitis, pulmonary emboli, gangrene, respiratory infections, malnutrition and gastrointestinal disturbances, musculoskeletal dysfunction, trauma, and psychosis.

Diagnosis

Diagnosis depends largely on a history that shows a pattern of pathologic use of a substance, related impairment in social or occupational function, and duration of abnormal use and impairment for at least 1 month. A urine or blood screen can determine the amount of the substance present.

Treatment

Treatment of acute drug intoxication depends on the drug ingested. (See *Treatment of Drug Intoxication*, pages 119 and 120.) It includes fluid replacement therapy, and nutritional and vitamin supplements, if indicated; detoxification with the same drug or a pharmacologically similar drug (ex-

SIGNS AND SYMPTOMS OF DRUG ABUSE

DRUG	CLINICAL FEATURES	COMPLICATIONS
Opioids codeine, heroin, meperidine, morphine, opium (butorphanol and pentazocine, though not narcotics, have similar effects and addictive potential)	*Acute:* coma, hypotension, tachycardia, pinpoint pupils *Chronic* (after injection): needle marks, scars from skin abscesses, thrombophlebitis *Withdrawal:* sweating, nausea, vomiting, diarrhea, anxiety, insomnia, dilated pupils, runny nose, tearing eyes, yawning, goosebumps, persistent back and abdominal pain, anorexia, cold flashes; spontaneous orgasm (in women) or ejaculation (in men), fever, tachycardia, rising blood pressure and respiration rate. Symptoms subside within 7 to 10 days after the last dose.	Viral hepatitis (resulting in hepatic dysfunction), osteomyelitis, pulmonary edema, bacterial endocarditis, coma (resulting in organic brain damage or seizures), secondary infection Physical and psychological dependence
Amphetamines amphetamine, dextroamphetamine, methamphetamine	*After high doses:* anxiety, hyperactivity, irritability, insomnia, muscle tension, repeated compulsive movement, tooth grinding, aggressive or violent behavior, paranoia, psychotic symptoms resembling schizophrenia, fever, hypertension, dilated pupils, tachycardia, convulsions, cardiovascular collapse, malnutrition, and threatening visual, auditory, and tactile hallucinations *After injection:* needle marks, scars from skin abscesses, thrombophlebitis *Withdrawal:* depression, overwhelming fatigue. Long-term use yields a rapidly developing delusional syndrome resembling paranoid schizophrenia.	Little or no physical dependence, but tolerance and psychological dependence possible
Cocaine	*Acute intoxication* (after I.V. injection): tremors, seizures, convulsions, delirium, potentially fatal cardiovascular or respiratory failure *Chronic intoxication:* hallucinations, formication, dilated pupils, tachycardia, muscle twitching, violent behavior, tachycardia, elevated respiratory rate, perforation of the nasal septum *Withdrawal:* depression, irritability, disorientation, tremors, muscle weakness	Psychological dependence
Barbiturates amobarbital, pentobarbital, secobarbital (methaqualone is not a barbiturate, but symptoms and treatment are similar)	*Acute intoxication:* progressive central nervous system and respiratory depression *Chronic intoxication:* slurred speech, impaired coordination, decreased mental alertness and attention span, impaired social and occupational judgment, memory disturbances, depressed pulse rate and tendon reflexes, mood swings, nystagmus or strabismus, diplopia, dizziness, hypotension, dehydration, and aggressive, combative, or suicidal behavior *Withdrawal:* jitteriness, anxiety, irritability, grand mal seizures, status epilepticus, orthostatic hypotension, tachycardia, auditory and visual disturbances. Symptoms subside within 1 week.	Apnea, shock, coma, death Physical and psychological dependence

(continued)

SIGNS AND SYMPTOMS OF DRUG ABUSE *(continued)*

DRUG	CLINICAL FEATURES	COMPLICATIONS
Phencyclidine (PCP)	*Acute intoxication:* apnea, status epilepticus, coma, death "Bad trip": paralysis, numbness, frightening hallucinations (may mimic schizophrenia), anxiety, dissociative reaction, feeling of imminent death, paranoid or violent behavior, uncontrollable rage *Chronic intoxication:* confusion, fatigue, irritability, depression, hallucinations	Psychological dependence
Cannabis hashish, marijuana, tetrahydrocannabinol (THC)	*Acute transient reaction* (rare): panic and paranoid reactions (with first-time use); pseudo-psychotic reaction (with THC)	Psychological dependence
Hallucinogens LSD, mescaline, psilocybin	*Acute intoxication ("bad trip"):* anxiety, frightening hallucinations, depression (possible suicidal tendencies)	Psychological dependence
Tobacco	*Acute intoxication:* none known *Withdrawal:* craving for tobacco, irritability, anxiety, difficulty concentrating, restlessness, headache, drowsiness, gastrointestinal disturbance	Physical and psychological dependence

ceptions: cocaine, hallucinogens, and marijuana are not used for detoxification); sedatives to induce sleep; anticholinergics and antidiarrheal agents to relieve GI distress; antianxiety drugs for severe agitation, especially in cocaine abusers; and symptomatic treatment of medical complications.

Treatment of drug dependence commonly involves a triad of care: detoxification, long-term rehabilitation, and aftercare; the latter means a lifetime of abstinence, possibly aided by participation in Narcotics Anonymous or a similar self-help group.

Detoxification, the controlled and gradual withdrawal of an abused drug, is achieved through substitution of a drug with similar action. Such gradual replacement of the abused drug controls the effects of withdrawal, reducing the patient's discomfort and associated risks. Depending on the abused drug, detoxification is managed on an inpatient or an outpatient basis. For example, withdrawal from general de-

pressants can produce hazardous effects, such as grand mal seizures, status epilepticus, and hypotension; the severity of these effects determines whether the patient can be safely treated as an outpatient or requires hospitalization. Withdrawal from depressants usually doesn't require detoxification. Opioid withdrawal causes severe physical discomfort; to minimize it, chronic opioid abusers are frequently detoxified with methadone.

To ease withdrawal from opioids, general depressants, and other drugs, useful nonchemical measures may include psychotherapy, exercise, relaxation techniques, and nutritional support. Sedatives and tranquilizers may be administered temporarily to help the patient cope with insomnia, anxiety, and depression.

After withdrawal, rehabilitation is needed to prevent recurrence of drug abuse. Rehabilitation programs are available for inpatients and outpa-

Continued on page 121

TREATMENT OF DRUG INTOXICATION

DRUG	TREATMENT	NURSING INTERVENTION
Opioids	• The immediate goal is to prevent shock and maintain respirations by endotracheal intubation and mechanical ventilation and administration of oxygen, I.V. fluids, and plasma expanders. • Naloxone (Narcan) is administered until central nervous system depressant effects are reversed.	• Observe the patient continuously and closely; monitor for hypoxia since narcotics may impair respiratory drive. Auscultate the lungs frequently for rales, possibly indicating pulmonary edema in the patient receiving I.V. fluids and plasma expanders. • Before giving naloxone, apply secure restraints. Patient may be disoriented and agitated as he emerges from coma. • Monitor cardiac rate and rhythm, being alert for atrial fibrillation. • Be alert for signs of withdrawal.
Amphet-amines	• If the drug was taken orally, treatment may include induction of vomiting or gastric lavage; then activated charcoal and a sodium or magnesium sulfate cathartic. • Ammonium chloride or ascorbic acid may be added to the patient's I.V. to acidify his urine and lower its pH to 5 • Mannitol may be given to force diuresis. • A short-acting barbiturate, such as pentobarbital, may be given to control stimulant-induced seizure activity. • Haloperidol (Haldol) I.M. may be administered to treat agitation or assaultive behavior. • An alpha-adrenergic blocking agent, such as phentolamine (Regitine), may be given for hypertension.	• Restrain the patient to keep him from injuring himself and others, especially if he's paranoid or hallucinating. • Watch for cardiac dysrhythmias. Notify the doctor if these develop, and expect to give propranolol or lidocaine to treat tachydysrhythmias or ventricular dysrhythmias, respectively. • Treat hyperthermia with tepid sponge baths or a hypothermia blanket, as ordered. • Provide a quiet environment to avoid overstimulation. • Be alert for signs and symptoms of withdrawal. • Observe suicide precautions, especially if the patient shows signs of withdrawal. • Closely monitor neurologic status, since haloperidol and chlorpromazine lower seizure threshold.
Cocaine	• If cocaine was ingested, treatment may include induction of vomiting or gastric lavage; then activated charcoal followed by a saline cathartic. • Other drugs may include an antipyretic to reduce fever; an anticonvulsant, such as diazepam (Valium), to prevent seizures; and propranolol to treat tachycardia.	• Monitor respirations and blood pressure closely. • Monitor cardiac rate and rhythm—ventricular fibrillation and cardiac standstill can occur as a direct cardiotoxic result of cocaine. Defibrillate and initiate CPR, if indicated. • Calm the patient by talking to him in a quiet room. • Observe for seizures, take seizure precautions, and administer ordered medication.

(continued)

TREATMENT OF DRUG INTOXICATION *(continued)*

DRUG	TREATMENT	NURSING INTERVENTION
Barbiturates	• Initial treatment aims to restore CNS and respiratory function and prevent shock. Treatment usually includes inducing vomiting or gastric lavage, if the patient ingested the drug within the past 4 hours; endotracheal intubation; I.V. fluids to correct hypotension and dehydration; vasopressors for phenobarbital overdose; and I.V. sodium bicarbonate to promote diuresis and counteract intoxication. • Gastric lavage or administration of activated charcoal followed by a cathartic is usually recommended to eliminate the toxic drug. Extreme intoxication may require dialysis. • During detoxification, a pentobarbital-challenge test determines the patient's tolerance level. An appropriate pentobarbital dose lessens withdrawal symptoms until the dosage can be gradually reduced and finally totally withdrawn.	• Perform frequent neurologic assessments, and check pulse rate, temperature, skin color, and reflexes often. • Notify the doctor if you observe signs of respiratory distress or pulmonary edema. • Watch for and report signs of withdrawal. • Protect the patient from injuring himself, and provide symptomatic relief of withdrawal symptoms, as ordered.
Phencyclidine (PCP)	• If the drug was taken orally, vomiting is induced or gastric lavage performed; activated charcoal is repeatedly instilled and removed. • Acidic diuresis is performed by acidifying the patient's urine with ascorbic acid to increase excretion of the drug. This is continued for 2 weeks, because symptoms may recur when fat cells release their stores of PCP. • Diazepam and haloperidol may be given to control agitation or psychotic behavior. • Diazepam may be given to control seizures. • Propranolol (Inderal) may be given for hypertension and tachycardia; nitroprusside, for severe hypertension. • If the patient develops renal failure, hemodialysis is performed.	• Provide a quiet, safe, dimly lit environment. • Be aware that overt attempts to reassure an aggressive patient often provoke aggressive behavior. • Closely monitor the patient's intake and output; maintain adequate hydration to promote PCP excretion; report diminished urinary output or abnormal renal function tests. • Take suicide precautions as needed.
Hallucinogens	• If the drug was taken orally, vomiting is induced or gastric lavage performed; activated charcoal and a cathartic are given. • Diazepam may be given to control seizures.	• Reorient the patient repeatedly to time, place, and person. • Restrain the patient, as ordered, to protect him from injuring himself and others. • Calm the patient by maintaining a quiet environment and talking in a soothing voice.

tients; they usually last a month or longer and may include individual, group, and family psychotherapy. During and after rehabilitation, participation in a drug-oriented self-help group may be helpful. The largest such group is Narcotics Anonymous. Three new groups were formed recently: Potsmokers Anonymous, Pills Anonymous, and Cocaine Anonymous.

Naltrexone (Trexan), a newly released drug, is used to help outpatients maintain abstinence. By blocking the opiate euphoria, it helps prevent readdiction. It is said to be more useful in middle-class patients.

Nursing intervention

Nursing care for drug abusers must focus not only on restoring physical health but also on educating the patient and family about drug abuse and dependence, providing support, and encouraging participation in drug treatment programs and self-help groups. Specific nursing interventions vary, depending on the drug abused, but commonly include the following:

• Observe the patient for signs and symptoms of withdrawal.

• During the patient's withdrawal from any drug, maintain a quiet, safe environment. Remove harmful objects from the room and use restraints judiciously. Use side rails for the comatose patient. Reassure the anxious patient that medication will control most symptoms of withdrawal.

• Closely monitor visitors who might bring the patient drugs from the outside.

• Develop self-awareness and an understanding, positive attitude toward the patient; control your reactions to his undesirable behaviors—dependency, manipulation, anger, easy frustration, and alienation.

• Set limits for dealing with demanding, manipulative behavior.

• Maintain and promote adequate nutrition.

• Administer medications carefully to prevent hoarding by the patient.

• Refer the patient for detoxification and rehabilitation, as appropriate.

• Encourage family members to seek help whether or not the abuser seeks it. You can suggest private therapy or community mental health clinics.

SANDRA SCHULER, RN, MSN

Infantile autism

Infantile autism (a pervasive developmental disorder, according to *DSM-III*) is a severe disorder marked by unresponsiveness to human contact, gross deficits in language development, and bizarre responses to various aspects of the environment. It becomes apparent before the child reaches age 30 months.

Severe autism is rare, affecting 2 to 4 children per 10,000 births. It affects three to four times more males than females, most commonly the firstborn male. Prognosis is poor.

Causes and incidence

The causes of infantile autism remain unclear but are thought to include psychological, physiologic, and sociologic factors. The autistic child's parents are commonly intelligent, educated people of high socioeconomic status whose behavior toward their autistic child may appear distant and lack affection. However, because autistic children are clearly different from birth, and are unresponsive or respond with rigid, screaming resistance to touch and attention, parental remoteness may be merely a frustrated, helpless reaction to this disorder, not its cause. However, some theorists consider autism related to early understimulation that causes the child to seek contact with the world through self-stimulating behaviors; or to overwhelming overstimulation that leads to regression, muteness, and unresponsiveness to external stimuli. Some autistic children show abnormal but nonspecific EEG findings that sug-

SYMBIOTIC PSYCHOSIS

This *pervasive developmental disorder*, similar to autism in its causes and treatment, has a later onset and becomes manifest at ages 30 months to 12 years.

Signs and symptoms
This condition is marked by abnormal development of ego, language and communication, and relationships with others. The child with this psychosis doesn't see himself as a separate person. His ego is fused with that of a significant other, usually his mother. He can express himself verbally but doesn't need language to convey his ideas to her. (They seem to know each other's thoughts.) He functions at an immature level unless his mother is present; then, the two function as one (when she is cold, both put on a sweater).

Nursing intervention
• Treatment is characteristically difficult and prolonged. Plan your interventions to support the child and mother in developing separate interests, ideas, and goals.
• Help each to develop a separate identity. Encourage separate activities. Point out individual successes.
• Practice reality therapy with both. Point out separate body parts. ("This is your hand. This is your mother's hand." Or, "I'm going to bandage your foot. This is your foot. Your mother's foot has no cut.")

gest brain dysfunction, possibly resulting from trauma, disease, or structural abnormality.

Signs and symptoms

A primary characteristic of infantile autism is unresponsiveness to people. Parents report that these children beome rigid or flaccid when held, cry when touched, and show little or no interest in human contact. The child's smiling response is delayed or absent; he does not lift his arms in anticipation of being picked up and doesn't "mold" himself to the adult's body when held. The result is mutual withdrawal by the parents and the child.

The autistic child treats everyone with equal indifference, showing no sign of recognition or affection to parents or caretakers. In later infancy, the child doesn't show the anxiety about strangers that's typical in the 8-month-old. Such a child doesn't learn the usual socialization games (peek-a-boo, pat-a-cake, or bye-bye). He's likely to relate to others only to fill a physical need and then without eye contact or speech (for example, by dragging the adult to the sink when he's thirsty). An autistic child is typically said to "look right through" people.

Severe language impairment is also characteristic. The child may be mute or may use immature speech patterns. For example, he may use a single word to express a series of activities; he may say "ground" when referring to any step in the use of a playground slide. His speech commonly shows echolalia (meaningless repetition of words or phrases) and pronoun reversal ("you go walk" when he means "I want to go for a walk.") When answering a question, he may simply repeat the question to mean yes and will remain silent if he means no.

The autistic child also shows characteristically bizarre behavior patterns, such as screaming fits, rituals, rhythmic rocking, arm flapping, or crying without tears, and disturbed sleeping and eating patterns. His behavior may also be self-destructive, with hand biting, eye gouging, hair pulling, or head banging. His bizarre responses to his environment include an extreme compulsion for sameness—the slightest change in arrangement of furniture can cause the child to return it immediately to its original place or, if he's unsuccessful, to fall into a panic state, marked by head banging, screaming, or biting himself.

In response to sensory stimuli, the autistic child may overreact or underreact; he may totally ignore objects—dropping objects he's given to hold or not looking at them at all—or become excessively absorbed in them—endlessly watching the motion of objects that spin or the movement of his own fingers. Commonly, he will respond to stimuli by head banging, rocking, whirling around, and hand flapping. He appears to rely more on smell, taste, and touch, which don't require him to reach out to the environment, and tends to avoid using sight and hearing to respond to or interact with the environment.

Diagnosis

The Denver Developmental Screening Test shows the autistic child to have delayed development, especially of social and language skills. IQ testing shows retardation in 70% of autistic children, but low IQ scores may simply reflect inability to cooperate during the test. In autistic children who do cooperate, IQ tests often show average or superior intelligence.

Treatment

Treatment of autism is difficult and prolonged. It must begin early, continue for years (through adolescence), and involve the child, parents, teachers, and therapists in coordinated efforts to encourage social adjustment and speech development and to reduce self-destructive behavior. Positive reinforcement, using food and other rewards, can promote language and social skills. Providing pleasurable sensory and motor stimulation (jogging, playing with a ball) encourages appropriate behavior and helps eliminate inappropriate behavior. In children with a biochemical disorder (excessive dopamine blood levels), haloperidol often mitigates withdrawn and stereotypical behavior patterns, making the child more amenable to behavior modification therapies.

Treatment may take place in a psychiatric institution, in a specialized school, or in a day-care program, but the current trend is to train parents to use behavioral techniques at home. Helping family members to develop strong one-to-one relationships with the autistic child often initiates responsive, imitative behavior. Family members often feel inadequacy and guilt, and may need family counseling.

Nursing intervention

• Encourage development of self-esteem. Show the child that he's acceptable as a person. For example, if he sits on the floor, sit on the floor with him.

• Reduce self-destructive behaviors. Physically stop the child from harming himself, while firmly saying "no." When he responds to your voice, give a primary reward (food); later, substitute a secondary reward (verbal, "good;" or physical, a hug or pat on the back).

• Encourage appropriate use of language. Give positive reinforcement when the child indicates his needs correctly. Give verbal reinforcement at first ("good, O.K., great"). Later, give physical reinforcement (a hug or pat on his hand or shoulder).

• Encourage self-care. For example, place a brush in his hand and guide his hand to brush his hair. Similarly, teach him to wash his hands and face.

• Encourage acceptance of minor environmental changes. Prepare the child for the change by telling him about it. Make the change minor: change the color of his bedspread or the placement of food on his plate. When he's accepted minor changes, move on to bigger ones.

• Support and assist parents. Refer the family to the National Society for Autistic Children for further assistance.

BARBARA WALSH CLARK, RN, MSN

Depression

Major depression, a recurring syndrome of persistent sad, dysphoric mood with accompanying symptoms, may be a primary disorder, a response to systemic disease, or a drug reaction. Major depression occurs in about 1 of 10 Americans, affecting all races and ethnic and socioeconomic groups. It affects both sexes but is more common in women. About 50% of depressed persons recover completely; the others experience recurrences. Depression is difficult to treat, especially in children, adolescents, elderly persons, or those with a history of chronic disease, but improved effectiveness of treatment is offering new hope.

Causes

The multiple causes of depression are controversial and not completely understood. Research suggests possible genetic, familial, biochemical, physical, psychological, and social causes. Psychological causes, the focus of many nursing interventions, may include feelings of helplessness and vulnerability, anger, pessimism, and low self-esteem; they may be related to abnor-

mal character and behavior patterns and troubled relationships. In many patients, the history identifies a specific loss or severe stress that probably interacts with an individual's predisposition to provoke major depression.

Signs and symptoms

According to the *DSM-III* classification, the primary feature of major depression is a relatively persistent and prominent dysphoric mood with loss of interest in usual activities and pastimes. The sad, hopeless, or apathetic mood may shift periodically to anger or anxiety. The second diagnostic requirement is the daily presence of at least four of the following symptoms for at least 2 weeks:
- appetite disturbance (weight loss of at least 1 lb/week without dieting, or significant appetite or weight increase)
- sleep disturbance (insomnia or hypersomnia)
- energy loss, fatigue
- psychomotor agitation or retardation (hyperactive or slowed behavior)
- loss of interest or pleasure in activities, decreased sex drive
- feelings of worthlessness, self-reproach, excessive guilt
- difficulty with concentration, decision making, or ability to think
- recurrent suicidal thoughts, suicide attempts, or death wishes.

Acute depression involves recent onset of four or five of these behaviors and dysphoric mood. Chronic depression involves the same symptoms in milder form, present for 2 or more months.

Diagnosis

Diagnosis of major depression rests primarily on observations and history of persistent or recurrent dysphoric mood, with a review of social, personal, family, and neuropsychiatric history for sources of grief and stress, drug toxicity, or medical problems.

Beck's Depression Scale and other psychological tests, as well as the dexamethasone suppression test and EEG evidence of sleep disturbance, may be

---

SUICIDE PREVENTION GUIDELINES

- **Assess for clues to suicide.** These include suicidal thoughts, threats, or messages; hoarding medication; talking about death; expressions of futility; giving away prized possessions; and changing behavior, especially as depression lifts.
- **Provide a safe environment.** Check patient areas and correct dangerous conditions: exposed pipes, windows without safety glass, and access to the roof or open balconies.
- **Remove dangerous objects.** Belts, razors, suspenders, light cords, glass, knives, nail files, and clippers.
- **Consult with staff.** Recognize and document both verbal and nonverbal suicidal behaviors; keep doctor informed; share data with all staff; clarify patient's specific restrictions; assess risk and plan for observation; clarify day and night staff responsibilities and frequency of consultation.
- **Observe suicidal patients.** Be alert when patients are using sharp objects (as in shaving); taking medication; or using the bathroom (to prevent hanging or other injury). Assign patient to a room near the nurses' station and with another patient. Observe acutely suicidal patients continuously.
- **Maintain personal contact with patient.** Suicidal patients feel alone and without resources or hope. Encourage continuity of care and consistency of primary nurses. Building emotional ties to others is the ultimate technique for preventing suicide.

OTHER AFFECTIVE DISORDERS

Dysthymic disorder (depressive neurosis)
This common affliction is marked by feelings of depression that have persisted at least 2 years in adults (and at least 1 year in children and adolescents). It causes persistent depression symptoms that are not sufficiently severe or prolonged to meet the criteria for major depression.

These symptoms may be relatively continuous or separated by intervening periods of normal mood that last a few days to a few weeks but not longer than a few months. At least three of the following symptoms are present:
• insomnia or hypersomnia
• low energy level or chronic tiredness
• feelings of inadequacy, loss of self-esteem, or self-deprecation
• decreased effectiveness or productivity at home, work, or school
• decreased attention, concentration, or ability to think clearly
• social withdrawal
• loss of interest in or enjoyment of pleasurable activities
• irritability or excessive anger (in children, hostility to parents or caretakers)
• inability to respond with apparent pleasure to praise or rewards

• less active or talkative than usual, or feelings of sluggishness or restlessness
• pessimistic attitude toward the future, brooding about past events
• tearfulness or crying, self-pity
• recurrent thoughts of death or suicide.

Cyclothymic disorder
This disorder describes patients who have moderate or transient symptoms of bipolar disorder, major depression, or mania. These patients have normal moods for months at a time. The essential feature of cyclothymic disorder is a chronic mood disturbance of at least 2 years' duration, involving numerous periods of depression and hypomania that aren't sufficiently severe or prolonged to meet the criteria for a major depressive or manic episode.

Cyclothymic disorder commonly precedes a bipolar disorder. Psychotic features, such as delusions and hallucinations, are absent.

Atypical affective disorder
This disorder produces manic symptoms that are less severe and less prolonged than those required for a diagnosis of bipolar or cyclothymic disorders.

used to support this diagnosis. Careful nursing assessment of the patient's mood and behavior also supports this diagnosis. Obtain an accurate account of the onset, severity, duration, and progression of all feelings, symptoms, and changes in daily activities. Pay special attention to recent changes in diet, appetite or sleep patterns; sexual activity; constipation; and use of alcohol. Ask about recent losses and unusual stress.

Treatment
The primary treatments—psychotherapy, drug and somatic therapy (including electroconvulsive therapy [ECT])—and adjuvant therapies aim to relieve the depressive symptoms. Research confirms the effectiveness of antidepressant drug therapy, which, when combined with psychotherapy, is more effective than either method alone. Drug therapy usually includes

tricyclic antidepressants (TCAs) and monoamine oxidase (MAO) inhibitors. TCAs produce fewer side effects and so are usually the preferred drugs. Treatment may also include sedatives if the patient suffers insomnia, but this requires careful monitoring to prevent hoarding of doses.

In severely depressed or suicidal patients who do not respond to other treatments, ECT may improve mood dramatically. However, ECT should be prescribed only after a complete evaluation—history, physical examination, chest X-ray, and EKG. ECT may cause such side effects as dysrhythmias, fractures, confusion, drowsiness, temporary memory loss, respiratory depression and, occasionally, permanent memory loss or learning difficulties. Consequently, before ECT, safety, long-term risk, and patients' rights should be discussed thoroughly with the patient and his family.

Nursing intervention

The depressed patient needs a therapeutic relationship with encouragement to talk and boost self-esteem.

• Encourage the patient to express his feelings. Show him he's important by setting aside time each day to listen attentively and respectfully, allowing time for sluggish responses.

• Provide a structured routine, including noncompetitive activities, to build confidence and encourage social interaction. Help him avoid isolation by involving him in group activities.

• Reassure him that he can help ease his depression by expressing his feelings, participating in activities, and improving grooming and hygiene.

• Ask the patient if he thinks of death or suicide. Such thoughts signal an immediate need for consultation and assessment (see *Suicide Prevention Guidelines*, page 124). Failure to detect suicidal thoughts early may encourage a patient to attempt suicide.

• Record all observations of and conversations with the patient; they are valuable for evaluating his response to treatment.

• While caring for the patient's psychological needs, don't forget his physical needs. If he's too depressed to take care of himself, help him with personal hygiene. Encourage him to eat, or feed him if necessary. If he's constipated, add high-fiber foods to his diet, offer small portions, and encourage physical activity and fluid intake. Offer warm milk or back rubs at bedtime to improve sleep.

• If drug treatment fails, the doctor may order ECT. A course of ECT usually includes two to three treatments per week for 3 to 4 weeks. Before each ECT, give the patient a sedative, and insert a nasal or oral airway. Monitor vital signs. Afterward, the patient may be drowsy and have transient amnesia, but he should be alert, with a good memory, within 30 minutes (or, at the latest, 6 to 8 hours).

SHARON MCBRIDE VALENTE, RN, MN, CS, FAAN

Obsessive-compulsive disorder

Obsessive thoughts and compulsive behaviors represent recurring efforts to control overwhelming anxiety, guilt, or unacceptable impulses that persistently enter the consciousness. Accordingly, *DSM-III* classifies obsessive-compulsive disorder as an anxiety disorder.

The word obsessive or obsession refers to a recurrent idea, thought, or image. Compulsive or compulsion, the action component, refers to a ritualistic, repetitive, and involuntary defensive behavior. This disorder is relatively rare in the general population (0.05%); it occurs in both sexes, with typical onset in adolescence or young adulthood. Recent studies indicate a greater incidence in upper-class persons with higher-than-average intelligence.

Obsessions and compulsions cause significant distress and may severely impair occupational and social functions. Generally, an obsessive-compulsive disorder is chronic, often with remissions and flare-ups. The prognosis is better than average when symptoms are quickly identified, diagnosed, and treated, and when the resulting environmental stress is recognized and adjusted.

Causes

The cause of obsessive-compulsive disorder is unknown. Some studies suggest the possibility of brain lesions, but the most useful research and clinical studies lead to an explanation based on psychological theories. These studies list four major theories of causation; of these, the psychoanalytic theory is accepted by most psychiatrists. (See *Causes of Obsessive-Compulsive Disorder.*) In addition, major depression, organic brain syndrome, and schizophrenia may contribute to the onset of obsessive-compulsive disorder.

CAUSES OF OBSESSIVE-COMPULSIVE DISORDER

PSYCHOANA-LYTIC THEORY	LEARNING THEORY	INTERPERSONAL THEORY	EXISTENTIALIST THEORY
Psychodynamic factors (ego defenses): • Isolation • Undoing • Reaction-formation	• Obsession—conditioned stimulus to anxiety • Compulsion—reduces anxiety, reinforces behavior	• Irrational coping strategies (inflexible) to handle intense anxiety or guilt • Unrealistic (rigid) view of self (self-hate, self-contempt—"bad me")	• Inability to live with uncertainty or ambiguity • Wish to flee situation of great anxiety • Threat of nonexistence
Psychogenic factors: • Preoccupation with aggression • Preoccupation with dirt • Disturbed growth/development pattern related to anal/sadistic phase	• Approach avoidance—reduces conflict • Emphasis on cognitive change to alter behavior	• Avoidance of anxiety-laden relationships (withdrawal) • Defenses (sublimation, selective inattention, substitution, dissociation) • Inferiority feelings (to gain control of others) • Threat to autonomy and loss of individuality	• Religious rituals • Excessively high morals
Regression: • Fixation at earlier level of development (anal stage) • Ambivalence • Magical thinking		• Family patterns and coping styles that reinforce obsessions • Inability to enjoy life	

Signs and symptoms

This disorder may be manifested physically or behaviorally as ideas or impulses, and may refer either to actions completed or to future anticipated events. These ideas or actions may be simple, mild, and uncomplicated or dramatic, elaborately complex, and ritualized. Their meanings may be obvious or may reflect inner psychological distortions that are unraveled only through intensive psychotherapy.

Obsessive symptoms are those in which thoughts, words, or mental images persistently and involuntarily invade the conscious awareness. Some common obsessions include thoughts of violence, thoughts of contamination, and repetitive doubts and worry about a traumatic event.

The dominant feature in compulsions is an irrational and recurring impulse to repeat a certain behavior as an expression of anxiety. Common compulsions include repetitive touching, doing and undoing (opening and closing doors, rearranging things), washing (especially hands), and checking (to be sure no tragedy has occurred).

Often, the patient's anxiety is so strong that he will avoid the situation or the object that evokes the impulse. For example, John had the recurring urge to push people down long flights of stairs, so he avoided climbing stairs in any building and lived in a one-story house, thus modifying his behavior so he wouldn't be tempted to act on this compulsion.

When the obsessive-compulsive phenomena are mental, no one knows that anything unusual is occurring unless the patient talks about these private ex-

---

BEHAVIORAL THERAPIES

Aversion therapy—application of a painful stimulus to create an aversion to the stimulus that leads to undesirable behavior.

Thought stopping—a technique to break the habit of fear-inducing anticipatory thoughts. Patient is taught to stop unwanted thoughts by saying the word "stop," and then to focus attention on achieving calmness and muscle relaxation.

Thought switching—a technique to replace fear-inducing self-instructions with competent self-instructions. Patient is taught to place negative thoughts with positive ones until the positive ones become strong enough to replace the anxiety-provoking ones.

Flooding—frequent full-intensity exposure—through use of imagery—to an object that triggers a symptom. Used with caution because it produces extreme discomfort.

Implosion therapy—a form of desensitization through repeated exposure to a highly feared object.

Response prevention—prevention of compulsive behavior by distraction, persuasion, or redirection of activity.

---

periences. Because of shame, anxiety, or embarrassment, the patient usually tries to limit compulsive actions to his own private time.

Obsessive-compulsive states seem to develop in certain personality types and under certain conditions. The obsessional personality is usually rigid and conscientious, and has great aspirations; he has a formal, reserved manner, with precise and careful movements and posture; he takes responsibility seriously and finds decision-making difficult. He lacks creativity and the ability to find alternate solutions to his problems. Such a person has a tendency to be painfully accurate and complete—carefully qualifying his statements to avoid making a mistake and anticipating every move and gesture of the person to whom he speaks. His affect is flat and unemotional, except for controlled anxiety.

Self-awareness is totally intellectual, without accompanying emotion or feeling.

Diagnosis

This diagnosis rests on evidence of compulsively repetitive patterns of thought or behavior. A careful history may identify previous obsessive-compulsive personality traits. Often, the patient's own description of his behavior offers the best clues to this diagnosis. However, the patient also needs evaluation for other physical or psychiatric disorders. One telling difference between obsessive-compulsive states and schizophrenia, which may produce similar behavior patterns, is that schizophrenics have less visible anxiety.

Treatment

Treatment of obsessive-compulsive states aims to reduce anxiety, resolve inner conflicts, relieve depression, and teach more effective ways of dealing with stress. Such treatment (especially during an acute episode) may include tranquilizers and antidepressants. But intensive long-term psychotherapy, brief supportive psychotherapy, or group therapy is the preferred treatment.

Behavioral therapies—aversion therapy, thought stopping, thought switching, flooding, implosion therapy, and response prevention—have also been effective in some cases.

Nursing intervention

Nursing care should focus on reducing the associated anxiety, fears, and guilt; building the patient's self-esteem; and helping him understand why he needs the compulsive behavior.

● Approach the patient unhurriedly.

● Provide an accepting atmosphere; don't show shock, amusement, or criticism of the ritualistic behavior.

● Allow the patient time to carry out the ritualistic behavior (unless it's dangerous) until he can be distracted into some other activity. Blocking this behavior raises anxiety to an intolerable level.

• Encourage the patient to express his feelings about the anxiety that causes the compulsive behavior, especially when he seems fearful.

• Explore patterns leading to the behavior or recurring problems.

• Listen attentively, offering feedback.

• Encourage the use of appropriate defense mechanisms to relieve loneliness and isolation.

• Engage the patient in activities that raise his self-esteem and confidence.

• Encourage active diversionary resources, such as whistling or humming a tune, to divert attention from the unwanted thoughts and to promote a pleasurable experience.

• Assist the patient with new ways to solve problems and to develop more effective coping skills by setting limits on unacceptable behavior (for example, by limiting the number of times per day he may indulge in compulsive behavior). Gradually shorten the time allowed. Help him attend to other feelings or problems for the remainder of the time.

• Help the patient identify progress and set realistic expectations of himself and others.

• Explain how to channel emotional energy to relieve stress (sports, creative endeavors, etc.)

• Identify insight and improved behavior (reduced compulsive behavior and/ or fewer obsessive thoughts). Evaluate behavioral changes by your own and the patient's self-reports.

• Identify disturbing topics of conversation that reflect underlying anxiety or terror.

• Observe when interventions do not work; reevaluate and recommend alternative strategies.

• Find ways to deal with the anger and frustration the patient often arouses.

• Keep the patient's physical health in mind. For example, compulsive hand-washing may cause skin breakdown, and rituals or preoccupations may cause inadequate intake of food and fluids and exhaustion.

• Make reasonable demands and set reasonable limits; make their purpose clear. Avoid creating situations that increase frustration and provoke anger, which may interfere with treatment.

MARY LOU L. HAMILTON, RN, MS

Personality disorders

Personality disorders are individual traits that reflect chronic, inflexible, and maladaptive patterns of behavior that cause discomfort and impair social and occupational function. Personality disorders are widespread, though no actual statistics exist. Persons with these disorders don't usually receive treatment; when they do, they're managed on an outpatient basis.

Prognosis is variable. Personality disorders are self-limiting in that most appear at adolescence and wane during middle age.

Causes

Only recently have personality disorders been categorized in detail, and research continues to identify their causes. Biologic theories hold that these disorders may stem from chromosomal and neuronal abnormalities. Social theories hold that they reflect learned responses, having much to do with reinforcement, modeling, and aversive stimuli as contributing factors. Psychodynamic theories hold that they reflect deficiencies in ego and superego development and are related to poor mother-child relationships fraught with unresponsiveness, inappropriate responsiveness, or early separation.

Signs and symptoms

Signs and symptoms of personality disorders are varied and differ depending on the diagnosis. (See *Characteristics of Personality Disorders*, page 130.) They differ among individuals and within the same individual at different

CHARACTERISTICS OF PERSONALITY DISORDERS

PARANOID	SCHIZOID AND SCHIZOTYPAL
• Suspicion; concern with hidden motives • Inability to relax; hypervigilance • Social isolation, inability to collaborate • Poor self-image • Coldness and detachment • Need to feel in control • Hostility; fault-finding with resultant anger • Argumentativeness, overt antagonism • Hypersensitivity, jealousy • Poor sense of humor	• Flat or depressed affect • Coldness, detachment, aloofness • Hypersensitivity or indifference • Social withdrawal • Poor self-image, depersonalization • Odd, elaborative speech • Magical thinking, ideas of reference, illusions • Suspicion • Inability to relax

HISTRIONIC	NARCISSISTIC
• Dramatic, emotional, or erratic behavior • Craving for stimulation and attention • Intolerance of being alone • Manipulative, divisive behavior • Inability to put others' needs first • Multiple physical complaints • Tantrums and angry outbursts • Superficial attachments	• Craving for stimulation and attention • Intolerance of being alone • Manipulative and exploitative behavior • No capacity for empathy • Self-centeredness; exaggeration of achievements and talents • Grandiosity; preoccupation with fantasies of unlimited success, power, or beauty

ANTISOCIAL	BORDERLINE
• Superficial charm, wit, and intelligence; manipulative, often seductive, behavior • Inability or refusal to accept responsibility for self-serving, destructive behavior • Failure at school and work; delinquency, rules violations, inability to keep a job • Promiscuity, desertion, two or more divorces or separations • Repeated substance abuse • Thefts, vandalism, multiple arrests • Inability to function as a responsible parent • Fights, assaults, abuse of others • Impulsiveness, recklessness, Inability to plan ahead	• Impulsive and unpredictable behavior in self-damaging areas: spending, sex, gambling, substance abuse, overeating • Unstable and intense interpersonal relationships: rapid attitude shifts, idealization, devaluation, or manipulation • Inappropriate, intense anger • Identity disturbance with uncertain self-image and imitative behavior • Unstable affect with rapid mood swings • Intolerance of being alone, chronic feelings of emptiness or boredom • Self-destructive behavior: suicidal gestures, self-mutilation, frequent accidents and fights

AVOIDANT	DEPENDENT
• Social withdrawal; mistrustful but desirous of close relationships • Hypersensitivity to rejection • Low self-esteem • Dependency in relationships	• Passivity and self-consciousness • Overly compliant, clinging behavior; avoiding independence, leaving major decisions to others, subordinating own needs to those of others

COMPULSIVE	PASSIVE-AGGRESSIVE
• Perfectionism • Confident attitude with others • Coldness, inability to express affection • Need for control; rigidity • Procrastination, indecisiveness	• Intentional inefficiency (social and occupational), chronic lateness, procrastination • Complaining and blaming behavior; feelings of confusion and mistreatment • Fear of authority

times. Generally, these disorders produce difficulties in interpersonal relationships and occupational function.

Diagnosis
Central and essential to diagnosis is a history that shows maladaptive personality traits as characteristic of lifelong behavior, and not just as part of an illness. (During illness, temporary regression causes negative personality traits to become exaggerated.) Symptoms of personality disorder impair social or occupational functioning or cause internal distress. Psychological evaluation must rule out similar personality or psychiatric disorders.

Treatment
Treatment depends on the patient's symptoms but requires a trusting relationship in which the therapist can use a directive approach. Drug therapy is generally ineffective but may be used to relieve severe distress, such as acute anxiety or depression. Family and group therapy are effective. Hospital inpatient milieu therapy can sometimes be effective in crisis situations and possibly for long-term treatment of borderline personality disorders. However, in-patient treatment is controversial.

Nursing intervention
First, know your own feelings and reactions as the basis for assessing the patient's overt responses. Keep in mind that many of these patients don't respond well to interviewing; others are charming masters of deceit. Offer patient, persistent, consistent, and flexible care. Follow a direct, involved approach to engage the patient's trust.

Nursing goals are teaching social skills; reinforcing appropriate behavior; setting limits on inappropriate behavior; encouraging expression of feelings; self-analysis of behavior and accountability for actions; and finally, helping the patient seek appropriate employment.

SANDRA SCHULER, RN, MSN

Phobias
(Phobic disorder, phobic neurosis)

Classified as a form of anxiety disorder, a phobia is a persistent, irrational fear of places or things that compels the patient to avoid them. Although he knows that his fear is out of proportion to any actual danger, the patient can't control it or explain it away. Many people harbor irrational fears, such as the fear of harmless insects, which make no major impact on their lives. In contrast, the phobic patient's irrational fear causes severe distress and impairment of function.

IDENTIFYING PHOBIC DISORDERS

Phobic disorders can take three forms and can even coexist in some patients. To help identify phobias, review the following information.

Agoraphobia affects 60% of all phobic patients who seek help. This severe phobia commonly affects women and tends to be chronic, with occasional remissions and flare-ups. Patients with agoraphobia fear being alone and losing control in public places where escape is difficult or where help isn't available. Typically, they fear *situations,* such as being in crowds, tunnels, or elevators. These fears can dominate their lives, restricting their normal activities and even confining them to their homes.

Social phobias are similar to agoraphobia. The central fear is one of self-embarrassment, which compels the patient to avoid the scrutiny of others. But most of these fears involve specific *functions,* such as using public lavatories or speaking in public. Characteristically, social phobias affect adolescents.

Simple phobias are the most common, easiest to identify, and most thematic. The patient fears certain objects or situations, such as animals, lightning, or high places. Usually, these fears begin in childhood and follow a chronic course with no remissions. They almost always stem from an actual or anticipated confrontation with the feared object or situation.

MECHANISMS OF ANXIETY DISORDERS

In generalized anxiety disorder or panic disorder, anxiety is the primary feature.

In phobic disorder, anxiety results when the individual *confronts* a threatening situation.

In obsessive-compulsive disorder, anxiety results when the individual *resists* threatening thoughts and feelings.

In posttraumatic stress disorder, the individual *reexperiences* anxiety related to an exceptionally traumatic event.

Three types of phobia exist: agoraphobia, social phobia, and simple phobia. (See *Identifying Phobic Disorders*, page 131.) Of the milder forms of mental illness, phobias are among the most persistent.

Causes and incidence

A phobia develops when anxiety about an object or situation compels the patient to avoid it. Phobic disorders may result from drug withdrawal, drug abuse, and anxiety-related behaviors, such as the inability to cope with anger and dependence.

Phobic disorders affect less than 1% of the population and account for less than 5% of all neurotic disorders in patients over age 18. These patients usually have no family history of psychiatric illness or of the same phobia. Because phobias tend to be chronic and resistant to treatment, the prognosis is only fair.

Signs and symptoms

Phobias produce severe anxiety—often panic—and discomfort that's out of proportion to the threat of the feared object or situation. Physically, the patient suffers profuse sweating, poor motor control, tachycardia, and elevated blood pressure.

In a *simple phobia*, the patient anticipates his anxiety and so avoids facing the perceived danger. If he suddenly confronts the object or situation, he may suffer a panic attack. (See *Recognizing a Panic Attack*, page 109.)

With a *social phobia*, the patient feels shameful, inept, or stupid in social interaction and expects others to criticize or laugh at him. His anxiety isn't focused.

In *agoraphobia*, anxiety causes a patient to restrict his movements to an increasingly smaller area, eventually leading to the inability to leave home without suffering a panic attack. To avoid leaving the familiar setting of his home, his behavior may become pleading, demanding, manipulative, or even infantile. A feeling of helplessness predominates, and obsessional behavior often occurs.

When a patient avoids the object of his phobia, he may feel loss of self-esteem and feelings of weakness, cowardice, or ineffectiveness. If he doesn't master the phobia, he may develop mild depression.

Diagnosis

Most often, diagnosis is based on careful history taking, observation, and a description of his behavior by the patient, his family, and friends. Interviews and a mental status examination help to confirm the diagnosis.

Treatment

The effectiveness of treatment depends on the severity of the patient's phobia. Because phobic behavior may never be completely cured, the goal of treatment is to help the patient function effectively in society. Although antianxiety drugs may help control the phobia, they must be prescribed with caution to prevent addiction. Antidepressants may help patients with agoraphobia, but they can't cure it completely.

Systematic desensitization, a behavior therapy, may be more effective than drugs, especially if it includes encouragement, instruction, and suggestion.

Such therapy should help the patient understand that his phobia is symbolic of a more fundamental anxiety and that he must tackle it directly.

In some cities, phobia clinics and group therapy are available. People who have recovered from phobias can often help other phobic patients.

Nursing intervention

• Stay with the patient until he feels comfortable alone.

• Work in an unhurried, reassuring manner. To make the atmosphere conducive to expression of feelings, intervene calmly, listen actively, and reinforce and encourage the patient constantly. Provide privacy, if needed.

• Give feedback and reliable information about the feared object or situation. Support a realistic view of the situation to reduce fear.

• Ask the patient how he normally copes with the fear. When he's able to face the fear, encourage him to verbalize and explore his personal strengths and resources with you.

• Prevent unpleasant surprises that could intensify the patient's fear.

• Reduce demands on the patient, so he has more energy available for coping.

• Teach the patient to use a systematic desensitization technique, such as deep breathing or relaxation exercises. Then bring the feared object closer until he can tolerate it with less anxiety.

• Suggest ways to channel the patient's energy and relieve stress (such as running and creative activities).

• Recommend relaxation methods, such as listening to music and meditating.

• Because many patients try to relieve their fears with alcohol, barbiturates, or antianxiety medications, teach them about the danger of addiction.

• Educate the patient's family and friends about the phobia and help them become a support system.

• Refer the patient to a doctor for medical intervention, if necessary.

MARY LOU L. HAMILTON, RN, MS

Posttraumatic stress disorder

The psychological consequence of a traumatic event that occurs outside the range of usual human experience is identified as posttraumatic stress disorder (PTSD). This is classified in *DSM-III* as an anxiety disorder.

Such a disorder can be acute, chronic, or delayed, and can follow a natural disaster (flood, tornado), a man-made disaster (war, imprisonment, torture, car accidents, large fires), or an assault or rape. Such extraordinary events produce stress in anyone. Psychological trauma always accompanies physical trauma and involves feelings of intense fear, helplessness, loss of control, and threat of annihilation. The acute subtype of PTSD occurs when symptoms appear within 6 months of the event and persist as long as 6 months. The acute subtype is similar to shell shock or combat fatigue. The chronic or delayed subtype occurs when symptoms persist longer than 6 months (chronic) or appear 6 months or more after the event (delayed). Chronic PTSD is less common but more debilitating; it has special relevance for veterans of the Vietnam war. These war veterans, victims of fires or airplane crashes, and survivors of earthquakes or volcanic eruptions are all vulnerable to this disorder, which often has a concomitant physical aspect to the trauma (direct damage to the central nervous system from malnutrition or head trauma). Apparently, the resulting disorder is more severe and persistent when the precipitating trauma is of human design.

Causes and incidence

PTSD can occur at any age (including childhood), but the very young and very old have more difficulty coping with unusual stressors. Preexisting psychopathology can also predispose to this disorder. Sex-related and familial patterns of incidence are unknown.

In most persons with PTSD, the stressor is a necessary but insufficient cause of the persisting symptoms. Even the most severe stressors do not produce PTSD in everyone, so psychological, physical, genetic, and social factors may also contribute to it (for example, a preexisting organic mental disorder, such as failing memory, difficulty in concentration, emotional lability, and/or depression with anxiety).

Theories of causation include the survivor theory, consisting of a latency or detachment phase, a denial-numbing phase, and an intrusive-repetitive phase, in which the survivor must work through the traumatic experiences and put the event into perspective.

In 1981, Arthur Egendorf and others released results of a comprehensive study on veterans and their postwar adjustment. This study encompassed all socioeconomic classes, geographic regions, and ethnic groups and analyzed responses from 1,400 persons directly or indirectly involved in the Vietnam conflict. Results show that unemployment, low educational attainment, minority status, instability in the family, and the amount and intensity of combat interact to influence the severity of PTSD. Veterans who have strong support systems (wives, friends, and family) are less likely to develop PTSD. Over 25% of all Vietnam veterans still show symptoms of delayed stress.

Signs and symptoms

Most common effects include pangs of painful emotion and unwelcome thoughts; a traumatic reexperiencing of the tragic event; insomnia, difficulty falling asleep, nightmares of the traumatic event, and aggressive outbursts upon awakening; emotional numbing—diminished or constricted response; chronic anxiety or panic attacks (with physical symptoms); rage and survivor guilt; use of violence to solve problems; depression and sui-

cidal thoughts; phobic avoidance of situations that arouse memories of trauma (for example, hot weather and tall grasses for the Vietnam veteran); memory impairment or difficulty in concentrating; and feelings of detachment or estrangement that destroy interpersonal relationships. Some patients also experience organic symptoms, fantasies of retaliation, and substance abuse.

Diagnosis

Characteristic symptoms that persist after unusual trauma confirm this diagnosis. A careful history identifies the subtype (acute or chronic). The history should include early life experiences, educational and vocational histories, and relationships with family, peers, and authority figures, as well as a careful military history and extensive psychosocial history in war veterans.

A psychiatric examination should include a mental status assessment and tests for organic impairment and should focus on other psychiatric syndromes that accompany PTSD, such as depression, generalized anxiety, and phobia).

Treatment

Goals of treatment include reducing the target symptoms, preventing chronic disability, and promoting occupational and social rehabilitation. Specific treatment may emphasize behavior techniques (relaxation therapy to decrease anxiety and induce sleep, or progressive desensitization); antianxiety and antidepressant drugs, prescribed with caution to avoid possible dependence; or brief psychotherapy (supportive, insight, or cathartic) to minimize risks of dependence and chronicity.

Support groups are highly effective and are provided through many Veterans Administration Centers and Crisis Clinics. These groups provide a forum in which victims of PTSD can work through their feelings with others who have had similar conflicts. Group settings are appropriate for most degrees of symptoms presented. Some group programs include spouses and families in their treatment process. Rehabilitation in physical, social, and occupational areas is also available for victims of chronic PTSD. Many patients need treatment for depression, alcohol or drug abuse, or medical conditions before psychological healing can take place.

Nursing intervention

The goal of intervention is to encourage the victim of PTSD to express his grief and complete the mourning process so he can go on with his life. Keep in mind that such a patient tends to sharply test your commitment and interest. So first examine your feelings about the event (war or other trauma) so you won't react with disdain and shock. This hampers the working relationship and reinforces the patient's poor self-image and sense of guilt.

To develop an effective therapeutic relationship:

• Know and practice crisis intervention techniques as appropriate.

• Establish trust by accepting the patient's current level of function and assuming a positive, consistent, honest and nonjudgmental attitude.

• Help the patient to regain control over angry impulses by identifying situations where he lost control and by talking about past and precipitating events (conceptual labeling) to help with later problem-solving skills.

• Give approval as the patient shows commitment to work on his problem.

• Deal constructively with anger. Encourage joint assessment of angry outbursts (identify how anger escalates, explore preventive measures that family members can take to regain control). Provide a safe, staff-monitored room in which the patient can safely deal with violent urges by displacement (such as pounding and throwing clay, destroying selected things). Encourage him to move from physical to verbal expressions of anger.

• Relieve shame and guilt precipitated by real actions, such as killing and mutilation, that violated a consciously held moral code through clarification (putting behavior into perspective); atonement (helping the patient see that he has atoned by social isolation and engaging in self-destructive behavior); and restitution (having clergy help him conquer guilt once authority and trust in others is accepted).

• Provide for or refer the patient to group therapy with other victims for peer support and forgiveness.

• Refer the patient to appropriate community resources.

MARY LOU L. HAMILTON, RN, MS

Psychogenic pain disorder

The striking feature of psychogenic pain is a persistent complaint of pain without appropriate physical findings. Although psychogenic pain has no physical cause, it's as real to the patient as organic pain. Psychogenic pain can occur in either sex at any age and is generally related to psychological stress. Such pain is usually chronic with exacerbations at times of stress. Its complications, including loss of work, interference with interpersonal relationships, drug dependence, extensive evaluations, and surgical procedures, can make the prognosis grim.

Causes

Psychogenic pain has no specific cause. A severe psychological stress or conflict is evident, but may not be as clearly time-related to the pain as in conversion disorders. The pain may have special significance, such as leg pain in the same leg a parent lost through amputation. The pain provides the patient with a means to settle upsetting psychological issues. For example, a person with dependency needs may develop psychogenic pain as an acceptable way to receive care and gain attention. The life history of the patient with psychogenic pain commonly shows aggression, violence, and organic or psychogenic pain. The patient may have learned to gain attention through pain.

Signs and symptoms
The cardinal feature is chronic, consistent complaints of pain without confirming physical disease. Such pain does not follow anatomical pathways. A helpful clue to psychogenic pain is a long history of evaluations and procedures at multiple settings without much pain relief. Such a patient speaks of health care professionals with anger and resentment because they've failed to relieve his pain. Because of frequent hospitalizations, the patient is familiar with pain medications and tranquilizers; he may ask for a specific drug and know its correct dosage and route of administration. The patient may not show typical nonverbal signs of pain, such as grimacing or guarding, but this isn't necessarily a clue to psychogenic pain, since such reactions are sometimes absent in patients with chronic organic pain.

An important feature in psychogenic pain disorder is secondary gain. The pain may allow the patient to avoid a stressful situation or receive attention not otherwise available. This secondary gain is essential to the persistence of the pain. Unfortunately, the patient does not usually acknowledge any psychological basis for his pain.

Diagnosis
Pain must be the overriding complaint; it must involve some psychological stress, either conscious or unconscious. The diagnosis of psychogenic pain disorder requires complete evaluation to rule out organic causes. Medical evaluation must consider organic diseases that cause persistent pain (such as multiple sclerosis, neuropathy, or tension headaches).

Psychiatric evaluation must rule out malingering (using the complaint to re-

ceive narcotics), depressive disorder, somatization disorder, hypochondriasis, schizophrenia, or personality disorders. Pain that subsides with suggestion, hypnosis, or placebo therapy is not necessarily psychogenic, since organic pain may also respond to these measures.

Treatment
The goal of treatment isn't necessarily to eradicate the pain, but rather to ease it and help the patient live with it. Treatment should avoid long, invasive evaluations and surgical interventions. Treatment at a comprehensive pain center may be helpful. Supportive measures for pain relief may include hot or cold packs, physical therapy, distraction techniques, or cutaneous stimulation with massage or transcutaneous electrical nerve stimulation (TENS). Measures to reduce the patient's anxiety may also be helpful. A continuing supportive relationship with an understanding health care professional is essential for effective management; regularly scheduled follow-up appointments are helpful.

Analgesics generally become an issue as the patient feels "I have to fight for everything I get." The patient should clearly be told what medication he will receive and should receive other supportive pain relief measures as well. Regularly scheduled analgesic doses can be more effective than p.r.n. scheduling; regular doses reduce pain by reducing anxiety about asking for medication. The use of placebos will destroy trust if the patient discovers the deceit.

Nursing intervention
● Provide a caring, accepting atmosphere where the patient's complaints are taken seriously and every effort is made to provide relief. This doesn't mean providing increasing amounts of narcotics on demand; rather, it means communicating to the patient that you'll collaborate in a treatment plan, and clearly stating the limitations. For example, you might say "I can stay with

you now for 15 minutes, but you can't receive another dose until 2 p.m."
• Don't tell the patient he's imagining the pain or can wait longer for medication that's due. Assess the patient's complaints and help him understand what's contributing to the pain. You might ask "I've noticed you complain of more pain after your doctor visits. What are his visits like for you?" to elicit contributing perceptions and fears.
• Teach the patient noninvasive, drug-free methods of pain control, such as guided imagery, relaxation techniques, or distraction.
• Encourage the patient to maintain independence despite his pain.
• Offer attention at times other than during the patient's complaints of pain, to weaken the link to secondary gain.
• Avoid confronting the patient with the psychogenic nature of his pain; this is rarely helpful because such pain is his means of avoiding psychological conflict. Psychiatric care can be useful, so consider psychiatric referrals; realize, however, that such patients usually resist psychiatric intervention and don't expect it to replace analgesic measures.
JEAN A. SHOOK, RN, MS, CS

Schizophrenic disorders

This group of disorders is marked mainly by withdrawal into self and failure to distinguish reality from fantasy. *DSM-III* recognizes five types of schizophrenia: catatonic, paranoid, disorganized, undifferentiated, and residual. Schizophrenic disorders are equally prevalent among males and females. According to current statistics, an estimated 2 million Americans may suffer from this disease.

Schizophrenic disorders produce varying degrees of impairment. As many as a third of such patients have just one psychotic episode. Some patients have no disability between periods of exacerbation; others need continuous institutional care. Prognosis worsens with each acute episode.

Causes and incidence

Various theories—both biologic and psychological—have been proposed to explain the development of schizophrenia. Some evidence supports a genetic predisposition to this disorder. Close relatives of schizophrenic patients are 2 to 50 times more likely to develop schizophrenia; the closer the degree of biologic relatedness, the higher the risk. One biochemical hypothesis holds that schizophrenia is a hyperdopaminergic condition. Another holds that schizophrenics have a deficiency or disturbance of β endorphins. Numerous psychological and sociocultural causes, such as disturbed family patterns, have also been proposed. Schizophrenic disorders have a higher incidence among lower socioeconomic groups, possibly related to downward social drift or lack of upward socioeconomic mobility, and to high stress levels that may be brought on by poverty, social failure, illness, and inadequate social resources. Higher incidence is also linked to low birth weight and congenital deafness.

Signs and symptoms

According to the *DSM-III* classification, schizophrenic disorders have these essential features: presence of psychotic features during the acute phase; deterioration from a previous level of functioning; onset before age 45; and presence of symptoms for at least 6 months, with deterioration in work, social relations, or self-care. Characteristically, symptoms involve several of the following areas: content and form of thought, perception, affect, sense of self, volition, relationship to the external world, and psychomotor behavior. No single symptom or characteristic is present in all schizophrenic disorders. There must be no symptoms that suggest organic disorder, substance abuse, or affective disorder.

Catatonic schizophrenia is most recognizable by its characteristic motor disturbances: stupor, negativism, rigidity, excitement, or posturing. The catatonic patient may be unable to move around or take care of his personal needs. Commonly, he doesn't even feed himself or talk and may show bizarre, stereotyped mannerisms (facial grimacing or sucking mouth movements). He may also exhibit waxy flexibility, in which the body, especially the extremities, will rigidly hold any placed position for prolonged periods. Diminished sensitivity to painful stimuli and rapid swings between excitement and stupor may also occur. The excitement phase may include extreme psychomotor agitation with excessive senseless or incoherent talking or shouting and with increased potential for destructive, violent behavior. This behavior is not influenced by environmental stimuli. Because many medical conditions may induce catatonia, careful differential diagnosis is essential.

Paranoid schizophrenia is characterized by persecutory or grandiose thought content and possible delusional jealousy. This condition may be associated with unfocused anxiety, anger, argumentativeness, and violence. It may also involve gender-identity problems, including fears of being thought of as homosexual or being approached by homosexuals. Paranoid schizophrenia may cause only minimal impairment of function if the patient doesn't act upon the delusional thoughts. His affective responsiveness may remain intact, but interactions with others commonly show stilted formality or intensity. This type of schizophrenia tends to develop in later life; its features tend to be stable over time.

See *Other Subtypes of Schizophrenia* for characteristics of disorganized, undifferentiated, and residual subtypes.

Diagnosis

The diagnosis of schizophrenia remains difficult and controversial. Psychiatrists in the United States have tended to diagnose schizophrenia more often than their English counterparts. Psychiatrists consider the following features important for diagnosing schizophrenia with greater accuracy: developmental background, genetic and family history, current environmental stressor, relationship of patient to interviewer, premorbid adjustment, course of illness, and response to treatment. Psychological tests may help, although none clearly confirms this diagnosis.

Some psychiatrists may use the dexamethasone suppression test to aid diagnosis, but others question its accuracy. Computed tomography scans may help establish an accurate diagnosis: they have shown enlarged ventricles in some schizophrenics. The ventricular brain ratio (VBR) determination may also support diagnosis. Some studies have reported an elevated VBR in schizophrenics.

Treatment

The goals of treatment for patients with schizophrenic disorders include equipping them with the skills they need to live in an unrestrictive environment that offers opportunity for meaningful interpersonal relationships. Another major aim of treatment is the control of schizophrenic symptoms through continuous administration of carefully selected neuroleptic drugs. Drug treatment should be continuous to prevent relapse after discontinuation.

Clinicians disagree about the effectiveness of psychotherapy in schizophrenics. Some consider it a useful adjunct through reducing loneliness, isolation, and withdrawal and enhancing productivity.

Nursing intervention

Management varies according to symptoms and type of schizophrenia.

For catatonic schizophrenia:
• Assess for physical illness. Remember that the mute patient won't com-

OTHER SUBTYPES OF SCHIZOPHRENIA

TYPE OF SCHIZOPHRENIA	NURSING INTERVENTIONS FOR ALL TYPES
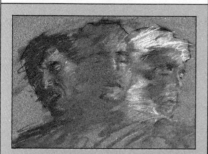	• Distinguish adult behavior from regressed behavior; reward adult behavior. Work with patient to increase sense of his own responsibility to improve level of functioning. • Engage patient in reality-oriented activities that involve human contact, such as inpatient social skills training groups, outpatient day care, and sheltered workshops. Provide reality-based explanations for distorted body images or hypochondriacal complaints. • Avoid promoting dependency. Meet patient's needs, but only do for patient what he cannot do for himself.
Disorganized • Marked incoherence; regressive, chaotic speech • Flat, incongruous, or silly affect • Delusions not systematized into coherent theme • Hallucinations fragmented • Unpredictable laughter • Grimaces • Mannerisms • Hypochondriacal complaints • Extreme social withdrawal • Oddities of behavior • Regressive behavior	• Remember, institutionalization may produce symptoms and handicaps that are not part of illness; evaluate symptoms carefully. • Clarify private language, autistic inventions, or neologisms. Give patient feedback that what he said is not understood. • Help patient engage in meaningful interpersonal relationships; do not avoid patient; maintain and convey to patient a sense of hope for possible improvement. • Expect patient to put you through rigorous period of testing before he shows evidence of trust. • Mobilize all resources to provide support system for patient to reduce vulnerability to stress.
Undifferentiated • Prominent psychotic symptoms that meet criteria for more than one subtype	
Residual • Previous history of episode of schizophrenia with prominent psychotic symptoms • Present clinical picture without prominent psychotic symptoms • Continuing evidence of illness, such as inappropriate affect, social withdrawal, eccentric behavior, illogical thinking, or loosening of associations	• Encourage compliance with neuroleptic medication regimen. Patients relapse when medication is discontinued. • Involve family in treatment; teach family the symptoms associated with relapse and suggest ways to manage symptoms. These include tension, nervousness, insomnia, decreased concentration ability, and loss of interest. • Provide continued support in helping patient learn social skills.

plain of pain or physical symptoms from a bizarre posture and consequently is at risk for pressure sores or decreased circulation to a body area.
• Meet physical needs for adequate food, fluid, exercise, and elimination; follow orders with respect to nutrition, urinary catheterization, and enema.
• Provide range-of-motion exercises or ambulate the patient every 2 hours.

• Prevent physical exhaustion and injury during periods of hyperactivity.
• Tell the patient directly, specifically, and concisely what needs to be done. Don't offer the negativistic patient a choice. For example, you might say: "It's time to go out. Let's go."
• Spend some time with the patient even if he's mute and unresponsive. The patient is acutely aware of his environ-

ment even though he seems not to be. Your presence can be reassuring and supportive. Avoid mutual withdrawal.

• Verbalize for the patient the message his nonverbal behavior seems to convey, and encourage him to do so as well.

• Offer reality orientation. You might say: "The leaves on the trees are turning colors and the air is cooler. It's fall!" Emphasize reality in all contacts to reduce distorted perceptions.

• Stay alert for violent outbursts; get help promptly to intervene safely for yourself and the patient.

For paranoid schizophrenia:

• When the patient is newly admitted, minimize his contact with staff.

• Don't crowd the patient physically or psychologically; he may strike out to protect himself.

• Be flexible; allow the patient some control. Approach him in a matter-of-fact, calm, and unhurried manner; let him talk about anything he wishes at first. Keep your conversational topics light and social; avoid power struggles.

• Respond to condescending attitudes (arrogance, put-downs, sarcasm, or open hostility) with neutral remarks; don't let the patient put you on the defensive and don't take his remarks personally. If he tells you to leave him alone, do leave, but return soon. Brief contacts with the patient may be most useful at first.

• Don't try to combat delusions with logic. Instead, respond to feelings, themes, or underlying needs: "It seems you feel you've been treated unfairly" (persecution).

• Build trust; be honest and dependable. Don't threaten, and don't promise what you can't fulfill.

• Don't tease, joke, argue with, or confront the patient. Remember, the patient's distorted perception will misinterpret such action in a way that's derogatory to himself.

• Make sure the patient's nutritional needs are met. Monitor his weight if he isn't eating. If he feels food is poisoned, let him fix his own food when possible, or offer foods in closed containers he can open. If giving liquid medication in a unit dose container, allow the patient to open the container. Monitor carefully for side effects of neuroleptic drugs: drug-induced parkinsonism, acute dystonia, akathisia, tardive dyskinesia, and malignant neuroleptic syndrome. Always document and report adverse effects promptly.

• If the patient is hallucinating, explore the content of his hallucinations. If he hears voices, find out if he feels that he must do what they command. Tell the patient you don't hear the voices but you know they're real to him.

• If he's expressing suicidal thoughts, take suicide precautions. Document his behavior and your precautions.

• If he's expressing homicidal thoughts (for example: "I have to kill my mother"), notify the doctor and document the patient's comments and who was notified.

• Decode the patient's autistic inventions and other private language; ask him to explain things that you don't understand.

• Don't touch the patient without telling him first exactly what you're going to do. For example: "I'm going to put this cuff on your arm so I can take your blood pressure."

• Postpone procedures that require physical contact with hospital personnel until the patient is less suspicious or agitated. For information on management of other forms of schizophrenia, see *Other Subtypes of Schizophrenia*, page 139.

ANNA P. MOORE, RN, BSN, MS

Somatization disorder

Somatization disorder is present when multiple signs and symptoms that suggest physical disorders exist without a verifiable disease or pathophysiologic condition to account for them. Commonly, the patient with somatization disorder undergoes repeated medical evaluations, which—unlike the symptoms themselves—can be potentially damaging and debilitating. Such a patient can always find just one more hospital or doctor to do another diagnostic workup. However, unlike the hypochondriac, he's not preoccupied with the belief that he has a specific disease.

Causes

This disorder has no specific cause. Its symptoms can begin or worsen after many kinds of losses (job security or personal relationship).

Characteristically, patients with this disorder have a lifelong pattern of sickliness—sometimes beginning in adolescence. They don't relate well to other people except by using their symptoms. They're locked into a pattern of getting attention and meeting their needs through physical complaints.

Signs and symptoms

The essential feature of this disorder is the pattern of recurrent, multiple symptoms and complaints. These complaints can involve any body system but most frequently involve the gastrointestinal tract, with nausea, vomiting, and abdominal pain; the neurologic system, with weakness, paresthesias, and headaches; and the cardiopulmonary system, with dizziness, chest pain, and palpitations. These symptoms can involve multiple body systems or can shift from one system to another.

An important clue to somatization disorder is a history of multiple medical evaluations at different institutions without significant findings.

Patients with somatization disorder typically relate their present complaints and their previous evaluations in great detail. They may be quite knowledgeable about tests, procedures, and medical jargon. They don't discuss other aspects of their lives without including their many symptoms. In fact, any attempts to explore areas other than their medical history may cause them to show noticeable

anxiety. They tend to disparage previous health care professionals and previous treatment, often with the comment, "No one seems to understand. Everyone thinks I'm imagining these things."

These patients' symptoms are not under voluntary control and they want to feel better. However, they are never symptom-free. The course of symptoms is chronic, with exacerbations during times of stress.

Diagnosis

No specific test or procedure verifies somatization disorder. The patient's complaints require careful evaluation for organic causes. This does not mean extensive invasive procedures, but rather a thorough history and review of previous evaluations. When reviewing the patient's history, listen for clues of recent losses or severe stress. Onset of somatization symptoms generally occurs before age 30.

Diagnostic evaluation should rule out physical causes that typically cause vague, confusing symptoms, such as multiple sclerosis, hypothyroidism, systemic lupus erythematosus, or porphyria. Psychological evaluation should rule out depression, schizophrenia with somatic delusions, hypochondriasis, psychogenic pain, and malingering.

Treatment

The goal of treatment is not to eradicate the patient's symptoms, but rather to help him learn to live with them. After diagnostic evaluation has ruled out organic causes, the patient should be told that he has no serious illness but will continue to receive care to ease his symptoms.

The most important aspect of treatment is a continuing supportive relationship with a sympathetic health care provider who acknowledges the patient's symptoms and is willing to help him live with them. The patient should have regularly scheduled appointments for review of symptoms and basic physical evaluation, but the main aspect of follow-up is review of the patient's coping. Follow-up appointments should last approximately 20 to 30 minutes and should focus on new symptoms or any change in old symptoms to avoid missing a developing physical disease. As many as 30% of patients initially diagnosed with somatization disorder eventually develop an organic disease. Patients with somatization disorder rarely acknowledge any psychological aspect of their illness and reject psychiatric treatment.

Nursing interventions
• Acknowledge the patient's symptoms and support his efforts to function and cope despite distress. Under no circumstances should you tell the patient his symptoms are imaginary. But do tell him the results and meanings of tests.
• Emphasize the patient's strengths. "It's good that you can still work with this pain." Gently point out the time relationship between stress and physical symptoms.
• Help the patient to manage stress, not eradicate symptoms. Typically, his relationships are linked to his symptoms; remedying them can impair his interactions with others.
• Develop a care plan with some input from the patient. The care plan should include participation of the patient's family. Encourage and help them to understand the patient's need for troublesome symptoms.

The danger in working with these patients is that the anger, irritation, and frustration they understandably generate may interfere with nursing care. It's not unusual to develop an attitude that says: "These people don't want to get better, so why should I waste my time?" Deal with these feelings first by acknowledging them. Consulting a psychiatric clinical nurse specialist can help nursing staff discuss their feelings and develop effective means of dealing with them.

JEAN A. SHOOK, RN, MS, CS

MISCELLANEOUS DISORDERS

Alport's syndrome

Alport's syndrome is a hereditary nephritis characterized by recurrent gross or microscopic hematuria. It's associated with deafness, albuminuria, and variably progressive azotemia.

Cause and incidence
Alport's syndrome is transmitted as an X-linked autosomal trait and affects males more often and more severely than females. Men with hematuria and proteinuria often develop end-stage renal disease in their 30s or 40s. Respiratory infection often precipitates recurrent bouts of hematuria; however, streptococcal infection isn't linked to Alport's syndrome.

Signs and symptoms
The primary clinical feature of Alport's syndrome is recurrent gross or microscopic hematuria, which typically appears during early childhood. The next most common symptom is deafness (especially to high-frequency sounds). Other associated findings may include proteinuria, pyuria, red cell casts in urine, and possibly flank pain or other abdominal symptoms; however, many patients are initially asymptomatic. Ocular features may include cataracts and, less commonly, keratoconus, microspherophakia, myopia, retinitis pigmentosa, and nystagmus. Hypertension is often associated with progressive renal failure.

Diagnosis
A family history of recurrent hematuria, deafness, and renal failure (especially in males) suggests Alport's syndrome. Laboratory tests include

urinalysis of all family members, blood studies to detect immunoglobulins and complement components, and audiometry testing. Renal biopsy confirms diagnosis.

Treatment and nursing intervention

Effective treatment is supportive and symptomatic. Treatment may include antibiotic therapy for associated respiratory or urinary tract infection, a hearing aid for hearing loss, eyeglasses or contact lenses to improve vision, antihypertensive drug therapy for associated hypertension, and dialysis or kidney transplantation for end-stage renal failure.

Refer the patient and his family for genetic counseling, as appropriate.

MARCIA GOLDSTEIN, RN, BSN, CHN

Hypoglycemia

Hypoglycemia is an abnormally low glucose level in the bloodstream. It occurs when glucose burns up too rapidly, when the glucose release rate falls behind tissue demands, or when excessive insulin enters the bloodstream. The disorder is classified into two types: *reactive* and *fasting*. Reactive hypoglycemia results from the reaction to the disposition of meals or the administration of excessive insulin. Fasting hypoglycemia causes discomfort during fasting periods—for example, in the early morning hours before breakfast. Although hypoglycemia is a specific endocrine imbalance, its symptoms are often vague and depend on how quickly the patient's glucose levels drop. If not corrected, severe hypoglycemia may result in coma and irreversible brain damage.

Causes

Reactive hypoglycemia may take several forms. In a diabetic patient, it may result from administration of too much insulin or—less commonly—too much oral hypoglycemia medication. In a mildly diabetic patient (or one in the early stages of diabetes mellitus), reactive hypoglycemia may result from delayed and excessive insulin production after carbohydrate ingestion. Similarly, a nondiabetic patient may suffer reactive hypoglycemia from a sharp increase in insulin output after a meal. Sometimes called *postprandial hypoglycemia*, this type of reactive hypoglycemia usually disappears when the patient eats something sweet. In some patients, reactive hypoglycemia may have no known cause (idiopathic reactive) or may result from hyperalimentation due to gastric dumping syndrome or from impaired glucose tolerance.

Fasting hypoglycemia usually results from an excess of insulin or insulin-like substance or from a decrease in counterregulatory hormones. It can be *exogenous,* resulting from such external factors as alcohol or other drug ingestion, or *endogenous,* resulting from organic problems.

Endogenous hypoglycemia may result from tumors or liver disease. Insulinomas, small islet cell tumors in the pancreas, secrete excessive amounts of insulin, which inhibits hepatic glucose production. They are generally benign (in 90% of patients). Extrapancreatic tumors, though uncommon, can also cause hypoglycemia by increasing glucose utilization and inhibiting glucose output. Such tumors occur primarily in the mesenchyma, liver, adrenal cortex, gastrointestinal system, and lymphatic system. They may be benign or malignant. Among nonendocrine causes of fasting hypoglycemia are severe liver diseases, including hepatitis, cancer, cirrhosis, and liver congestion associated with congestive heart failure. All of these conditions reduce the uptake and release of glycogen from the liver. Some endocrine causes include destruction of pancreatic islet cells; adrenocortical insufficiency, which contributes to hypoglycemia by reducing the production of cortisol and cortisone needed for gluconeogenesis; and pituitary insufficiency, which reduces the levels of adrenocorticotropic hormone/growth hormone.

Hypoglycemia is at least as common in newborns and children as it is in adults. Usually, infants develop hypo-

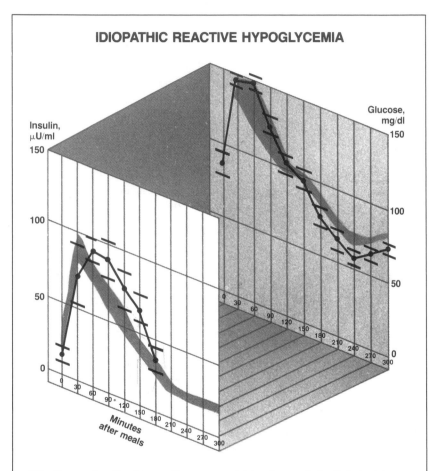

IDIOPATHIC REACTIVE HYPOGLYCEMIA

This often puzzling disorder, sometimes dubbed "non-hypoglycemia" because of its vague symptoms and difficult diagnosis, produces symptoms about 2 to 5 hours after eating. The reason for this is unclear, however; in some patients, insulin levels rise, while in others, intestinal glucose absorption increases.

Nonspecific symptoms suggesting epinephrine release (such as sweating, tremor, rapid heartbeat, dizziness, and confusion) arise and subside spontaneously in 15 to 20 minutes. The syndrome is easily

mistaken for an actual pathologic state unless the patient's blood glucose level is measured while he is experiencing symptoms.

The curves on the diagram above reflect postprandial blood glucose and blood insulin responses in 44 patients with idiopathic reactive hypoglycemia. The responses are compared with a series of normal controls (shaded areas). Short dashes above and below points indicate the range of individual responses, plotted at 30-minute intervals.

glycemia because of an increased number of cells per unit of body weight and because of increased demands on stored liver glycogen to support respirations, thermoregulation, and muscular activity. In full-term infants, hypoglycemia may occur 24 to 72 hours after birth and is usually transient. In infants who are premature or small for gestational age, onset of hypoglycemia is much more rapid—it can occur as soon as 6 hours after birth—due to their small, immature livers, which produce much less glycogen. Maternal factors that can produce hypoglycemia in infants within 24 hours after birth include diabetes mellitus, toxemia, erythroblastosis, and glycogen storage disease.

Signs and symptoms

Signs and symptoms of reactive hypoglycemia include fatigue and malaise, nervousness, irritability, trembling, tension, headache, hunger, cold sweats, and rapid heart rate. These same clinical effects usually characterize fasting hypoglycemia. In addition, fasting hypoglycemia may also cause central nervous system (CNS) disturbances; for example, blurry or double vision, confusion, motor weakness, hemiplegia, convulsions, or coma.

In infants and children, signs and symptoms of hypoglycemia are vague. A newborn's refusal to feed may be the primary clue to underlying hypoglycemia. Associated CNS effects include tremors, twitching, weak or high-pitched cry, sweating, limpness, convulsions, and coma.

Diagnosis

Dextrostix or Chemstrip provides a quick screening method for determining blood glucose level. A color change that corresponds to < 45 mg/dl indicates the need for a venous blood sample.

Laboratory blood testing confirms diagnosis of hypoglycemia by showing decreased blood sugar values. The following values indicate hypoglycemia:

Full-term infants:
  < 30 mg/dl before feeding
  < 40 mg/dl after feeding

Preterm infants:
  < 20 mg/dl before feeding
  < 30 mg/dl after feeding

Children and adults:
  < 40 mg/dl before meal
  < 50 mg/dl after meal.

In addition, a 5-hour glucose tolerance test may be administered to provoke reactive hypoglycemia. Following a 12-hour fast, laboratory testing to detect plasma insulin and plasma glucose levels may identify fasting hypoglycemia.

Treatment

Effective treatment of reactive hypoglycemia requires dietary modification to help delay glucose absorption and gastric emptying. Usually, this includes small, frequent meals; ingestion of complex carbohydrates, fiber, and fat; and avoidance of simple sugars, alcohol, and fruit drinks. The patient may also receive anticholinergic drugs to slow gastric emptying and intestinal motility and to inhibit vagal stimulation of insulin release.

For fasting hypoglycemia, surgery and drug therapy are usually required. In patients with insulinoma, removal of the tumor is the treatment of choice. Drug therapy may include the nondiuretic benzothiadiazine, diazoxide to inhibit insulin secretion, streptozocin, and hormones, such as glucocorticoids and long-acting glycogen.

Therapy for newborn infants who have hypoglycemia or risk developing it includes preventive measures. A hypertonic solution of 10% to 25% dextrose, calculated at 2 to 4 ml/kg of body weight and administered I.V., should correct a severe hypoglycemic state in newborns. To reduce the chance of developing hypoglycemia, high-risk infants should receive feedings—either breast milk or a solution of 5% to 10% glucose and water—as soon after birth as possible.

Nursing intervention

• Watch for and report signs of hypoglycemia (such as poor feeding) in high-risk infants.

• Monitor infusion of hypertonic glucose in the newborn to avoid hyperglycemia, circulatory overload, and cellular dehydration. Terminate glucose solutions gradually to prevent hypoglycemia caused by hyperinsulinemia.

• Explain the purpose and procedure for any diagnostic tests. Collect blood samples at the appropriate times, as ordered.

• Monitor the effects of drug therapy, and report the development of side effects to the doctor.

• Teach the patient which foods to include in his diet (complex carbohydrates, fiber, fat) and which foods to avoid (simple sugars, alcohol). Refer the patient and family for dietary counseling, as appropriate.

JOYCE LEFEVER KEE, RN, MSN

Primary degenerative dementia

(Alzheimer's disease)

Primary degenerative dementia accounts for over half of all dementias. An estimated 5% of persons over age 65 have a severe form of this disease; 12% suffer from mild to moderate dementia. Because this is a primary progressive dementia, prognosis is poor.

Causes

The cause of primary degenerative dementia is unknown. However, several factors are implicated in this disease: *neurochemical factors,* such as deficiencies in neurotransmitter substances of acetylcholine, somatostatin, substance P, and norepinephrine; *environmental factors,* such as exposure to aluminum and manganese; *viral factors,* such as slow-growing central nervous system viruses; *trauma;* and *genetic immunologic factors.* The brain tissue of affected patients has three hallmark features: neurofibrillary tangles, neuritic plaques, and granulovascular degeneration.

Signs and symptoms

Onset is insidious. Initially, the patient experiences almost imperceptible changes, such as forgetfulness, recent memory loss, difficulty learning and remembering new information, deterioration in personal hygiene and appearance, and an inability to concentrate. Gradually, tasks that require abstract thinking and activities that require judgment become harder. Progressive difficulty in communication and severe deterioration in memory, language, and motor function results in a loss of coordination and an inability to write or speak. Personality changes (restlessness, irritability) and nocturnal awakenings are common. Eventually, the patient becomes disoriented, and emotional lability and physical and intellectual disability progress. The patient becomes very susceptible to infection and accidents. Usually, death results from infection.

Diagnosis

Early diagnosis is difficult, because of the subtlety of the patient's signs and symptoms. Diagnosis relies on an accurate history from a reliable family member, mental status and neurologic examination, and psychometric testing. A positron emission transaxial tomography scan measures the metabolic activity of the cerebral cortex and may help confirm early diagnosis. An electroencephalogram and a computed tomography scan may help diagnose later stages of primary degenerative dementia. Currently, primary degenerative dementia is diagnosed by exclusion; a variety of tests are performed to rule out other disorders. True diagnosis cannot be confirmed until death, when pathologic findings are found at autopsy.

Treatment

Therapy consists of cerebral vasodilators, such as ergoloid mesylates (Hydergine), isoxsuprine (Vasodilan), and cyclandelate (Cyclospasmol) to enhance the brain's circulation; hyperbaric oxygen to increase oxygenation to the brain; psychostimulators, such as methylphenidate (Ritalin), to enhance the patient's mood; and antidepressants if depression seems to exacerbate the patient's dementia. Most drug therapies currently being used are experimental. These include choline salts, lecithin, physostigmine, deanol enkephalins, and naloxone, which may slow the disease process. Another approach to treatment includes avoiding antacids, aluminum cooking utensils, and aluminum-containing deodorants to help decrease aluminum intake.

Nursing intervention

Overall care is focused on supporting the patient's abilities and compensating for those abilities he has lost.
• Establish an effective communication system with the patient and family to help them adjust to the patient's altered cognitive abilities.
• Offer emotional support to the patient and his family. Teach them about the disease, and listen to their concerns and special problems.
• Protect the patient from injury by providing a safe environment.
• Encourage the patient to exercise, as ordered, to help maintain mobility.
CONNIE A. WALLECK, RN, MS, CNRN

Sleep apnea syndrome

Sleep apnea syndrome is a disorder marked by recurrent episodes of apnea or hypoventilation during sleep. This syndrome has three forms: obstructive, central, or mixed. Sleep apnea occurs predominantly in males during the first, fifth, and sixth decades of life, and in postmenopausal women. Approximately 10% to 15% of the population of industrialized countries have some form of sleep disorder; of this percentage, 5% to 10% suffer from sleep apnea syndrome. The loss of sleep associated with sleep apnea syndrome can have severe physical and psychological consequences.

Causes

Obstructive sleep apnea, the syndrome's most common form, is the periodic cessation of airflow for at least 10 seconds due to complete upper airway occlusion despite respiratory effort. Occlusion occurs at the oropharynx and nasopharynx from an overrelaxed tongue and soft palate. The brief apnea disrupts sleep and activates the oropharyngeal muscles to move the tongue away from the oropharynx and nasopharynx, restoring airflow, Resumption of deep sleep begins the cycle again. With repeated episodes, the apneic periods grow more prolonged; the cycle eventually becomes self-perpetuating. Patients with obstructive sleep apnea may have as many as 80 episodes per hour.

Central sleep apnea is characterized by the absence of both airflow and respiratory effort resulting from disrupted central nervous system (CNS) stimulation of respiratory muscles.

Mixed sleep apnea involves alternating episodes of obstructive and central sleep apnea.

Sleep apnea syndrome may be associated with conditions that restrict the upper airways, including hypertrophy of the tongue or tonsils, tumor, velopharyngeal incompetence, retrognathia, and micrognathia. It can also be caused by conditions that depress respiratory drive: endocrine disorders, such as endogenous obesity, hypothyroidism, acromegaly, and Cushing's disease; neuromuscular disorders, such as poliomyelitis, muscular dystrophy, amyotrophic lateral sclerosis, kyphoscoliosis, and autonomic

HOW OBSTRUCTIVE SLEEP APNEA DEVELOPS

Loss of palatal, lingual, and pharyngeal muscle tone permits the airway to collapse as inspiratory effort produces a relative negative pressure within the oropharynx and nasopharynx. As the snorer moves into the stages of deep sleep, muscular relaxation increases. The tongue drops into the airway and vibrates against a limp soft palate and uvula and against the pharyngeal walls, which are drawn inward because of poor superior constrictor muscle tone.

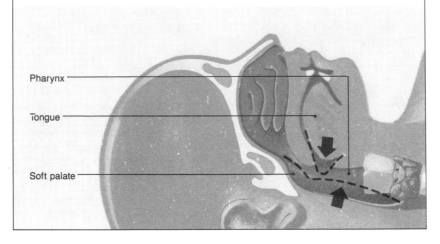

Pharynx

Tongue

Soft palate

dystrophy; CNS disorders, such as cerebrovascular accident, head trauma, encephalitis, and brain stem glioma; and cardiovascular disorders, such as ischemic heart disease and congestive or restrictive cardiomyopathy.

Signs and symptoms

Initial complaints in sleep apnea syndrome usually include snoring and daytime drowsiness from disrupted sleep. Snoring, which results from airway narrowing, may precede the onset of sleep apnea by many years. Other typical features include morning headaches, insomnia, dyspnea, exercise intolerance, sexual dysfunction, personality changes, hypnagogic hallucinations, and automatic behavior. Physical examination findings often include obesity (a history of recent weight gain is particularly significant, possibly pointing to pickwickian syndrome—a condition marked by obesity, somnolence, hypoventilation, and erythrocytosis); mild to moderate essential hypertension; and nasal obstruction, enlarged tonsils or tongue, or structural deformities in the upper airways.

Advanced sleep apnea syndrome can produce polycythemia, pulmonary hypertension, right heart failure, or cor pulmonale from progressive tissue hypoxia. Hypoxia can also cause cardiac dysrhythmias such as bradycardia, varying degrees of heart block, ventricular asystole, premature ventricular contractions, short bursts of ventricular tachycardia, and ventricular fibrillation, which can cause sudden nocturnal death.

Diagnosis

A history of persistent snoring and sleep disturbances suggests sleep apnea syndrome. Definitive diagnosis is made by polysomnography—the polygraphic recording of various physiologic parameters during sleep. Parameters commonly recorded are respiratory air flow, breath sounds, diaphragmatic movements, pulmonary gas exchange, and body movements. An electroencephalogram, right and left electrooculogram, submental electromyogram (EMG), and electrocardiogram are commonly recorded as well. Polysomnography can determine the number and duration of apneic episodes and of different sleep stages, as well as the effects of respiratory alterations on heart rate and rhythm. Rhythmic EMG activity in the diaphragm, intrathoracic pressure changes, and paradoxical rib cage movements indicate the presence of respiratory drive, pointing to obstructive sleep apnea. The typical pattern in obstructive sleep apnea consists of cyclical apneic periods, arterial oxygen desaturation, and bradycardia alternating with upper airway muscle movement and large tidal volumes. In central sleep apnea, the cessation of tidal volume excursion occurs simultaneously with quieting of the electrical activity in the diaphragm and intercostal muscles, no fluctuations in intrathoracic pressure, and the absence of rib cage and abdominal movement.

Treatment
Treatment for sleep apnea syndrome is still investigational and may include surgery, physical therapy, and drugs. Surgery is aimed at enlarging the upper airways and removing any structures that inhibit airflow through such procedures as adenoidectomy, tonsillectomy, nasal septal repair, and mandibular revisions.

Uvulopalatropharyngoplasty, a procedure that enlarges the oropharynx by removing uvular and palatal tissue, may be performed in patients with no obvious structural obstruction. In patients with obstructive sleep apnea, especially those who've developed cor pulmonale, cardiac dysrhythmias, and pickwickian syndrome, tracheostomy may be necessary. Use of a fenestrated tracheostomy tube allows normal swallowing and speech during the day when plugged, and normal breathing at night when unplugged.

Possible surgical interventions for patients with central sleep apnea include electrical pacing of the phrenic nerve or direct stimulation of the diaphragm by implanted electrodes to induce diaphragmatic movement.

Tracheostomy may still be necessary to prevent airway obstruction from collapsed upper airway muscles caused by diaphragmatic stimulation without simultaneous upper airway muscle activation.

Therapy for patients with sleep apnea syndrome includes mechanical ventilation—either positive or negative pressure—and diet therapy for obese patients. Oxygen therapy may help relieve hypoxemia during sleep and prevent complications, such as pulmonary hypertension and dysrhythmias. Continuous positive-pressure ventilation through a nosepiece or nasal cannula may help relieve symptoms of obstructive sleep apnea, as may an artificial airway.

Drug therapy for sleep apnea syndrome is limited and controversial. Drugs that have been used include medroxyprogesterone, the exact mechanism of which is still unknown; tricyclic antidepressants, such as protriptyline, which presumably decreases the duration of REM sleep; strychnine, which increases upper airway abductor and dilator muscles; and acetazolamide, which has a direct central effect and a stimulating effect by causing metabolic acidosis.

Nursing intervention
• Advise the patient to avoid substances, such as alcohol, antihistamines, and sedatives, that could depress the CNS and induce or prolong sleep apnea.
• Don't give hypnotics or sedatives to patients with sleep apnea syndrome; these drugs can further compromise respirations, possibly causing death.
• Teach a patient with a tracheostomy how to care for his stoma, how to clean and change the tracheostomy tube, and how to suction secretions if necessary.

TERRI E. WEAVER, RN, MSN, CS

Sexually transmitted diseases

A sexually transmitted disease (STD) is a contagious disorder that's trans-mitted and acquired by sexual inter-course or genital contact. STDs include the classic venereal diseases of syphilis and gonorrhea, as well as urethral and genital infections caused by bacteria, fungi, and viruses, such as herpes gen-italis, granuloma inguinale, and chan-croid; enteric infections, such as hep-

SEXUALLY TRANSMITTED DISEASES

DISEASE AND ETIOLOGY	CLINICAL MANIFESTATIONS	THERAPY
Chancroid *Hemophilus ducreyi,* a gram-negative bacillus	• Nonindurated, painful penile ul-cer (sometimes multiple) that may be necrotic with ragged borders; unilateral inguinal adenopathy with possible bubo formation • Females are usually asymptom-atic.	• Erythromycin or co-trimoxa-zole, P.O. • Aspiration of fluctuant lymph nodes
Condylomata acuminata (genital warts) Human papilloma virus	• Single or multiple soft, fleshy, papillary or sessile, painless growths around the anus, vulvova-ginal area, penis, urethra, or peri-neum	• Podophyllin 10% to 25% in compound tincture of benzoin, applied to warts • Cryotherapy, electrocautery, or curettage
Gonorrhea *Neisseria gonorrhoeae,* a gram-negative diplococ-cus	• Males: if symptomatic, usually dysuria, frequency, and purulent urethral discharge • Females: if symptomatic, abnor-mal vaginal discharge, dysuria, or abnormal menses possible • Both: anorectal and pharyngeal infections are common.	• Tetracycline or penicillin prep-aration P.O. (probenecid given to increase penicillin levels) • Spectinomycin I.M. for treat-ment failures, drug intolerance, or penicillinase-producing *N. gonorrhoeae* infections
Granuloma inguinale *Calymmatobacterium granulomatis,* a gram-neg-ative coccobacillus	• Single or multiple subcutaneous nodules that erode to form granu-lomatous, painless ulcers, which bleed on contact and enlarge slowly	• Chiefly tetracycline P.O. or streptomycin, I.M. (other anti-biotics may be used, but peni-cillins are not effective)

atitis, amebiasis, and shigellosis; and arthropod infestations, such as pediculosis pubis and scabies.

In most STDs, infection remains localized to the genitourinary tract, but in some STDs, it can spread to other structures and even become systemic. Often, asymptomatic carriers transmit a pathogen that eventually causes symptomatic infection in the recipient.

The chart below reviews some common and not so common, but dangerous, STDs and their causes, clinical manifestations, recommended treatments, and pertinent nursing considerations.

COMPLICATIONS	NURSING CONSIDERATIONS
• Secondary infection, fistulae, paraphimosis, or phimosis	• Apply compresses to ulcers to remove necrotic materials. • Ensure examination of sexual partners as soon as possible. • Encourage patient to return for evaluation 3 to 5 days after therapy begins and then weekly or biweekly, as ordered, until completely healed. • Teach males that the prepuce should remain retracted during therapy unless edema results and to clean the ulcerative lesions three times a day. • Teach patients that use of condoms will help prevent future infections.
• Malignant change • Obstruction of birth canal due to enlarging vascular warts	• Encourage patient to return for weekly or biweekly treatments until lesions are resolved. • Encourage patient to have sexual partners examined for warts. • Teach patient to abstain from sexual activity or to use condoms during therapy.
• Females: pelvic inflammatory disease (PID) and its sequelae • Males: epididymitis, sterility, urethral stricture, infertility • Newborns: ophthalmia neonatorum, scalp abscess from fetal monitor, rhinitis, pneumonia, anorectal infection • All: disseminated infection, including septicemia, arthritis, dermatitis, meningitis, and endocarditis	• Teach patient how to take any prescribed oral medication. Tetracycline should be taken 1 hour before or 2 hours after meals, avoiding dairy products, antacids, iron preparations, and direct sunlight. • Encourage patient to refer sexual partners for examination and treatment. • Teach patient to avoid sexual activity until cured and that use of condoms helps prevent future infections. • Encourage follow-up as ordered by doctor, usually 4 to 7 days after completing therapy, or earlier if symptoms persist.
• Secondary infection, keloid scar, necrosis of genitalia, toxic manifestations such as fever, malaise, anemia, cachexia, and death	• Teach patient how to take medications. Tetracycline should be taken 1 hour before meals or 2 hours after meals, avoiding dairy products, antacids, iron preparations, and direct sunlight. • Ensure examination of sexual partners as soon as possible. • Encourage return for follow-up 3 to 5 days after therapy begins and then weekly or biweekly until entirely healed.

(continued)

SEXUALLY TRANSMITTED DISEASES *(continued)*

DISEASE AND ETIOLOGY	CLINICAL MANIFESTATIONS	THERAPY
Herpes genitalis Herpes simplex virus (HSV) Types I and II	• Single or multiple vesicles appearing anywhere on the genitalia. Vesicles rupture to form shallow ulcers that may be very painful. Lesions resolve spontaneously with minimal scarring. • Recurrent infections are usually milder.	• No known cure • Acyclovir ointment 5% to cover all lesions (may be initiated as soon as possible) • Acyclovir P.O. for subsequent outbreaks
Lymphogranuloma venereum (LGV) *Chlamydia trachomatis,* an intracellular bacterium	• Primary lesion is painless vesicle or nonindurated ulcer, followed by regional adenopathy. • Feeling of stiffness and aching in the groin along with swelling may be the first indication in most patients.	• Chiefly tetracycline P.O. or erythromycin P.O.; possibly sulfisoxazole
Nongonococcal urethritis (NGU) • *Chlamydia trachomatis* • *Ureaplasma urealyticum*	• Urinary frequency, dysuria, urethral discharge that varies from mucoid to purulent • Some males may be asymptomatic.	• Tetracycline P.O. or, if contraindicated, erythromycin P.O.
Syphilis *Treponema pallidum,* a spirochete	• Primary: painless, indurated chancre at exposure site • Secondary: variable skin rash, mucous patches, condylomata lata, lymphadenopathy • Latent: no clinical signs	• I.M. benzathine penicillin (if allergic, tetracycline preparation P.O. or erythromycin P.O. as a second alternative)
Vulvovaginitis • *Trichomonas vaginalis,* a protozoan • *Gardnerella vaginalis,* a gram-negative coccobacillus • *Candida albicans,* a fungus that grows as oval budding yeast cells	• Trichomoniasis: asymptomatic to erythema and edema of external genitalia with frothy, greenish gray vaginal discharge • Gardnerella vaginitis: asymptomatic or vulvar irritation and thin grayish white vaginal discharge • Candidiasis: asymptomatic, but vulva is usually edematous and erythematous; thick, white vaginal discharge • Male sexual partners may be asymptomatic or may develop urethritis, balanitis, or cutaneous penile lesions	• Trichomoniasis: metronidazole P.O. • Gardnerella vaginitis: metronidazole or ampicillin P.O. • Candidiasis: nystatin or clotrimazole vaginal suppository or miconazole nitrate 2% intravaginal cream

COMPLICATIONS	NURSING CONSIDERATIONS
• Neuralgia, meningitis, ascending myelitis, urethral strictures • Females: possibly increased risk for cervical cancer and fetal wastage • Congenital herpes, which may be fatal or result in ocular or neurologic sequelae	• Teach patient to keep genital area clean and dry. • Teach patient to abstain from sexual activity while symptomatic, since lesions shed a high concentration of virus at this time; since a small amount of virus may be transmitted during asymptomatic periods, use of condoms is advised. • Encourage patient to have annual Pap smears. • Encourage women to inform their doctors of their history of herpes when pregnant.
• Dissemination with nephropathy, hepatomegaly, or phlebitis • Perineal abscess, rectovaginal fistulae, rectal stricture, elephantiasis	• Teach patient how to take medications. Tetracycline should be taken 1 hour before meals or 2 hours after meals, avoiding dairy products, antacids, iron preparations, and direct sunlight. • Ensure examination of sexual partners as soon as possible. • Encourage patient to return for follow-up 3 to 5 days after therapy begins and then weekly or biweekly, as ordered, until completely healed.
• Urethral strictures, prostatitis, epididymitis • Chlamydial NGU may lead to endocervitis, PID, neonatal ophthalmia, or neonatal pneumonia	• Teach patient how to take oral medications. Tetracycline should be taken 1 hour before meals or 2 hours after meals, avoiding dairy products, antacids, iron preparations, and bright sunlight. • Teach patient to refrain from sexual activity until cured and that use of condoms will prevent future infections. • Encourage patient to refer sexual partners for examination and treatment. • Encourage patient to return for evaluation 4 to 7 days after completion of therapy for follow-up, or earlier if symptoms persist.
• Late syphilis with its sequelae, including neurosyphilis, cardiovascular syphilis, and localized gumma formation • Congenital syphilis	• Teach patient how to take any prescribed oral medications. Tetracycline should be taken 1 hour before or 2 hours after meals, avoiding dairy products, antacids, iron preparations, and direct sunlight. • Encourage follow-up serologies at 3, 6, 12, and 24 months after therapy. • Teach patient to avoid sexual activity until cured and that using condoms will help prevent future infections.
• Secondary excoriations • Note: recurrent infections common	• Teach patient how to take prescribed medications. With metronidazole therapy, alcohol should be avoided until 3 days after completion of therapy. Tetracycline should be taken 1 hour before or 2 hours after meals, avoiding dairy products, antacids, iron preparations, and bright sunlight. Suppositories should be stored in the refrigerator and the patient should wash hands before and after inserting vaginal suppositories or cream. Medication should be continued during menstrual period. Sanitary pads can be worn with creams and suppositories to protect clothing. • Encourage patient to refer sexual partners for evaluation. • Use condoms to prevent future infections.

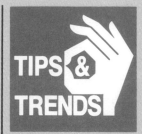

TIPS & TRENDS

Lyme disease

Lyme disease, a tick-borne bacterial infection that can produce recurrent arthritis and neurologic or cardiac complications, is on the rise in the northeast, midwest, and far west. Initial signs and symptoms typically include a characteristic skin lesion—erythema chronicum migrans—at the site of the tick bite, along with fever, chills, neck stiffness, sore throat, muscle and joint pain, and nausea and vomiting. If untreated, Lyme disease may eventually produce Bell's palsy, meningoencephalitis, peripheral neuritis, transverse myelitis, atrioventricular conduction defects, myocarditis, or chronic arthritis. Because Lyme disease is transmitted to humans through the bite of an infected tick, incidence is greatest in the summer months, when ticks are most active.

Cochlear implants

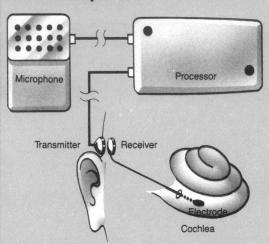

The FDA has approved a new bioelectronic cochlear implant that can restore hearing to people whose deafness has resulted from cochlear damage. The device consists of an implanted receiver and an external microphone, transmitter, and signal processor. Here's how it works: The microphone transmits sound impulses to the signal processor, worn on the patient's belt or tucked in his pocket. The processor then modifies these impulses and sends them through a slender cable to the external transmitter located above and behind the ear. Then, the transmitter sends the signal through the skin to the implanted receiver. Finally, the signal travels from the receiver to the cochlea through a wire electrode; current flowing between this electrode and a nearby ground electrode stimulates auditory nerve fibers, producing impulses that the brain interprets as sounds.

Cochlear implants are either single- or multi-channel. Single-channel implants, now available, allow the wearer to hear loud sounds, such as doorbells, telephone signals, and sirens, as well as subtler sounds, such as running water and voices—including the wearer's own voice, which helps his speech. The single-channel implant *doesn't* enable actual word discrimination, but it does pick up volume differences, which enhances lip-reading ability.

Multi-channel implants, currently under development, may eventually restore hearing to almost normal levels; studies indicate recognition of about 70% of vowels and 30% of consonants in wearers under experimental conditions.

Left ventricular assist device

A new electronically powered mechanical heart pump, the left ventricular assist device (LVAD), may give thousands of people renewed life. Designed to provide an alternative to total heart replacement with an artificial pump, the LVAD augments left ventricular function to help the heart pump more blood. Still somewhat experimental, LVADs have been implanted only temporarily in patients who are awaiting heart transplant, recovering from viral myocarditis, or being weaned from heart-lung machines. Ultimately, its most valuable application will be permanent implantation in the hundreds of thousands of patients with end-stage congestive heart failure (which usually results from left ventricular dysfunction).

The LVAD's pump is implanted in the patient's upper abdomen; hoses from the pump route blood directly from the left ventricle to the ascending or descending aorta. The pump is connected directly to a large power and control console at the patient's bedside or, for ambulatory patients, to a belt-mounted control and power packet that can be plugged in to an external console. Work is continuing on a completely portable device consisting of a permanently implanted controller and transformer driven by a belt-mounted power source.

The LVAD has several advantages over an artificial heart. Because the patient's heart is left in place, normal endocrine and nerve control of its function is preserved, the heart also acts as a back-up pump in case of LVAD malfunction. The LVAD is also less complex (and less costly) than an artificial heart, making it easier to implant and less prone to mechanical failure.

**PORTABLE
LVAD SYSTEM**

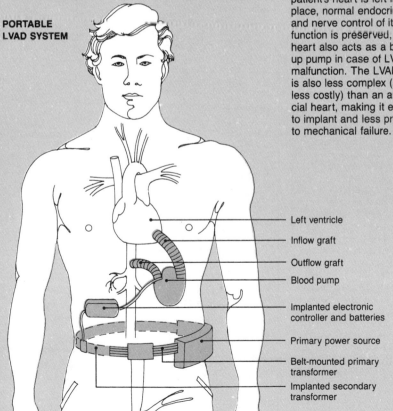

Left ventricle

Inflow graft

Outflow graft

Blood pump

Implanted electronic controller and batteries

Primary power source

Belt-mounted primary transformer

Implanted secondary transformer

Creutzfeldt-Jakob disease

One of the most mysterious human diseases—Creutzfeldt-Jakob disease (CJD)—is the subject of intense research interest as scientists search for clues to its origin. An invariably fatal subacute disorder that produces widespread neuronal degeneration and spongiform pathologic changes in the cerebrum and cerebellum, CJD strikes approximately one person per million population per year. Although so rare, CJD bears some important similarities to common brain disorders, such as Alzheimer's disease, and thus is of great research interest.

CJD, along with kuru in humans and scrapie and Aleutian mink disease in animals, make up a rare class of diseases known as slow or unconventional virus infections—so-called because many months or even years may pass between the time of infection and the appearance of disease symptoms. Scientists suspect that the slow infections may be caused by a previously unknown class of viruslike agents that somehow transmit disease despite not having any DNA or RNA, the two nucleic acids that govern transmission of genetic information in all known species of life. Research on the nature of these agents continues.

Computerized walking

A new therapeutic technique designed to enhance ambulation in some victims of spinal cord injury is currently undergoing clinical evaluation. This technique, known as spinal cord stimulation (SCS), involves neurophysiologic stimulation of the spinal cord through temporary or implanted epidural electrodes usually placed at the T1 to T2 level. The electrodes are connected to an in-line microcomputer and electrostimulator, which control the frequency and amplitude of SCS.

Not every spinal cord injury patient can benefit from SCS therapy. Very few patients with complete spinal cord transection ever regain useful motor control, because both anterior and posterior neuronal elements are necessary for neurologic control of locomotion. SCS is most promising for patients with incomplete lesions who retain some motor activity and locomotion ability. These patients have difficulty walking because of sensory loss and muscle spasticity; in such patients, SCS provides some control over the spasticity and a reduction in its severity and duration, improving volitional control of paralyzed muscles and, in some cases, restoring ambulation.

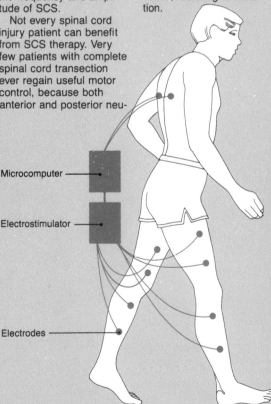

Microcomputer

Electrostimulator

Electrodes

Lasers in ophthalmology

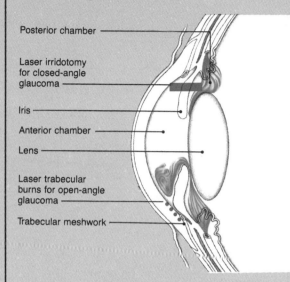

Posterior chamber

Laser irridotomy
for closed-angle
glaucoma

Iris

Anterior chamber

Lens

Laser trabecular
burns for open-angle
glaucoma

Trabecular meshwork

Lasers have many important therapeutic applications; nowhere are they more important than in ophthalmology.

The finely focused high-energy laser beam is ideally suited to the precision work required in ophthalmic surgery. As the beam comes in contact with tissue, light energy is absorbed and converted to heat, creating a burn (photocoagulation). The laser beam is used either to create small nonpenetrating scars or to burn completely through tissue, depending on the ocular disorder being treated.

Treatment of diabetic retinopathy involves photocoagulation of proliferating retinal vessels and focal leak points—requiring as many as 1,000 to 2,000 small retinal burns. Photocoagulation of subretinal or choroidal new vessel membranes can prevent the loss of central vision in age-related macular degeneration from neovascularization.

In open-angle glaucoma, the creation of multiple scars around the trabecular meshwork relieves aqueous humor buildup, reducing intraocular pressure. In closed-angle and chronic narrow-angle glaucoma, laser energy is used to burn through the peripheral iris, creating an opening between the anterior and posterior chambers for the outflow of excess aqueous humor.

Laser therapy can also prevent retinal detachment by repairing peripheral retinal thinning, holes, or tears. And surrounding an existing localized detachment with laser burn scars can limit its size and prevent further damage.

Diabetes developments

Curing or controlling diabetes mellitus continues to be a major research priority. Recent developments include pancreatic islet cell and segmental pancreatic transplantation to replace dysfunctioning tissue, cyclosporine therapy to combat antibodies that destroy islet cells in early stages of Type I diabetes, and an implantable probe and pump that monitors blood glucose levels and automatically delivers insulin.

Unfortunately, each of these techniques has inherent problems. Islet cell or pancreatic tissue transplantation requires massive doses of immunosuppressive agents to reduce the risk of organ rejection, and cyclosporine itself is a potent immunosuppressive agent. (The risks of immunosuppressive therapy include nephrotoxicity, hepatotoxicity, or lymphoma.) Indwelling probes and pumps have proved incompatible with the body's immune system.

So despite the excitement surrounding them, these new developments remain strictly experimental. For now, recent advances in more conventional diabetes treatment—purified insulin, second-generation oral hypoglycemic agents, blood glucose self-monitoring kits, and continuous subcutaneous insulin infusion—offer improved control and reduced side effects.

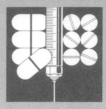

Drugs

Handling antineoplastic drugs safely

Most antineoplastic drugs are highly toxic compounds that cause mutagenic, carcinogenic, or teratogenic effects. For example, chemotherapy for Hodgkin's disease has been linked to an increased risk of leukemia; so has chemotherapy with alkylating agents for ovarian cancer. Some antineoplastic drugs are hazardous on direct contact, causing skin, eye, and mucous membrane irritation, or even tissue ulceration and necrosis. This toxicity causes potential hazards for doctors, pharmacists, and nurses during preparation and administration of parenteral antineoplastic drugs and is the subject of growing concern about occupational exposure. No study has yet irrefutably linked occupational exposure to antineoplastic drugs and increased incidence of cancer, but the known hazards of these agents have focused attention on the need for developing guidelines for handling them safely.

The hazards

The major sources of exposure during the preparation and administration of antineoplastic drugs are primarily through inhalation of the aerosolized drug and direct skin contact.

Various steps during preparation of the drug can cause splattering or spraying of droplets. Such steps include withdrawing needles from drug vials, transferring drugs with syringes or filter straws, breaking open ampules, and expelling air from a syringe to measure the drug volume.

During administration of these drugs, clearing air from a syringe or an I.V. infusion line and leakage at syringe or tubing connections present obvious opportunities for aerosol generation and accidental skin contact.

Improper disposal of waste antineoplastic drugs and of contaminated equipment is another possible source of exposure. Excreta from a patient receiving certain antineoplastic drugs (high-dose methotrexate, for example) may also contain high drug concentrations, posing a potential hazard to the nurses who care for him.

Occupational precautions

Nurses, doctors, and pharmacists can reduce the risk from contact with parenteral antineoplastic drugs by a combination of proper equipment and correct technique. The following guidelines are adapted from recommendations developed by the National Institutes of Health. Review them in light of your own institution's protocol.

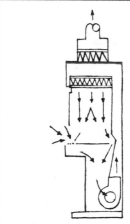

THE CLASS II BIOLOGICAL SAFETY CABINET

The safe preparation of parenteral antineoplastic drugs requires aseptic techniques and a sterile work environment. Many institutions provide this sterile environment by using a horizontal laminar flow work bench. But although this type of unit protects the drug from outside contaminants, it exposes the operator (and other persons in the room) to aerosols generated during drug preparation. In contrast, a Class II *vertical* laminar flow biological safety cabinet (shown above with a canopy that discharges exhaust air to the outdoors) protects both the drug and the operator by filtering incoming and exhaust air through high-efficiency particulate air (HEPA) filters.

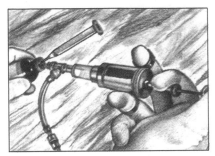

Vent vials.

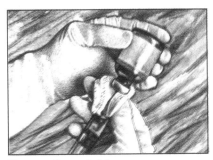

Wrap needles and vials.

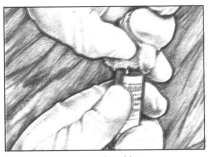

Wrap ampules before breaking.

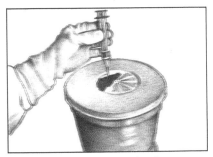

Dispose of used needles and syringes properly.

WHEN PREPARING PARENTERAL ANTINEOPLASTIC DRUGS

• Perform all procedures involved in the preparation of parenteral antineoplastic drugs in a Class II vertical laminar flow biological safety cabinet, if one is available. If you must use a horizontal flow cabinet, turn off the fan before starting drug preparation. If your facility doesn't have a biological safety cabinet, prepare parenteral antineoplastic drugs on a clean table or countertop in a quiet area with no air turbulence.

• Cover the work surface with plastic-backed absorbent paper. This will reduce the potential for dispersion of droplets and spills and will speed clean-up. Change the paper and wipe the work area thoroughly with 70% alcohol, using a disposable towel, after any spills and after each work shift.

• Before beginning drug preparation procedures, put on surgical gloves and either a washable or disposable closed-front surgical gown with knit cuffs. After preparing the drugs, remove and replace overtly contaminated gloves or gowns.

• Vent vials containing reconstituted drugs to reduce internal pressure. This will help reduce the possibility of spraying and spillage when you withdraw the needle from the septum.

• Carefully wrap a sterile, alcohol-dampened cotton swab around the needle and vial top as you withdraw the needle from the vial septum. Similarly, place an alcohol-dampened swab at the needle tip when ejecting air bubbles from a filled syringe. This practice will control the dripping and aerosol production that may occur during these procedures.

• Wipe the external surfaces of syringes and I.V. bottles clean of any drug contamination.

• When breaking the top off a glass ampule, wrap the ampule neck at the anticipated break point with a sterile, alcohol-dampened cotton swab to contain the aerosol produced and also to protect your fingers from laceration by broken glass.

• Make sure you properly identify and date all syringes and I.V. bottles containing antineoplastic drugs. When preparing drugs for other nurses, attachment of another label, such as "Caution: Cancer Chemotherapy—Dispose of Properly," is also recommended.

• When disposing of contaminated needles and syringes, keep them intact to prevent aerosol generation created by clipping needles. Place contaminated needles and syringes in a leakproof and puncture-resistant container. Then place this container, as well as any contaminated bottles, vials, gloves, disposable gowns, cotton swabs, absorbent paper, and other items, in an appropriately labeled, plastic bag–lined box for incineration. Washable gowns may be laundered normally.

• Dispose of waste antineoplastic drugs in accordance with federal and state requirements applicable to toxic chemical waste; check your institution's protocol for specific procedures.

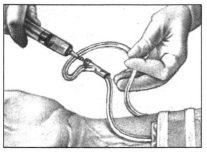

Wear gloves when handling tubing and syringes.

WHEN ADMINISTERING PARENTERAL ANTINEOPLASTIC DRUGS

• Put on a protective outer garment, such as a washable or disposable closed-front surgical gown with knit cuffs. Be sure to wear disposable surgical gloves during any procedures that may entail drug leakage, such as removing air bubbles from syringes and I.V. tubing, injecting drugs into the patient, disconnecting I.V. tubing, and fixing leaky tubing or syringe connections. (*Note:* Whenever possible, use syringes and I.V. sets with Luer-Lok fittings to minimize leakage.) Discard gloves after each use.

• When removing bubbles from syringes or I.V. tubing, carefully place a sterile, alcohol-dampened cotton swab over the tips of needles, syringes, or I.V. tubing to collect any inadvertent drug discharge.

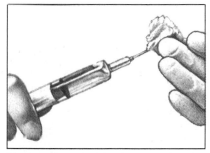

Wrap needles and vials when removing air bubbles.

• Dispose of contaminated needles and syringes intact to prevent aerosol generation created by clipping needles. Place them in a leakproof and puncture-resistant container, and follow the steps outlined above for disposing of contaminated equipment and waste antineoplastic drugs after preparation.

• Take care to avoid skin contact and minimize aerosol generation when handling the excreta of patients who've received antineoplastic drugs; wear disposable surgical gloves and follow standard and approved disposal procedures.

GENERAL PRECAUTIONS

• In case of skin contact with an antineoplastic drug, thoroughly wash the affected area with soap and water. Flush affected eyes with copious amounts of clean water for at least 15 minutes; then seek medical attention.

• *Avoid self-inoculation.* Take care when conducting any procedure that involves the use of needles.

• Wash your hands thoroughly after preparing or administering any antineoplastic drug. Surgical gloves are not a substitute for handwashing.

LARRY NEIL GEVER, RPh, PharmD

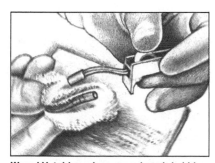

Wrap I.V. tubing when removing air bubbles.

New drugs overcome beta-lactamase resistance

A major problem with conventional antibiotic therapy is beta-lactamase resistance—destruction of the antibiotic's beta-lactam ring by the beta-lactamase enzyme, which resistant bacteria produce. This action disrupts the antibiotic's chemical structure, impairing its effectiveness against infection. Beta-lactamase–resistant bacteria include *Hemophilus influenzae, Staphylococcus aureus, Escherichia coli,* and *Klebsiella.* These organisms cause infections that commonly don't respond to conventional penicillins or cephalosporins. Two new antibiotic drugs— Augmentin (amoxicillin/potassium clavulanate) and Timentin (ticarcillin disodium/potassium clavulanate)— combat infection caused by beta-lactamase–resistant bacteria by attacking the bacteria and the beta-lactamase they produce.

The key ingredient in these new antibiotics is potassium clavulanate, a potent beta-lactamase inhibitor. Potassium clavulanate works by competitive inhibition. The drug's chemical structure contains a beta-lactam ring that has a strong affinity for the beta-lactamases produced by resistant bacteria. Consequently, the beta-lactamases bind with the potassium clavulanate instead of with the antibiotic molecule, blocking destructive enzyme activity

OVERCOMING BETA-LACTAMASE RESISTANCE

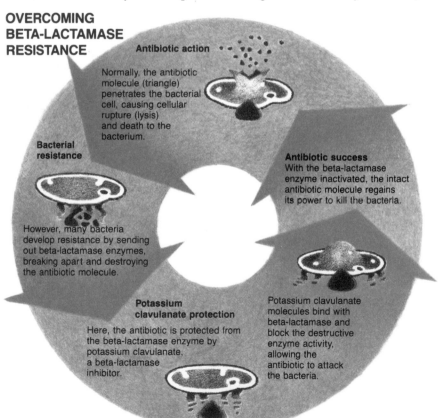

Antibiotic action
Normally, the antibiotic molecule (triangle) penetrates the bacterial cell, causing cellular rupture (lysis) and death to the bacterium.

Bacterial resistance
However, many bacteria develop resistance by sending out beta-lactamase enzymes, breaking apart and destroying the antibiotic molecule.

Potassium clavulanate protection
Here, the antibiotic is protected from the beta-lactamase enzyme by potassium clavulanate, a beta-lactamase inhibitor.

Potassium clavulanate molecules bind with beta-lactamase and block the destructive enzyme activity, allowing the antibiotic to attack the bacteria.

Antibiotic success
With the beta-lactamase enzyme inactivated, the intact antibiotic molecule regains its power to kill the bacteria.

TWO NEW ANTIBIOTICS

amoxicillin/potassium clavulanate
Augmentin, Clavulin♦

Indications
Treatment of lower respiratory tract infections, otitis media, sinusitis, skin and skin-structure infections, and urinary tract infections caused by susceptible strains of gram-positive and gram-negative organisms.

Dosage
Adults: 250 mg (based on the amoxicillin component) P.O. q 8 hours. For more severe infections, 500 mg q 8 hours.
Children: 20 to 40 mg/kg/day (based on the amoxicillin component) given in divided doses q 8 hours.

Adverse reactions
Blood: anemia, thrombocytopenia, thrombocytopenic purpura, eosinophilia, leukopenia.
GI: *nausea*, vomiting, *diarrhea*.
Other: *hypersensitivity (erythematous maculopapular rash, urticaria, anaphylaxis)*, overgrowth of nonsusceptible organisms.

Interactions
Probenecid: increases blood levels of penicillin.
Chloramphenicol, erythromycin, tetracyclines: antibiotic antagonism. Give penicillins at least 1 hour before bacteriostatic antibiotics.

Nursing considerations
• Both the "250" and "500" tablets contain the same amount of clavulanic acid (125 mg). Therefore, two "250" tablets are *not* equivalent to one "500" tablet.
• Particularly useful in clinical settings with a high prevalence of amoxicillin-resistant organisms.
• Give with food to prevent GI distress.
• Incidence of diarrhea is greater than with amoxicillin alone.

Unmarked trade names available in the United States only.
♦ Available in Canada only.
Italicized adverse reactions are common or life-threatening.

ticarcillin disodium/potassium clavulanate
Timentin

Indications
Treatment of septicemia and of lower respiratory tract, urinary tract, bone and joint, and skin and skin-structure infections caused by beta-lactamase–producing bacteria.

Dosage
Adults: 3.1-g vial (contains ticarcillin 3 g and potassium clavulanate 0.1 g) administered by I.V. infusion q 4 to 6 hours.

Adverse reactions
Blood: leukopenia, neutropenia, eosinophilia, *thrombocytopenia*, hemolytic anemia.
CNS: convulsions, neuromuscular excitability.
GI: nausea, diarrhea.
Metabolic: *hypokalemia.*
Local: pain at injection site, vein irritation, phlebitis.
Other: *hypersensitivity (rash, pruritus, urticaria, chills, fever, edema, anaphylaxis)*, overgrowth of nonsusceptible organisms.

Interactions
Chloramphenicol, erythromycin, tetracyclines: antibiotic antagonism. Give penicillins at least 1 hour before bacteriostatic antibiotics.
Probenecid: increases blood levels of penicillin.
Aminoglycoside antibiotics (e.g., gentamicin, tobramycin): chemically incompatible. Don't mix together in I.V. Give 1 hour apart, especially in patients with renal insufficiency.

Nursing considerations
• Dosage should be decreased in patients with impaired hepatic and renal functions.
• Check CBC frequently. Drug may cause thrombocytopenia.
• Monitor serum potassium.
• Administer by I.V. infusion over 30 minutes. Don't give by I.V. push or I.M.
• Particularly useful in clinical settings with a high prevalence of ticarcillin-resistant organisms.

and allowing the antibiotic to attack the bacteria. (See diagram).

Augmentin and Timentin offer new ammunition in the fight against the many bacterial infections that resist conventional penicillins and cephalosporins; they may eliminate the need for multiple antibiotic therapy in certain "mixed" infections.

LARRY NEIL GEVER, RPh, PharmD

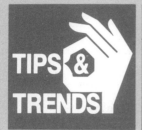

TIPS & TRENDS

IN EATING DISORDERS

Ipecac abuse growing

Syrup of ipecac is being abused by thousands of women who suffer from the eating disorders anorexia nervosa and bulimia, according to the American Pharmaceutical Association (APhA). The APhA estimates that as many as 30,000 young women are abusing ipecac syrup, and it has launched a campaign to increase professional and public awareness of this growing problem.

The substance, a nonprescription drug used to induce vomiting after ingestion of poisons, has been implicated in the deaths of at least four women, including recording artist Karen Carpenter. These women had reportedly misused ipecac—intended for one-time-only use—to induce vomiting after eating. Although nontoxic when used for single instances of poisoning, ipecac syrup can become deadly with chronic use. One of its constituents, the alkaloid emetine, can cause irreversible heart damage and possibly fatal myocarditis.

FOR PROTECTION AGAINST MENINGITIS

Hib vaccine approved

Sometime before age 5, 1 out of every 200 American children—a total of at least 20,000 children per year—becomes infected with a bacterium known as *Hemophilus influenzae* type B (Hib). Nearly two out of three infected children develop Hib meningitis, the most common form of childhood meningitis, which can result in blindness, deafness, seizures, partial paralysis, mental retardation, and, in 10% of cases, death. Hib has also been linked to the development of epiglottitis, pericarditis, cellulitis, pneumonia, and septic arthritis.

The insidious onset of Hib infection often delays diagnosis, reducing the effectiveness of antibiotic drug therapy. But now the FDA has approved a Hib vaccine. According to recent studies, the vaccine reduces the Hib attack rate by 90% and is virtually free of side effects.

Now, the Centers for Disease Control and the Public Health Service recommend that all children between ages 2 and 5 receive the Hib vaccination.

Vaccination at age 18 months is recommended for children in daycare centers and other group settings, and for children at high risk—those without a spleen or with sickle cell disease, leukemia, Hodgkin's disease, or an immunodeficiency. Children immunized at age 18 months may need a second vaccination 18 months later to ensure protection.

Unfortunately, the Hib vaccine doesn't protect children under age 18 months, who make up at least nearly half of Hib victims. But work is continuing on an effective Hib vaccine for this age group as well.

PRESCRIPTION POT

Therapeutic THC approved

Despite numerous studies demonstrating that marijuana effectively minimizes the side effects of cancer chemotherapy and may help in the treatment of other disorders, notably glaucoma and multiple sclerosis, the federal government has not legalized its use in medicine. But now the FDA has approved the manufacture of marijuana's key ingredient—tetrahydrocannabinol, or THC.

Efforts are continuing to legalize natural marijuana for medical use. But for now, the new pharmaceutical THC promises some relief for the approximately 75,000 patients currently undergoing chemotherapy.

NEW DEVELOPMENTS OFFER MANY ADVANTAGES

New drug delivery systems

Traditional drug delivery methods—injection, infusion, and oral administration—have many inherent disadvantages. Depending on the drug and the route of administration, such disadvantages include rapid loss of drug effect, adverse side effects from too much drug in the bloodstream, poor or unpredictable drug absorption, and—perhaps most importantly—inconvenience to patients who require frequent doses, which invites noncompliance with drug therapy. But recent breakthroughs in drug delivery technology promise to eliminate many of these problems.

Transdermal delivery
The new age of drug delivery technology began in 1979 with the development of Transderm-Scop, a skin-adherent patch that provides a constant controlled dose of the anti-motion sickness drug scopolamine. Before long, drug manufacturers began adapting the transdermal delivery method for other drugs. The method's most popular application is transdermal nitroglycerin patches, which continuously release nitroglycerin to prevent angina attacks. Newer applications include antihypertensive drugs (Catapres-TTS) and hormones (TTS-Estradiol).

Externally applied drug delivery isn't limited to transdermal patches. Elastomeric infusors are disposable I.V. pumps now used mainly to deliver

THE OROS SYSTEM

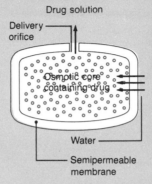

Drug solution

Delivery orifice

Osmotic core containing drug

Water

Semipermeable membrane

PROGESTASERT

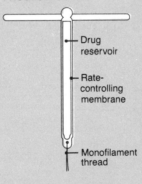

Drug reservoir

Rate-controlling membrane

Monofilament thread

cancer chemotherapy. Worn on the abdomen, this device frees a patient from attachment to a pole-mounted I.V. bottle. Another external delivery system helps treat patients with glaucoma. This system, known as Ocusert, is a thin, flexible wafer that's placed under the eyelid and delivers a weekly dosage of pilocarpine, a powerful miotic drug.

Oral delivery
The new drug delivery technology extends to oral

drugs as well. The OROS (oral osmotic) system consists of a solid drug core coated with a semipermeable polymer membrane that contains a single tiny orifice. After it's swallowed, the system functions as a minute osmotic pump, admitting water through the membrane and releasing medication through the orifice at a controlled rate for up to 24 hours.

In contrast, the Pennkinetic drug delivery system, now used for several liquid cough and cold medicines, employs the principle of ion exchange to control drug release. Drug molecules and an ion-exchange polymer are bound together to form a drug-polymer complex. This complex is coated with a semipermeable membrane of varying thickness, depending on the drug release rate. Sodium and potassium ions in body fluids penetrate the membrane and displace the drug molecules on the surface of the drug-polymer complex, releasing the drug at a controlled rate.

Implantable delivery
Implantable drug delivery systems also hold great promise. One of the first of these systems, an intra-uterine contraceptive known as Progestasert, releases controlled amounts of progesterone directly into the uterus. The tiny, flexible device prevents pregnancy for 1 year after insertion.

Beta blockers and hypertension

For years, the stepped-care approach to treating patients with hypertension almost always began with the use of thiazide diuretics. Beta blockers and other adrenergic inhibitors were reserved for Step 2 care, if the patient didn't respond to diuretic therapy. But recent findings in antihypertensive treatment are changing this traditional approach: now, more and more doctors are prescribing beta blockers instead of diuretics for Step 1 care of certain patients.

Why the change? Well, despite their effectiveness and relatively low cost, diuretics have been proven to cause serious adverse effects in some patients. And although beta blockers can also produce side effects, overall adverse effects seem less severe than those of diuretics.

So now, depending on the patient, you can expect to see either a diuretic or a beta blocker prescribed for Step 1 of antihypertensive therapy. Diuretics are still recommended for patients over age 50, patients with low-renin hypertension (a form of hypertension that predominantly affects blacks), and patients with peripheral vascular disease or chronic pulmonary disease. But for hypertensive patients under age 50 and those with ischemic heart disease, beta blockers are the new drugs of choice.

STEPPED-CARE HYPERTENSION TREATMENT

Step 1

| Begin with less than a full dose of a thiazide-type diuretic. | OR | Begin with less than a full dose of beta blockers. |

Proceed to a full dose if necessary and desirable.

If blood pressure control isn't achieved, proceed to Step 2.

Step 2

| Add a small dose of a beta blocker or another adrenergic inhibiting agent. | OR | Add a small dose of a thiazide-type diuretic. |

Proceed to a full dose if necessary and desirable; drug substitutions may be made at this point.

If blood pressure control isn't achieved, proceed to Step 3.

Step 3

Add a vasodilator—hydralazine, or minoxidil for resistant cases.

If blood pressure control isn't achieved, proceed to Step 4.

Step 4

Add guanethidine monosulfate.

Tissue plasminogen activator

An experimental drug—human tissue-type plasminogen activator (TPA)—may revolutionize the treatment of acute myocardial infarction (MI).

As reported in a major government-sponsored study, injecting TPA during the early stages of an acute MI quickly dissolves coronary artery blood clots, preventing extensive and often fatal myocardial damage.

According to the study, TPA dissolves blood clots twice as fast as streptokinase, a similar, commercially available drug that's been used for several years. TPA has other advantages as well: It's more specific for fibrin clots than streptokinase, less antigenic, and less likely to have systemic anti-clotting effects or to cause excessive bleeding. And unlike streptokinase, which is most effective when administered through cardiac catheterization—a time-consuming and sometimes risky procedure—TPA begins working almost immediately after simple intravenous injection, saving precious time.

Tocainide—the new oral lidocaine

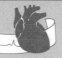

A new oral analog of lidocaine tocainide (Tonocard)—is now available to treat adults with symptomatic ventricular dysrhythmias. It's the first new oral antiarrhythmic to be approved by the FDA in almost a decade.

A class 1B antiarrhythmic, tocainide has been proven effective in treating premature ventricular contractions and ventricular tachycardia in patients with cardiac disorders, including myocardial infarction, congestive heart failure, and valvular heart disease.

Because tocainide is very similar in structure and properties to lidocaine, it's particularly valuable for patients being switched from intravenous lidocaine to oral antiarrhythmic therapy.

Side effects are usually mild and transient; most common reactions include dizziness, nausea, numbness or paresthesia, and tremors. But because tocainide may have a slight negative inotropic effect and may slightly increase peripheral resistance, it should be used cautiously in patients with heart failure, particularly when given with a beta blocker. In addition, it's contraindicated in any patient with second- or third-degree AV block who doesn't have an artificial pacemaker.

A new use for methotrexate

Conventional treatment of rheumatoid arthritis—mainly gold salt or corticosteroids—is often ineffective and sometimes produces unacceptable side effects. But recent studies suggest that low doses of methotrexate, a folic acid antagonist traditionally used with other drugs in cancer chemotherapy, also reduces pain and swelling in some cases of rheumatoid arthritis.

The serious side effects of long-term, high-dose methotrexate administration are well-known. Because more research is needed on the effects of chronic low-dose therapy, the FDA hasn't yet approved the clinical use of methotrexate to treat rheumatoid arthritis—even though the practice is already widespread.

Minoxidil abuse

A side effect of the antihypertensive drug minoxidil—hypertrichosis—has excited thousands of prematurely balding men—and shady entrepreneurs that exploit their lust for a hair restorer that works.

Although the FDA hasn't approved topical use of minoxidil ointment for hair restoration, advertising touting the drug as a "miracle" hair restorer has led to unauthorized sale and use.

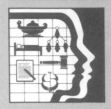

Law, ethics, and professional practice

MEETING THE
D.R.G.
CHALLENGE

"With a creative–and cost-conscious– attitude, you can meet the DRG challenge: providing quality patient care in less time at a lower cost."

BY LILLEE GELINAS, RNC, MSN

A
lthough the time and money you can spend on patients have decreased, your responsibilities...have increased.

In 1982, a Medicare patient admitted for cataract surgery could have been hospitalized for up to 6 days at a substantial cost. Now the same patient would be treated on an outpatient basis for a fraction of the cost. This shift to shorter patient stays and reduced costs began in 1983, with the passage of laws mandating a prospective payment system—a hospital reimbursement system designed to control soaring health care costs.

In the past, hospitals were reimbursed retrospectively for Medicare patients on a per diem basis, where the number of hospitalization days was multiplied by the hospital's daily rate. The newer prospective payment system reimburses hospitals based on a fixed rate for a specific illness, or diagnosis-related group (DRG).

DRGs: What they are and how they work
The DRG system helps classify a patient and determine how much his hospital stay should cost. Assignment of a patient to a particular DRG depends on six key factors:
• principal diagnosis
• principal surgical procedure and secondary diagnosis
• diagnostic and other therapeutic procedures
• age
• sex
• discharge status (routinely discharged to home, discharged against medical orders, transferred, or died).
These factors guide patient placement into one of 468 groups. Patients in each group should consume similar hospital

resources and, therefore, cost the same to treat.

Once the patient is assigned to a DRG, Medicare will pay a predetermined flat rate for all of his inpatient services. If the patient's care costs more than the flat rate, the hospital must absorb the difference. But if it costs less, the hospital keeps the difference—a reward for cost containment.

DRGs' effects on nursing
DRGs demand cost-consciousness, especially in nurses. All other effects of DRGs stem from this central concern. As a direct result of DRGs, you'll have to shift your focus from holistic patient care to separate body parts or diseases. Because of DRGs' restriction on length of stay, you'll be caring for patients who are more acutely ill when they enter the hospital—and when they leave. With shorter hospitalizations, you'll have to concentrate the care you give and rely on ancillary personnel to do nonnursing tasks, such as distributing linen or transporting specimens. Nurses aren't the only ones who will be affected so dramatically by DRGs. (See *DRGs' Effects on Health Care*, page 172.)

Although the time and money you can spend on patients have decreased, your responsibilities certainly haven't. They have *increased*. You may be directed to look after patients less comprehensively than before, but you'll still be legally responsible for their care. You'll be caring for more acutely ill patients in less time, yet you'll still be expected to give them comprehensive care. Earlier discharges will require more extensive patient teaching and

*H*ow do you cope with shrinking resources and growing responsibilities? You adapt.

will often require coordination of continuing care by a home health care nurse. You'll need to document all patient care *in detail* for proper reimbursement. You'll even have to conserve patient and unit supplies and help evaluate products for their ability to meet your needs at the best price.

Adapting to DRGs

So how do you cope with shrinking resources and growing responsibilities? You adapt. By adjusting some of your work habits and looking for creative ways to meet the DRG challenge, you may do more than adapt—you may even thrive. Here are some techniques you can use to start adapting now:

• *Work closely with nursing administrators to identify ways to give quality patient care economically.* Remember, as hospitals continue to trim costs, the minimal standards of care—the minimum amount of nursing intervention each patient receives—will be redefined. You can also expect redefinition of clinical death based on economic and ethical considerations. To make your opinions heard on these issues, participate in decision making as much as possible. This may mean anything from joining a Quality Circle to representing staff nurses on your hospital's committees.

• *Analyze problems and look for shortcuts.* For instance, detailed documentation is essential, but it consumes valuable time—time that you could spend with a patient. So try using charting forms instead of narrative notes and store them at the patient's bedside for easy access. You'll have bet-

ter documentation in less time. Another timesaving option for documenting patient care could be the use of computers.

• *Specialize.* Increased nursing specialization leads to increased nursing productivity. The more specialized you become, the better you can deal with a specific group of patients. You'll intervene faster and more efficiently because you'll know more about those patients.

To raise your level of nursing knowledge—and efficiency—discuss options for continuing education with your nursing administrators. You may want to suggest inservice sessions, seminars, and flexible hours for nurses who want to expand their education outside the hospital.

• *Work with other nurses and other departments more effectively.* Take full advantage of the specialized skills of other nurses. Collaborate with other departments to help your hospital deliver the most efficient and comprehensive care possible. Remember, if you lose a patient because of poorly coordinated care, everybody in your hospital loses, too.

• *Rethink your patient-teaching methods.* Who says patient teaching has to be one-on-one? Group teaching can be just as effective plus save time for other important nursing duties. Instead of writing out individual instructions, consider preparing and copying your own patient-teaching materials or obtaining them from such organizations as the American Heart Association, the American Red Cross, or the American Diabetes Association.

*N*urses aren't the only ones who will be affected so dramatically by DRGs.

D.R.G.s' EFFECTS ON HEALTH CARE

The major effect of DRGs on health care is *change*. Payment methods have already changed, promoting cost control and price competition. Because of this, access to health care and the quality of that care may also change. The chart below shows how DRGs will affect the four major parts of the health care system: the patients, hospitals, doctors, and *you*.

EFFECTS ON PATIENTS

- Benefits and eligibility will decrease for those in federally sponsored programs.
- Health care programs won't cover patients' extra expenses.

- Patients with private health insurance may have greater access to higher-quality care.
- Patients will have to lower their expectations of the health care system.

EFFECTS ON HOSPITALS

- Multi-hospital organizations will evolve to help smaller hospitals become more competitive.
- New types of health care providers, such as HMOs and alternative delivery systems, will compete with hospitals for less acutely ill outpatients.
- Emphasis on hospital care will shift to ambulatory and home health services.
- Capital financing will be harder to attract.
- Hospital staffs will favor lower-cost health care workers to cut costs.
- Contract nursing services will supplement hospital staffs more frequently.
- Hospitals will emphasize advertising and develop marketing strategies to remain competitive.

EFFECTS ON DOCTORS

- Incomes will diminish as DRGs regulate doctors' fees.
- Supply of doctors will increase, threatening nurses' independent practice in such roles as midwives and nurse practitioners.
- Hospitals will allow less autonomy as they enforce cost-containing standards for patient care.
- Doctors and other groups will redefine minimum standards of care and, possibly, clinical death.

EFFECTS ON NURSES

- Nursing services will be based on actual patient care rather than on a percentage of the room and board charge.
- Less expensive nursing delivery systems, such as team or functional nursing, will be more popular.
- Home health care will offer more job opportunities—especially in acute care—as hospitals' demand for nurses decreases.
- Patients will need "high touch" nursing skills in the high technology environment.
- Collective bargaining efforts will grow stronger as nurses resist staff cuts and try to maintain the quality of patient care.
- Increased specialization by nurses will help increase productivity.
- Nurses will develop a "bottom line" business orientation.

*D*RGs are here to stay. But there is life after DRGs.

- *Establish a support group.* Under the DRG system, your job may become more crucial, demanding, and even psychologically draining. A support group, coffee klatch, or journal club can give you a chance to share your concerns and help each other cope with pressures on the job.
- *Network with nurses from other units and other hospitals.* This not only offers additional support, but may also provide ideas that you can use in your unit or hospital.
- *Consider yourself an autonomous patient care manager.* Decentralized hospital management will make you more responsible for moment-to-moment decisions about your patient's care. As an autonomous patient care manager, you'll have greater individual accountability. So make sure your nurses' notes are clear and legible. You may also have more responsibility for discharging patients on time, according to their DRG classification. So use your resources wisely.
- *Relax after work.* Such activities as aerobics, jogging, and hobbies can help you deal with the stress of your demanding job—*and* make you more productive at work, too.
- *Be flexible.* Expect change, including hospital consolidation, restructuring, and reorganization, and be prepared to "go with it." These changes may even affect the brands of nursing supplies available on each unit, such as I.V. lines, Foley catheters, infusion pumps, and cardiac monitors. Here's why. In the budget-conscious times ahead, hospitals will band together to get substantial discounts on bulk purchases. If

your hospital joins such an alliance, you may have to get used to new brands of equipment and supplies.

Hospitals may hire agency nurses for extra coverage when the census is high. If your hospital does this, stay flexible. Help the agency nurses adjust by orienting them to the floor and by being available to help during the shift.
- *Be creative.* Creativity at all levels will help nursing survive the budget crunch ahead. Don't hesitate to try new strategies that could make your hospital run more efficiently or make your job easier. Work with others to develop more efficient nurses' notes, better ways to write care plans, quicker patient-teaching methods, faster discharge-planning strategies, and smoother ways to interface with home health care agencies. Here's a strategy you may want to try: Make rounds with home health care nurses before patients go home. This kind of idea can improve the continuity of quality care.

DRGs are here to stay

By October 1986, Medicare's prospective payment system and DRG plan will be phased in completely. Private insurers are expected to demand prospective payment rates as well. In some states, such as New Jersey and Massachusetts, *all* patients are classified by DRGs, and other states may begin to do this, too.

So it looks like DRGs are here to stay. But there *is* life after DRGs. With a creative—and cost-conscious—attitude, you can meet the DRG challenge: providing quality patient care in less time at a lower cost.

IS A NURSE A PROFESSIONAL?

"Education is
a major factor in the
courts' division
on whether registered
nurses are—
in the legal sense of
the term—
professionals."

BY ELEANOR TINTNER SEGAL, RN, BS, JD

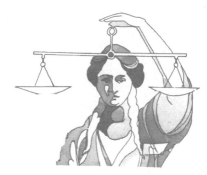

Are you a professional? If you're like most nurses, you'll answer a resounding *yes*. However, a court of law may not treat you as a professional. And that difference in treatment can make a *big* difference to you. Here's how.

Most lawsuits brought against nurses are for negligence, or acting in a manner that no reasonable person, guided by considerations that normally regulate human behavior, would act. Lawsuits against doctors, however, are usually for malpractice, or an act of negligence committed in the course of carrying out *professional* responsibilities—a charge with three advantages.

Statutes of limitations
These statutes ensure that lawsuits are brought within a reasonable time after an alleged act has occurred. Because of the growing number of malpractice suits, many states have enacted shorter statutes of limitations for professional negligence (about 1 year) than ordinary negligence (about 2 years). The courts are almost unanimous in rejecting a shorter statute of limitations for nurses. So if a patient sues a doctor (for malpractice) and a nurse (for ordinary negligence), the statute of limitations may protect the doctor from standing trial while the nurse remains liable—an advantage for the doctor.

Standards of care
In malpractice cases, the courts always use a professional standard of care to

evaluate a doctor's actions. This second legal advantage ensures that the court will compare the doctor's alleged actions with the actions of a prudent and competent peer (another doctor).

The conduct of a nurse charged with ordinary negligence isn't always compared to that of another nurse, but to that of any prudent person. That comparison is unfair. Hospital patients expect more than ordinary prudence; they expect to be cared for by a well-educated, experienced nurse.

In order for the courts to apply a professional standard of care to nursing, they need a clear definition of the scope of nursing practice. Nurse practice acts usually don't provide this. They vary from state to state and are often unclear, restrictive, and unrepresentative of the actual scope of nursing practice.

Medical practice acts, on the other hand, clearly define the three basic responsibilities of doctors—diagnosis, treatment, and prescription of medications. Unlike nurse practice acts, which often state what a nurse *can't* do, medical practice acts are not restrictive. Once licensed in a state, a doctor is granted unlimited authority to perform all medical acts.

Expert witnesses
As a rule, an expert witness is called to testify in a malpractice case so the jury can better evaluate the doctor's actions, which the jury's not qualified to

NURSE'S GUIDE TO B.S.N. PROGRAMS

If you want to earn a BSN degree, you can choose from 534 colleges and universities in the United States. As of 1984, 146 of these institutions offered programs designed *exclusively* for RNs. The schools listed below have these specialized programs and are accredited by the National League of Nurses (NLN)—a professional accreditation that ensures a high-quality program. For more information about educational opportunities, contact the school directly or get in touch with the NLN or your State Board of Nursing.

CALIFORNIA
California State College, San Bernardino
California State College Sonoma, Rohnert Park
California State University, Fullerton
Holy Names College, Oakland
The Consortium of the California State University, Long Beach
University of California, San Francisco
University of San Diego

COLORADO
Mesa College, Grand Junction
Metropolitan State College, Denver
University of Southern Colorado, Pueblo
University of Denver

CONNECTICUT
University of Hartford, West Hartford

FLORIDA
University of West Florida, Pensacola

IDAHO
Boise State University

ILLINOIS
Governors State University, Park Forest South
McKendree College, Lebanon
Sangamon State University, Springfield

INDIANA
Purdue University, Calumet Campus, Hammond
Purdue University, West Lafayette

IOWA
Briar Cliff College, Sioux City
University of Dubuque

KANSAS
Saint Mary College, Leavenworth

KENTUCKY
Northern Kentucky University, Highland Heights
Western Kentucky University, Bowling Green

LOUISIANA
Loyola University in New Orleans

MASSACHUSETTS
Worcester State College

MINNESOTA
Moorhead State University

MISSOURI
Maryville College, Saint Louis
Southwest Missouri State University, Springfield
University of Missouri at St. Louis

NEBRASKA
University of Nebraska at Omaha

NEVADA
University of Nevada at Las Vegas

NEW JERSEY
Felician College, Lodi
Jersey City State College
Kean College of New Jersey, Union
St. Peter's College, Jersey City

NEW YORK
Daemon College, Amherst
Dominican College, Orangeburg
Elmira College
Medgar Evers College of CUNY, Brooklyn
Mercy College, Dobbs Ferry
Pace University, New York
Pace University, Pleasantville
State University College at Utica/Rome, Utica

OHIO
Cleveland State University
Miami University, Oxford
Ohio University College of Health and Human Services, Athens
Otterbein College, Westerville
Youngstown State University
Xavier University, Edgecliff College, Cincinnati

OREGON
Southern Oregon State College, Ashland

PENNSYLVANIA
Gwynedd-Mercy College, Gwynedd Valley
Hahnemann Medical College and Hospital, Philadelphia
La Salle College, Philadelphia
Slippery Rock University of Pennsylvania

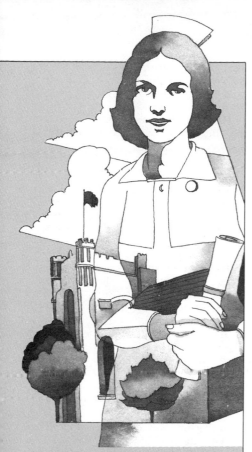

SOUTH CAROLINA
University of South Carolina, Spartanburg

TENNESSEE
Memphis State University
Southern Missionary College, Collegedale

TEXAS
Corpus Christi State University

VERMONT
Vermont College, Montpelier

VIRGINIA
Marymount College of Virginia, Division of
Nursing, Arlington

WASHINGTON
Gonzaga University, Spokane
Western Washington University, Bellingham

WEST VIRGINIA
Marshall University, Huntington

WISCONSIN
Viterbo College, La Crosse

judge for itself. Also, the calling of expert witnesses reflects the court's respect for the medical profession, acknowledging that only a doctor can correctly define the standards of behavior that apply to another member of this profession.

When it comes to judging nursing actions or decisions, however, the courts are inconsistent—sometimes calling expert witnesses, sometimes not.

Recent cases have used the technical level of the nursing action in question as a yardstick for determining the need for an expert witness. Usually, the more technical the act, the more likely an expert will be required to testify. But even then, the court sometimes accepts doctors, not nurses, as experts in nursing care. This practice presents two problems. First, doctors are not qualified to discuss nursing standards; they're experts in medical care, not nursing care. Second, if a nurse's attorney calls another nurse as an expert witness, the plaintiff's attorney can gain a subtle advantage by countering with an expert witness who's a doctor. Because juries tend to have a higher opinion of doctors, they may subconsciously give more credence to the doctor's testimony, even though the nurse knows much more about the nursing standards by which the nurse-defendant should be judged.

The legal concept of professionalism

To overcome these three serious disadvantages that nurses experience in court, we need to begin with the legal concept of professionalism. How do the courts determine whether a particular field is really a profession?

Historically, the most important factor has been a rigorous and systematic educational program for those who wish to enter the field. Other factors come into play—a code of ethics, an element of altruism, a strong research program, and a certain authority and prestige associated with the field.

Nursing immediately meets two of these criteria—a code of ethics and an element of altruism. Nursing research is progressing well. But nursing doesn't have the authority and prestige that the courts tend to associate with professions. Most of all, it doesn't have the one essential criterion, according to the courts—an intensive, systematic preparation for entry into the field.

Strict, consistent educational requirements are considered necessary for several reasons: they limit access to the field, weeding out the uncommitted and unqualified; they ensure that aspirants receive the specialized knowledge they'll need to work within the field; and they separate the professionals from workers in related but nonprofessional fields.

In nursing, three educational programs enable a graduate nurse to sit for state boards: the 2-year associate degree program; the 2- to 3-year hospital-based diploma program; and the 4-year baccalaureate degree program. (In contrast, medical and law schools essentially follow one program.) Once graduate nurses pass their state boards, they are registered and considered by statute to be professional nurses. However, because of these different educational paths, the courts continue to be split on the question of whether registered nurses arc— in the legal sense of the term—professionals.

A case for the entry-level BSN

The disparity between the educational curricula of nursing students and medical students is often viewed by the courts (and the public) as the difference between "training" and "education." It contributes significantly to the inferior image of nursing that is acted upon in courts of law. To dispel this image once and for all, nursing must consider standardizing the educational program for entrance into the field. If you think that's not possible, consider this: American medical education didn't become standardized until the beginning of this century when medical schools introduced a consistent curriculum requiring undergraduate and graduate education, as well as practicum.

Perhaps the time has come for nursing to take the same giant step that medicine took decades ago: standardize all nursing education—and make the bachelor's degree (BSN) the minimum educational requirement for registered nurses. The new standards could be implemented gradually over several decades. New bachelor's degree graduates could slowly replace nondegree nurses now in practice. And all current nondegree nurses could be protected by a grandfather clause, which would allow them to continue practicing without meeting the new qualifications.

Standardized nursing education at the BSN level can confer a professional status to nurses and remove legal handicaps in court. But a bachelor's program offers other benefits, too:
• exposure to a wide range of social and cultural experiences
• intellectual and academic standards equal to those of students in other fields
• a chance to study with a highly qualified nursing faculty
• *special* education in nursing theory and practice plus *general* education in humanities and sciences
• facilities for research
• the educational background needed for graduate study in nursing: a stepping stone to teaching, administration, expert practice, or research
• qualification to give high-standard nursing care and to direct the care given by others on the nursing team.

Nursing doesn't exist in a vacuum. In the harsh reality of the courtroom, nursing's present educational system comes off looking second-rate, deprives us of our professional status, and creates significant legal handicaps. BSN-level nursing education would compare more favorably with that of other professions. Maybe then the courts would unanimously agree that nurses *are* professionals.

Opportunities for nurse entrepreneurs

More and more nurses are starting their own businesses. These nurse entrepreneurs have found endless opportunities in child care, adult day care, home health care, private duty nursing, staff relief nursing, pain control, weight loss counseling, stress management, continuing nursing education, patient teaching, and health risk management.

A nurse entrepreneur can start a business alone, with other nurses, or in connection with a health care institution or corporation. If you'd like to be an entrepreneur, use these tips to get started.

Research your business
First, explore your area of interest by attending seminars or courses, doing research, and getting a special certificate or degree, if needed. Think about how to make your service unique or better than the competition. Next, check your state's nurse practice act to make sure your idea falls within the

realm of nursing practice. Join the local or state chapter of the American Nurses' Association to make contacts and to find out what others are doing that could help or hurt your business.

Contact your state health department or other agency to learn about specific regulations and legal requirements for your business. For example, day care regulations may require a specific staff-to-child ratio. Find out how to start your own business by attending a course or by asking your state employment agency or better business bureau for information. Before you open, be sure to get malpractice insurance.

Market your business
Now all you need are clients. If you sell your services through a hospital or related business, clients will come to you almost automatically. But if you're an independent entrepreneur, you'll have to work harder to market your services. Call on doctor's offices, head nurses, hospital social workers, and other health care professionals to get clients by referral. Advertise in local newspapers, nursing journals, newsletters of professional associations, or direct mail pieces targeted to your audience.

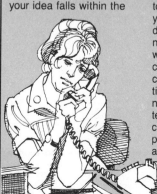

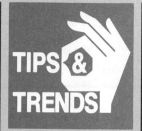

Home health care needs nurses

Since DRGs have taken effect, occupancy rates in hospitals have dwindled and staff members have been laid off. At the same time, home health care has grown and so have job opportunities for nurses in this field.

Basically, three types of home care organizations exist: local branches of public health services, independent agencies, and hospital-based programs, which are expanding most rapidly. All three have grown in response to the new reluctance to hospitalize patients and the tendency to encourage early discharge. Patients need home care more than ever before and are more likely to need complex nursing care as well. For these reasons, today's home health care nurses must be competent to use highly technical equipment, such as mechanical ventilators and I.V. infusion pumps. They must assess and manage patients independently and plan for their future health needs.

NEW LAWS REQUIRE DIRECT PAYMENTS TO NURSES

Support grows for third-party reimbursement

In 1948, the American Nurses' Association saw the need for direct, third-party reimbursement. Thirty years later, supporters finally convinced legislators to pass the first bills for direct reimbursement. Now 17 states have adopted laws that mandate direct third-party reimbursement from health insurers to different types of nurses. (See map below.)

And support continues to grow. In the wake of DRGs, patients and insurers want freedom of choice and quality health care that's less expensive. In many cases, nursing can meet these needs.

Direct third-party reimbursement can benefit nurses, too. It can raise the status of the nursing profession by recognizing the nurse's role in health care, making her contributions highly visible, and giving her more autonomy.

If your state doesn't allow third-party reimbursement, you can help lobby for legislation. Contact your state's nursing organization for more information.

KEY:
● Nurse midwives
■ Registered nurses
☐ Nurse practitioners
● Nurse anesthetists
■ Psychiatric nurse specialists

WHO RECEIVES THIRD-PARTY REIMBURSEMENT

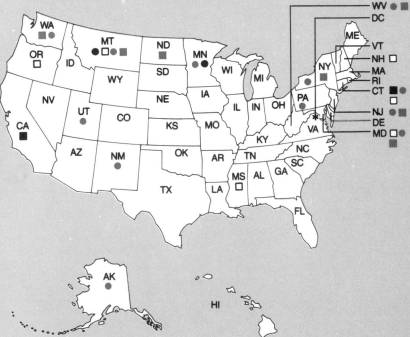

MAKING LIFE OR DEATH DECISIONS

D.R.G.s' IMPACT

Nurses liable for patient teaching

Now patient teaching is more important than ever. Why? Because as DRGs shorten hospital stays, patients are more likely to be discharged with complex equipment, such as mechanical ventilators, or with the need for skilled treatments, such as postoperative wound care. And if a patient is harmed because of lack of information about his condition, care, or treatment, he may sue *you* for negligence.

Here are some ways to make your patient teaching more efficient and to avoid the possibility of future litigation:

• When a patient can't monitor or perform treatments by himself, explain all discharge instructions to a responsible family member or friend. If a responsible "other" isn't available, refer the patient to a home care nursing agency.

• Use printed instruction forms, teaching plans, and oral directions.

• Review the information with the patient or "other" until he's comfortable with it. Check his learning with open-ended questions and return demonstrations.

• When you've completed your teaching, sign the instruction form along with the patient and "other."

• If you strongly believe that the patient won't receive proper follow-up care, notify the doctor.

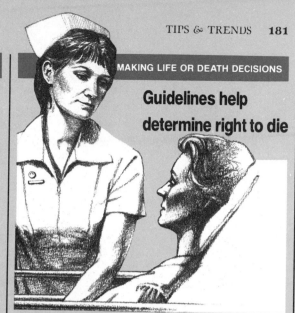

MAKING LIFE OR DEATH DECISIONS

Guidelines help determine right to die

As medical technology advances, it raises complex ethical and legal questions about the right to die. New guidelines provide some answers.

Harvard criteria

The Harvard criteria define death as loss of brain stem and spinal reflexes and isoelectric EEGs over at least 24 hours (brain death). They provide a legal definition of death that supersedes the traditional one—loss of cardio-respiratory function—and allows the health care team to stop advanced life support. About 40 states accept this definition.

Living wills

A seriously ill or terminally ill patient may choose to end his pain and his family's suffering and expense by making a living will. Usually, a living will is a written document signed by the patient and witnesses. It spells out exactly what the patient wants and doesn't want (such as resuscitation and advanced life support)

when he can no longer participate in discussions about his care. About 25 states accept living wills as legal guidance in life or death decisions.

Additional guidelines

For patients who aren't covered by these criteria, you may be held liable for any care you do *or* do not give. To protect yourself and provide the proper care, follow these guidelines:

• Discuss extraordinary measures with the patient's family. Explain their feelings to the doctor and pass his decision to the health care team.

• Talk to your nursing supervisor about situations that you're unsure of, such as doctor's orders to withhold feedings for a newborn, and family's and doctor's orders that conflict. If necessary, contact your state nurses' association or even the state attorney general's office to discuss the legal implications of your actions.

• Document all assessments and interventions.

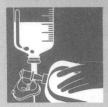

Nursing procedures

How to prepare a sterile field

Many procedures require surgical asepsis, which is the absence of microorganisms from an area. Before performing procedures that require surgical asepsis or sterile technique, you must prepare a sterile field, an organism-free area. The sterile field must include nearby furniture, which must have sterile drapes, and personnel, who must be properly dressed.

Expect to use sterile technique in the operating room, in the labor and delivery department, and for some bedside nursing and medical procedures. When you must prepare for a sterile procedure, such as urinary catheterization or central venous line insertion, check your hospital manual to review the steps involved and to determine the equipment you'll need.

Equipment

Sterile tray with reusable supplies or sterile package with disposable supplies; other sterile supplies, as needed; antiseptic cleansing solution; sterile mask, cap, and gown, as needed; sterile gloves; sterile solution, as needed; sterile basin or other container; sterile drapes.

Essential steps

• Gather all supplies before you start the procedure. Be sure to get a few extra supplies to replace any that may become contaminated. If possible, have another nurse stand by to get additional supplies or to help you during the procedure.

• Explain the procedure to the patient before you begin. This should reduce his fear and gain his cooperation.

• Check the sterilization tape, expiration date, and integrity of the sterile kit or package. If it's out of date, opened, or damaged, do *not* use it.

• Wash your hands thoroughly.

• Open the supplies on a clean, flat working area above waist level, such as an over-the-bed stand. Keeping your arm away from the sterile field, pick up the package's outermost flap and open it away from you. If the package has several flaps, unfold them one at a time, opening the last flap toward your body, so you don't have to reach over the sterile field. Avoid touching the inside of the wrapper, except for a 1″ border along the edges that's considered contaminated.

• Check your supplies to see if you need any others, such as an indwelling (Foley) catheter or cotton balls. To add sterile supplies to the sterile field, grasp the wrapper and peel—don't tear—it open. Without touching it or allowing it to slide over the wrapper, gently flip the object onto the sterile field.

• Wash your hands vigorously with an antiseptic solution, cleaning under the fingernails and between the fingers. Keep your hands up as you rinse, and let the water drip from your elbows.

• Put on a gown, cap, mask, and gloves, as directed in your hospital's procedure manual. Many procedures require only sterile gloves. (See *How to Put on Sterile Gloves*, page 184.)

• Pour a sterile solution with the help of another nurse. A sterile-gloved nurse must set or hold a sterile basin or other container at the edge of the sterile field. Without reaching across the sterile field, an ungloved nurse must pour the solution as she holds only the mouth of the container over the basin. Once you open a sterile solution bottle, you must use or discard its contents, because the cap can't be replaced without contaminating the pouring edges.

Outside of operating room procedures, you may have to pour a sterile solution by yourself. Remove the cap with ungloved hands (being careful not to touch the inside of the cap). Do not rest it on its lip or place it inside the sterile field. As you hold the solution bottle with the label facing the palm of your hand, pour a few milliliters of solution into a plastic cup or waste re-

HOW TO PUT ON STERILE GLOVES

All sterile procedures require you to wear sterile gloves. But if you put them on improperly, they won't remain sterile. Here's how to maintain sterility when donning these gloves:

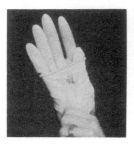 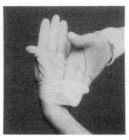 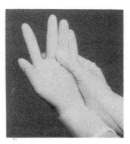

1. Using your left hand, pick up the right glove by the folded edge of the cuff. Insert your right hand into the glove and pull it down, leaving the cuff turned up.

2. To pick up the other glove, slip the fingers of your right hand under the left glove's turned up cuff. Next insert your left hand into the glove and pull it down over the fingers. Then unroll the left cuff by leaving the fingers of your right hand in the cuff fold and pulling down. Unroll the right cuff in the same way.

3. Finally, adjust both gloves so they fit properly. Be careful not to let the outside of your gloves touch your skin, or they could be contaminated.

ceptacle to eliminate contaminants around the lip. Then pour the required amount of solution into the sterile basin or container. The solution container can be reused.

• Drape your patient, as needed. After opening the sterile drape package using sterile technique, pick up a corner of the drape and let it unfold by gravity. Next, grasp the adjacent corner, and place the free edge where you want it. Then carefully lower the rest of the drape over the patient without touching him or his linens, which could contaminate your gloves.

Special considerations
Remember these principles when preparing for sterile procedures:
• All items in a sterile field must be sterile. A sterile object or field will be contaminated if an unsterile object touches it.
• If you can't see it, it's contaminated. Consider any sterile object or field that's out of your range of vision or held below the waist contaminated. So keep sterile objects in front of you.
• Microorganisms can travel through air and contaminate sterile material. Therefore, minimize all movement to prevent air currents around the sterile field, and wear a mask as needed.
• Contact with a wet surface can contaminate a sterile field or object. Never set up a sterile field near a damp area. Discard sterile supplies with wet wrappers.
• A sterile field's edges are considered contaminated. So avoid placing sterile supplies within 1″ of its border.
• When in doubt, throw it out. Consider any sterile item that touches an area of questionable cleanliness or dryness contaminated.

Complications
Any lapse in sterile technique may cause contamination and an infection.
SANDRA LUDWIG NETTINA, RN, BSN

A new look at isolation precautions

In the past, the isolation precautions in most hospitals were based on *broad categories of diseases*. Now many hospitals are using a newer system based on *specific diseases*. With this new system, you can save money because you don't have to take unnecessary precautions that waste supplies. You may also save time because you won't don masks, gowns, and gloves if they're not needed.

The guidelines below show disease-specific isolation precautions for common infectious agents and diseases. (Hand washing isn't listed as a specific precaution because it's important for all patients, whether or not they have an infection.) As always, check your hospital's procedure manual for specific precautions required in your institution.

NURSE'S GUIDE TO ISOLATION PRECAUTIONS FOR SPECIFIC DISEASES

DISORDER AND INFECTIVE MATERIAL	PRECAUTIONS NEEDED	SPECIAL CONSIDERATIONS
Abscess		
Draining, major* • Pus	• Private room • Gown, if soiling is likely • Gloves for touching infective material	• Take precautions throughout illness.
Draining, minor or limited** • Pus	• Gown, if soiling is likely • Gloves for touching infective material	• Take precautions throughout illness.
No draining • No infective material	• None	• None
Acquired immunodeficiency syndrome (AIDS) • Blood • Body fluids • Feces may be infective if gastrointestinal bleeding is present.	• Private room, if patient has poor hygiene • Gown, if soiling is likely • Gloves for touching infective material	• Take precautions throughout illness. • Avoid needle stick injuries.
Actinomycosis, all lesions • No infective material	• None	• None
Adenovirus infection, respiratory, in infants and young children • Respiratory secretions • Feces	• Private room • Gown, if soiling is likely	• Take precautions throughout hospitalization. • Have infected patients share rooms during an epidemic, if needed.

*Major refers to draining with no dressing or with a dressing that doesn't contain the pus.

**Minor or limited refers to draining with a dressing that controls or contains the pus, or to draining from a very small infected area.

(continued)

NURSE'S GUIDE TO ISOLATION PRECAUTIONS
FOR SPECIFIC DISEASES *(continued)*

DISORDER AND INFECTIVE MATERIAL	PRECAUTIONS NEEDED	SPECIAL CONSIDERATIONS
Amebiasis		
Dysentery • Feces	• Private room, if patient has poor hygiene • Gown, if soiling is likely • Gloves for touching infective material	• Take precautions throughout illness.
Liver abscess • No infective material	• None	• None
Anthrax		
Cutaneous • Pus	• Gloves for touching infective material	• Take precautions throughout illness.
Inhalation • Respiratory secretions may be infective.	• Gown, if soiling is likely • Gloves for touching infective material	• Take precautions throughout illness.
Anthropod-borne viral encephalitides, such as eastern equine encephalomyelitis and California encephalitis • No infective material	• None	• None
Anthropod-borne viral fevers, such as dengue, yellow fever, and Colorado tick fever • Blood	• Gloves for touching infective material	• Take precautions throughout hospitalization.
Ascariasis • No infective material	• None	• None
Aspergillosis • No infective material	• None	• None
Babesiosis • Blood	• Gloves for touching infective material	• Take precautions throughout illness.
Blastomycosis, North American—cutaneous or pulmonary • No infective material	• None	• None
Botulism See *Food poisoning.*		

**NURSE'S GUIDE TO ISOLATION PRECAUTIONS
FOR SPECIFIC DISEASES** *(continued)*

DISORDER AND INFECTIVE MATERIAL	PRECAUTIONS NEEDED	SPECIAL CONSIDERATIONS
Bronchiolitis, etiology unknown, in infants and young children		
• Respiratory secretions	• Private room • Gown, if soiling is likely	• Take precautions throughout illness. • Take precautions to prevent spread of possible causative agents, such as respiratory syncytial virus, parainfluenza and influenza viruses, and adenoviruses.
Bronchitis, infective, etiology unknown		
Adults • Respiratory secretions may be infective.	• None	• Dispose of respiratory secretions carefully.
Infants and young children • Respiratory secretions	• Private room • Gown, if soiling is likely	• Take precautions throughout illness.

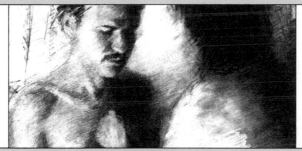

Brucellosis (undulant, Malta, or Mediterranean fever)		
Draining lesions, minor or limited** • Pus	• Gown, if soiling is likely • Gloves for touching infective material	• Take precautions throughout illness.
Other • No infective material	• None	• None
Campylobacter See *Gastroenteritis.*		
Candidiasis, all forms • No infective material	• None	• None

**Minor or limited refers to draining with a dressing that controls or contains the pus, or to draining from a very small infected area.

(continued)

NURSE'S GUIDE TO ISOLATION PRECAUTIONS FOR SPECIFIC DISEASES *(continued)*

DISORDER AND INFECTIVE MATERIAL	PRECAUTIONS NEEDED	SPECIAL CONSIDERATIONS
Cat-scratch fever (benign inoculation lymphoreticulosis) • No infective material	• None	• None
Cellulitis Draining, minor or limited** • Pus	• Gown, if soiling is likely • Gloves for touching infective material	• Take precautions throughout illness.
Intact skin • No infective material	• None	• None
Chancroid (soft chancre) • No infective material	• None	• None
Chicken pox (varicella) • Respiratory secretions • Lesion secretions	• Private room with special ventilation, if possible, to control outbreaks • Mask for those who are susceptible • Gown • Gloves	• Take precautions until all lesions are crusted. • Keep susceptible people out of patient's room, if possible. • Take isolation precautions at birth for neonates born to mothers with active chicken pox. • Place exposed susceptible patients on isolation precautions from day 10 to day 21 after exposure.
***Chlamydia trachomatis* infection** Conjunctivitis • Purulent exudate	• Gloves for touching infective material	• Take precautions throughout illness.
Genital infection • Genital discharge	• Gloves for touching infective material	• Take precautions throughout illness.
Respiratory infection • Respiratory secretions	• Gloves for touching infective material	• Take precautions throughout illness.

**Minor or limited refers to draining with a dressing that controls or contains the pus, or to draining from a very small infected area.

NURSE'S GUIDE TO ISOLATION PRECAUTIONS
FOR SPECIFIC DISEASES *(continued)*

DISORDER AND INFECTIVE MATERIAL	PRECAUTIONS NEEDED	SPECIAL CONSIDERATIONS
Cholera • Feces	• Private room, if patient has poor hygiene • Gown, if soiling is likely • Gloves for touching infective material	• Take precautions throughout illness.
Closed-cavity infection Draining, minor or limited** • Pus	• Gown, if soiling is likely • Gloves for touching infective material	• Take precautions throughout illness.
No draining • No infective material	• None	• None
Clostridium perfringens Food poisoning • No infective material	• None	• None
Gas gangrene • Pus	• Gown, if soiling is likely • Gloves for touching infective material	• Take precautions throughout illness.
Other • Pus	• Gown, if soiling is likely • Gloves for touching infective material	• Take precautions throughout illness.
Coccidioidomycosis (valley fever) Draining lesions • Drainage may be infective if spores form.	• None	• Handle drainage carefully.
Pneumonia • No infective material	• None	• None
Colorado tick fever See *Anthropod-borne viral fevers.*		
Common cold Adults • Respiratory secretions may be infective.	• None	• Dispose of respiratory secretions carefully.

**Minor or limited refers to draining with a dressing that controls or contains the pus, or to draining from a very small infected area.

(continued)

NURSE'S GUIDE TO ISOLATION PRECAUTIONS
FOR SPECIFIC DISEASES *(continued)*

DISORDER AND INFECTIVE MATERIAL	PRECAUTIONS NEEDED	SPECIAL CONSIDERATIONS
Common cold *(continued)*		
Infants and young children • Respiratory secretions	• Gown, if soiling is likely	• Take precautions throughout illness. • Rhinoviruses can cause severe infections in infants and children. • Take precautions to prevent the spread of viral agents, such as parainfluenza viruses, which can also cause the common cold.
Congenital rubella See *Rubella.*		
Conjunctivitis, acute bacterial (sore eye, pink eye) • Purulent exudate	• Gloves for touching infective material	• Take precautions throughout illness.
Conjunctivitis, chlamydia See *Chlamydia trachomatis* infection.		
Conjunctivitis, gonococcal		
Adults • Purulent exudate	• Gloves for touching infective material	• Take precautions for 24 hours after treatment begins.
Newborns • Purulent exudate	• Private room • Gloves for touching infective material	• Take precautions for 24 hours after treatment begins.
Conjunctivitis, viral, etiology unknown • Purulent exudate	• Private room, if patient has poor hygiene • Gloves for touching infective material	• Take precautions throughout illness.
Coronavirus infection, respiratory		
Adults • Respiratory secretions may be infective.	• None	• Dispose of respiratory secretions carefully.
Infants and young children • Respiratory secretions	• Private room • Gown, if soiling is likely	• Take precautions throughout illness.
Coxsackievirus disease • Feces • Respiratory secretions	• Private room, if patient has poor hygiene • Gown, if soiling is likely • Gloves for touching infective material	• Take precautions for 7 days after onset.

NURSE'S GUIDE TO ISOLATION PRECAUTIONS
FOR SPECIFIC DISEASES *(continued)*

DISORDER AND INFECTIVE MATERIAL	PRECAUTIONS NEEDED	SPECIAL CONSIDERATIONS
Creutzfeldt-Jakob disease • Blood • Brain tissue • Spinal fluid	• Gloves for touching infective material	• Take precautions throughout hospitalization.

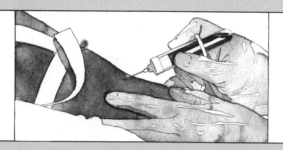

DISORDER AND INFECTIVE MATERIAL	PRECAUTIONS NEEDED	SPECIAL CONSIDERATIONS
Croup • Respiratory secretions	• Private room • Gown, if soiling is likely	• Take precautions throughout illness. • Take precautions to prevent the spread of viral agents, such as parainfluenza viruses and influenza A virus.
Cryptococcosis • No infective material	• None	• None
Cysticercosis • No infective material	• None	• None
Cytomegalovirus infection, neonatal or immunosuppressed • Urine may be infective. • Respiratory secretions may be infective.	• None	• Make sure pregnant women avoid contact with patient.
Decubitus ulcer, infected Draining, major* • Pus	• Private room • Gown, if soiling is likely • Gloves for touching infective material	• Take precautions throughout illness.
Draining, minor** • Pus	• Gown, if soiling is likely • Gloves for touching infective material	• Take precautions throughout illness.

*Major refers to draining with no dressing or with a dressing that doesn't contain the pus.

**Minor or limited refers to draining with a dressing that controls or contains the pus, or to draining from a very small infected area.

(continued)

**NURSE'S GUIDE TO ISOLATION PRECAUTIONS
FOR SPECIFIC DISEASES *(continued)***

DISORDER AND INFECTIVE MATERIAL	PRECAUTIONS NEEDED	SPECIAL CONSIDERATIONS
Dengue See *Anthropod-borne viral fevers.*		
Diarrhea, acute, possibly infective • Feces	• Private room, if patient has poor hygiene • Gown, if soiling is likely • Gloves for touching infective material	• Take precautions throughout illness.
Diphtheria Cutaneous • Lesion secretions	• Private room • Gown, if soiling is likely • Gloves for touching infective material	• Take precautions until two cultures from skin lesions (taken at least 24 hours apart, after completion of antimicrobial therapy) are negative for *Corynebacterium diphtheriae.*
Pharyngeal • Respiratory secretions	• Private room • Mask • Gown, if soiling is likely • Gloves for touching infective material	• Take precautions until two cultures from the nose and throat (taken at least 24 hours apart, after completion of antimicrobial therapy) are negative for *Corynebacterium diphtheriae.*
Echinococcosis (hydatidosis) • No infective material	• None	• None
Echovirus disease • Feces • Respiratory secretions	• Private room, if patient has poor hygiene • Gown, if soiling is likely • Gloves for touching infective material	• Take precautions for 7 days after onset.
Eczema vaccination See *Vaccinia.*		
Encephalitis or encephalomyelitis, infection suspected • Feces	• Private room, if patient has poor hygiene • Gown, if soiling is likely • Gloves for touching infective material	• Take precautions throughout illness or for 7 days after onset, whichever is less. • Take precautions against enteroviruses until the doctor can make a definite diagnosis.

NURSE'S GUIDE TO ISOLATION PRECAUTIONS
FOR SPECIFIC DISEASES *(continued)*

DISORDER AND INFECTIVE MATERIAL	PRECAUTIONS NEEDED	SPECIAL CONSIDERATIONS
Endometritis		
Group A *Streptococcus* • Vaginal discharge	• Private room, if patient has poor hygiene • Gown, if soiling is likely • Gloves for touching infective material	• Take precautions for 24 hours after therapy begins.
Other • Vaginal discharge	• Gown, if soiling is likely • Gloves for touching infective material	• Take precautions throughout illness.
Enterobiasis (pinworm disease, oxyuriasis) • No infective material	• None	• None
Enterocolitis, due to *Clostridium difficile* or *Staphylococcus* • Feces	• Private room, if patient has poor hygiene • Gown, if soiling is likely • Gloves for touching infective material	• Take precautions throughout illness.
Enteroviral infection • Feces	• Private room, if patient has poor hygiene • Gown, if soiling is likely • Gloves for touching infective material	• Take precautions for 7 days after onset.
Epiglottitis due to *Hemophilus influenzae* • Respiratory secretions	• Private room • Mask for those close to patient	• Take precautions for 24 hours after therapy begins.
Epstein-Barr virus infection, including infectious mononucleosis • Respiratory secretions may be infective.	• None	• Dispose of respiratory secretions carefully.
Erysipeloid • No infective material	• None	• None
Erythema infectiosum • Respiratory secretions	• Private room • Mask for those close to patient	• Take precautions for 7 days after onset.
***Escherichia coli* infection** See *Gastroenteritis.*		

(continued)

NURSE'S GUIDE TO ISOLATION PRECAUTIONS FOR SPECIFIC DISEASES *(continued)*

DISORDER AND INFECTIVE MATERIAL	PRECAUTIONS NEEDED	SPECIAL CONSIDERATIONS
Fever of unknown origin (FUO)		• Take isolation precautions *only* if the patient has other signs and symptoms that suggest a disease warranting these precautions.
Food poisoning		
Botulism • No infective material	• None	• None
Clostridium perfringens (or *C. welchii*) food poisoning • No infective material	• None	• None
Salmonellosis • Feces	• Private room, if patient has poor hygiene • Gown, if soiling is likely • Gloves for touching infective material	• Take precautions throughout illness.
Shigellosis • Feces	• Private room, if patient has poor hygiene • Gown, if soiling is likely • Gloves for touching infective material	• Take precautions until three consecutive fecal cultures (taken after completing antimicrobial therapy) are negative for *Shigella*.
Staphylococcal food poisoning • No infective material	• None	• None

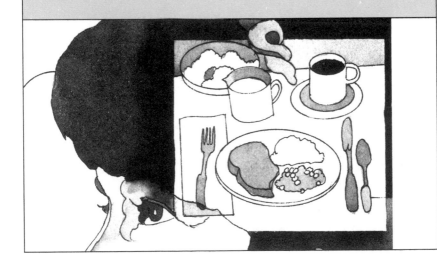

NURSE'S GUIDE TO ISOLATION PRECAUTIONS FOR SPECIFIC DISEASES *(continued)*

DISORDER AND INFECTIVE MATERIAL	PRECAUTIONS NEEDED	SPECIAL CONSIDERATIONS
Furunculosis, staphylococcal		
Newborns • Pus	• Private room • Gown, if soiling is likely • Gloves for touching infective material	• Take precautions throughout illness. • Have ill and colonized infants room together during a nursery outbreak, if needed.
Others • Pus	• Gown, if soiling is likely • Gloves for touching infective material	• Take precautions throughout illness.
Gangrene, gas • Pus	• Gown, if soiling is likely • Gloves for touching infective material	• Take precautions throughout illness.
Gastroenteritis *Campylobacter* species, *Clostridium difficile, Cryptosporidium* species, *Dientamoeba fragilis, Escherichia coli, Giardia lamblia,* Norwalk agent, rotavirus, *Salmonella* species, *Shigella* species, *Vibrio parahaemolyticus,* viral, *Yersinia enterocolitica,* or unknown etiology		
• Feces	• Private room, if patient has poor hygiene • Gown, if soiling is likely • Gloves for touching infective material	• Take precautions throughout illness. • For rotavirus infection, use precautions throughout illness or for 7 days after onset, whichever is less.
See also *Food poisoning.*		
German measles See *Rubella.*		
Giardiasis • Feces	• Private room, if patient has poor hygiene • Gown, if soiling is likely • Gloves for touching infective material	• Take precautions throughout illness.
Gonococcal ophthalmia See *Conjunctivitis, gonococcal.*		
Gonorrhea • Discharge may be infective.	• None	• Handle discharge carefully.
Granulocytopenia • No infective material	• None	• Wash hands well *before* caring for patient.
Granuloma inguinale (donovanosis, granuloma venereum) • Drainage may be infective.	• None	• Handle drainage carefully.

(continued)

NURSE'S GUIDE TO ISOLATION PRECAUTIONS
FOR SPECIFIC DISEASES *(continued)*

DISORDER AND INFECTIVE MATERIAL	PRECAUTIONS NEEDED	SPECIAL CONSIDERATIONS
Guillain-Barré syndrome • No infective material	• None	• None
Hand, foot, and mouth disease • Feces	• Private room, if patient has poor hygiene • Gown, if soiling is likely • Gloves for touching infective material	• Take precautions for 7 days after onset.
Hemorrhagic fever, such as Lassa fever • Blood • Body fluids • Respiratory secretions	• Private room, with special ventilation • Mask • Gown • Gloves	• Take precautions throughout illness. • Call the state health department and the Centers for Disease Control (CDC) for further advice.
Hepatitis, viral Type A (infectious) • Feces may be infective.	• Private room, if patient has poor hygiene • Gown, if soiling is likely • Gloves for touching infective material or when gross soiling is likely	• Take precautions for 7 days after onset of jaundice. However, hepatitis A is most contagious before signs and symptoms appear.
Type B (serum hepatitis), including hepatitis B antigen (HBsAg) carrier • Blood • Body fluids • Feces, if gastrointestinal bleeding occurs	• Private room, if profuse bleeding could contaminate the room • Gown, if soiling is likely • Gloves for touching infective material	• Take precautions until patient is HBsAg-negative. • Avoid needle stick injuries. • Make sure pregnant personnel seek special counseling.
Non-A, non-B • Blood • Body fluids	• Gown, if soiling is likely • Gloves for touching infective material	• Take precautions throughout illness. • Length of infective period is unknown.
Unspecified viral type		• Take precautions for the infection that's most likely.
Herpangina • Feces	• Private room, if patient has poor hygiene • Gown, if soiling is likely • Gloves for touching infective material	• Take precautions for 7 days after onset.

**NURSE'S GUIDE TO ISOLATION PRECAUTIONS
FOR SPECIFIC DISEASES** *(continued)*

DISORDER AND INFECTIVE MATERIAL	PRECAUTIONS NEEDED	SPECIAL CONSIDERATIONS
Herpes simplex *(Herpesvirus hominis)*		
Encephalitis • No infective material	• None	• None
Mucocutaneous, severe (disseminated or primary) • Lesion secretions from infected site	• Gown, if soiling is likely • Gloves for touching infective material	• Take precautions throughout illness.
Mucocutaneous, recurrent (skin, oral, and genital) • Lesion secretions from infected site	• Gloves for touching infective material	• Take precautions until all lesions have crusted.
Neonatal • Lesion secretions	• Private room • Gown, if soiling is likely • Gloves for touching infective material	• Take precautions throughout illness. • Use the same isolation procedures for infants born to women with active genital herpes simplex infections.
Herpes zoster (varicella zoster)		
Disseminated or localized in an immunocompromised patient • Lesion secretions • Respiratory secretions may be infective.	• Private room with special ventilation, if possible • Mask for people who are susceptible • Gown • Gloves for touching infective material	• Take precautions throughout illness. • Keep susceptible people out of the room. • Place exposed susceptible patients on isolation precautions from day 10 after first exposure to day 21 after last exposure.
Localized in other patients • Lesion secretions	• Private room, if patient has poor hygiene • Gloves for touching infective material	• Take precautions until all lesions have crusted. • Keep susceptible people out of the room. • Make sure roommates aren't susceptible to chicken pox.
Histoplasmosis • No infective material	• None	• None
Hookworm disease (ancylostomiasis, uncinariasis) • No infective material	• None	• None

(continued)

NURSE'S GUIDE TO ISOLATION PRECAUTIONS
FOR SPECIFIC DISEASES (continued)

DISORDER AND INFECTIVE MATERIAL	PRECAUTIONS NEEDED	SPECIAL CONSIDERATIONS
Immunocompromised status • No infective material	• None	• Wash hands well *before* caring for patient.
Impetigo • Lesions	• Private room, if patient has poor hygiene • Gown, if soiling is likely • Gloves for touching infective material	• Take precautions for 24 hours after starting therapy.
Infectious mononucleosis See *Epstein-Barr virus infection*.		
Influenza Adults • Respiratory secretions may be infective.	• None	• Most patients recover by the time a diagnosis is made, so precautions may not be practical. • Have patients with influenza share rooms during an epidemic, if necessary.
Infants and young children • Respiratory secretions	• Private room • Gown, if soiling is likely	• If no epidemic exists, influenza can be hard to diagnose. • Have patients with influenza share rooms during an epidemic, if needed.
Kawasaki disease • No infective material	• None	• None
Keratoconjunctivitis, infective • Purulent exudate	• Private room, if patient has poor hygiene • Gloves for touching infective material	• Take precautions throughout illness.
Lassa fever See *Hemorrhagic fever*.		
Leprosy • No infective material	• None	• None
Leptospirosis • Blood • Urine	• Gloves for touching infective material	• Take precautions throughout hospitalization.
Listeriosis • No infective material	• None	• None

**NURSE'S GUIDE TO ISOLATION PRECAUTIONS
FOR SPECIFIC DISEASES** *(continued)*

DISORDER AND INFECTIVE MATERIAL	PRECAUTIONS NEEDED	SPECIAL CONSIDERATIONS
Lyme disease • No infective material	• None	• None
Lymphocytic choriomeningitis • No infective material	• None	• None
Lymphogranuloma venereum • Drainage may be infective	• None	• Handle drainage carefully.
Malaria • Blood	• Gloves for touching infective material	• Take precautions throughout illness.
Marburg virus disease • Blood • Body fluids • Respiratory secretions	• Private room with special ventilation • Mask • Gown • Gloves	• Take precautions throughout illness. • Call the state health department and the CDC for further advice.

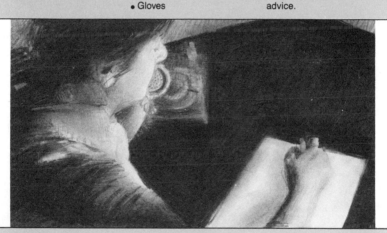

Measles (rubeola) • Respiratory secretions	• Private room • Mask for those who are susceptible and must be close to the patient	• Take precautions for 4 days after rash begins or throughout illness for immunocompromised patient. • Keep susceptible people out of the room.
Melioidosis • Respiratory secretions may be infective. • Sinus drainage, if present, may be infective.	• None	• Dispose of secretions and drainage carefully.

(continued)

NURSE'S GUIDE TO ISOLATION PRECAUTIONS
FOR SPECIFIC DISEASES *(continued)*

DISORDER AND INFECTIVE MATERIAL	PRECAUTIONS NEEDED	SPECIAL CONSIDERATIONS
Meningitis		
Aseptic (nonbacterial or viral) • Feces	• Private room, if patient has poor hygiene • Gown, if soiling is likely • Gloves for touching infective material	• Take precautions for 7 days after onset. • Enteroviruses commonly cause aseptic meningitis.
Bacterial, gram-negative enteric in neonates • Feces may be infective	• Gown, if soiling is likely during nursery outbreak • Gloves for touching feces during nursery outbreak	• Have ill and colonized infants share rooms during a nursery outbreak, if needed.
Fungal • No infective material	• None	• None
Hemophilus influenzae • Respiratory secretions	• Private room • Mask for those close to patient	• Take precautions for 24 hours after starting therapy.
Listeria monocytogenes • No infective material	• None	• None
Neisseria meningitidis (meningococcal) • Respiratory secretions	• Private room • Mask for those close to patient	• Take precautions for 24 hours after starting therapy. • Receive prophylaxis after exposure, as required.
Pneumococcal • No infective material	• None	• None
Tuberculous • No infective material	• None	• Check patient for signs of active pulmonary tuberculosis. If present, take precautions. (See *Tuberculosis.*)
Other bacterial • No infective material	• None	• None
Meningococcal pneumonia See *Pneumonia.*		
Meningococcemia (meningococcal sepsis) • Respiratory secretions	• Private room • Mask for those close to patient	• Take precautions for 24 hours after starting therapy. • Receive prophylaxis after exposure, as required.

NURSE'S GUIDE TO ISOLATION PRECAUTIONS
FOR SPECIFIC DISEASES *(continued)*

DISORDER AND INFECTIVE MATERIAL	PRECAUTIONS NEEDED	SPECIAL CONSIDERATIONS
Molluscum contagiosum • No infective material	• None	• None
Mucormycosis • No infective material	• None	• None
Multiply resistant organisms, infection or colonization†		
Gastrointestinal • Feces	• Private room • Gown, if soiling is likely • Gloves for touching infective material	• Take precautions until patient is off antimicrobials and has a negative culture. • Have infected and colonized patients share rooms, if necessary, during an outbreak.
Respiratory • Respiratory secretions • Feces may be infective.	• Private room • Mask for those close to the patient • Gown, if soiling is likely • Gloves for touching infective material	• Take precautions until patient is off antimicrobials and has a negative culture. • Have infected and colonized patients share rooms, if necessary, during an outbreak.
Skin, wound, or burn • Pus • Feces may be infective.	• Private room • Gown, if soiling is likely • Gloves for touching infective material	• Take precautions until patient is off antimicrobials and has a negative culture. • Have infected and colonized patients share rooms, if necessary, during an outbreak.
Urinary • Urino • Feces may be infective.	• Private room • Gloves for touching infective material	• Take precautions until patient is off antimicrobials and has a negative culture. • Handle urine and urine measuring devices carefully to prevent infection, especially in a patient with an indwelling (Foley) catheter. • Have infected and colonized patients share rooms, if necessary, during an outbreak.
Mumps (infectious parotitis) • Respiratory secretions	• Private room • Mask for those who are susceptible and must be close to the patient	• Take precautions for 9 days after swelling begins.

† Multiply-resistant organisms include: aminoglycoside-resistant gram-negative bacilli; methicillin-resistant *Staphylococcus aureus;* penicillin-resistant *Pneumococcus;* ampicillin and chloramphenicol-resistant *Haemophilus influenzae;* and other bacteria judged resistant by the infection control team.

(continued)

NURSE'S GUIDE TO ISOLATION PRECAUTIONS
FOR SPECIFIC DISEASES *(continued)*

DISORDER AND INFECTIVE MATERIAL	PRECAUTIONS NEEDED	SPECIAL CONSIDERATIONS
Mycobacteria, nontuberculous (atypical)		
Pulmonary • No infective material	• None	• None
Wound • Drainage may be infective.	• Gown, if soiling is likely • Gloves for touching infective material	• Take precautions until drainage stops.
Mycoplasmal pneumonia See *Pneumonia.*		
Necrotizing enterocolitis • Feces may be infective.	• Gown, if soiling is likely • Gloves for touching infective material	• Have sick infants share rooms in nurseries, if needed.
Neutropenia • No infective material	• None	• Wash hands well *before* caring for patient.
Nocardiosis		
Draining lesions • Drainage may be infective.	• None	• Dispose of drainage carefully.
Other • No infective agent	• None	• None
Orf • Drainage may be infective.	• None	• Dispose of drainage carefully.
Parainfluenza virus infection, respiratory, in infants and young children		
• Respiratory secretions	• Private room • Gown, if soiling is likely	• Take precautions throughout illness. • Have infected patients share rooms, if necessary, during an epidemic.
Pediculosis • Infested area	• Private room, if patient has poor hygiene • Gown for close contact • Gloves for close contact	• Take precautions for 24 hours after starting therapy.
Pertussis (whooping cough) • Respiratory secretions	• Private room • Mask for those close to the patient	• Take precautions for 7 days after starting therapy. • Receive prophylaxis after exposure, as required.

NURSE'S GUIDE TO ISOLATION PRECAUTIONS
FOR SPECIFIC DISEASES (continued)

DISORDER AND INFECTIVE MATERIAL	PRECAUTIONS NEEDED	SPECIAL CONSIDERATIONS
Pharyngitis, infective Adults • Respiratory secretions may be infective.	• None	• Dispose of respiratory secretions carefully.
Infants and young children • Respiratory secretions	• Private room, if patient has poor hygiene • Gown, if soiling is likely	• Take precautions throughout illness. • Take precautions to prevent spread of adenoviruses, influenza viruses, and parainfluenza viruses associated with pharyngitis.
Pinworm disease See *Enterobiasis.*		
Plague Bubonic • Pus	• Gown, if soiling is likely • Gloves for touching infective material	• Take precautions for 3 days after starting therapy.
Pneumonic • Respiratory secretions	• Private room • Mask • Gown, if soiling is likely • Gloves for touching infective material	• Take precautions for 3 days after starting therapy.
Pleurodynia • Feces	• Private room, if patient has poor hygiene • Gown, if soiling is likely • Gloves for touching infective material	• Take precautions for 7 days after onset. • Enteroviruses often cause infection.

(continued)

NURSE'S GUIDE TO ISOLATION PRECAUTIONS FOR SPECIFIC DISEASES *(continued)*

DISORDER AND INFECTIVE MATERIAL	PRECAUTIONS NEEDED	SPECIAL CONSIDERATIONS
Pneumonia		
Bacterial not listed below, including gram-negative • Respiratory secretions may be infective.	• None	• Dispose of respiratory secretions carefully.
Chlamydia • Respiratory secretions	• Gloves for touching infective material	• Take precautions throughout illness.
Fungal • No infective material	• None	• None
Hemophilus influenzae Adults • Respiratory secretions may be infective.	• None	• Dispose of respiratory secretions carefully.
Infants and children • Respiratory secretions	• Private room • Mask for those close to patient	• Take precautions for 24 hours after starting therapy.
Legionella • Respiratory secretions may be infective.	• None	• Dispose of respiratory secretions carefully.
Meningococcal • Respiratory secretions	• Private room • Mask for those close to patient	• Take precautions for 24 hours after starting therapy. • Receive prophylaxis after exposure, as required.
Multiply resistant bacterial • Respiratory secretions • Feces may be infective.	• Private room • Mask for those close to the patient • Gown, if soiling is likely • Gloves for touching infective material	• Take precautions until patient is off antimicrobials and has a negative culture. • Have infected and colonized patients share rooms, if necessary, during an outbreak.

NURSE'S GUIDE TO ISOLATION PRECAUTIONS
FOR SPECIFIC DISEASES *(continued)*

DISORDER AND INFECTIVE MATERIAL	PRECAUTIONS NEEDED	SPECIAL CONSIDERATIONS
Pneumonia *(continued)*		
Mycoplasmal (primary atypical or Eaton agent pneumonia) • Respiratory secretions may be infective.	• Private room may be useful for children.	• Dispose of respiratory secretions carefully.
Pneumococcal • Respiratory secretions may be infective for 24 hours after starting therapy.	• None	• Dispose of respiratory secretions carefully.
Pneumocystis carinii • No infective material	• None	• None
Staphylococcus aureus • Respiratory secretions	• Private room • Mask for those close to the patient • Gown, if soiling is likely • Gloves for touching infective material	• Take precautions for 48 hours after starting therapy.
Streptococcus, group A • Respiratory secretions	• Private room • Mask for those close to the patient • Gown, if soiling is likely • Gloves for touching infective material	• Take precautions for 24 hours after starting therapy.
Unknown etiology		• Take precautions for type of pneumonia that is most likely.
Viral (see also specific etiologic agents)		
Adults • Respiratory secretions may be infective.	• None	• Dispose of respiratory secretions carefully.
Infants and young children • Respiratory secretions	• Private room • Gown, if soiling is likely	• Take precautions throughout illness. • Take precautions to prevent the spread of agents, such as parainfluenza viruses, influenza viruses, and respiratory syncytial virus, which can cause viral pneumonia.

NURSE'S GUIDE TO ISOLATION PRECAUTIONS
FOR SPECIFIC DISEASES *(continued)*

DISORDER AND INFECTIVE MATERIAL	PRECAUTIONS NEEDED	SPECIAL CONSIDERATIONS
Poliomyelitis • Feces	• Private room, if patient has poor hygiene • Gown, if soiling is likely • Gloves for touching infective material	• Take precautions for 7 days after onset.
Psittacosis (ornithosis) • Respiratory secretions may be infective.	• None	• Dispose of respiratory secretions carefully.
Q fever • Respiratory secretions may be infective.	• None	• Dispose of respiratory secretions carefully.
Rabies • Respiratory secretions	• Private room • Mask for those close to the patient • Gown, if soiling is likely • Gloves for touching infective material	• Take precautions throughout illness. • Receive prophylaxis after exposure, as required.
Rat-bite fever *(Streptobacillus moniliformis* disease or *Spirillum minus* disease) • Blood	• Gloves for touching infective material	• Take precautions for 24 hours after starting therapy.
Relapsing fever • Blood	• Gloves for touching infective material	• Take precautions throughout illness.
Respiratory infectious disease, acute (not covered elsewhere) Adults • Respiratory secretions may be infective.	• None	• Dispose of respiratory secretions carefully.
Infants and young children • Respiratory secretions may be infective.		• Take precautions for the bacterial or viral infection that's most likely.
Respiratory syncytial virus (RSV) infection, in infants and young children • Respiratory secretions	• Private room	• Take precautions throughout illness. • Have patients with RSV infections share rooms during an epidemic, if needed.
Reye's syndrome • No infective material	• None	• None
Rheumatic fever • No infective material	• None	• None

NURSE'S GUIDE TO ISOLATION PRECAUTIONS
FOR SPECIFIC DISEASES *(continued)*

DISORDER AND INFECTIVE MATERIAL	PRECAUTIONS NEEDED	SPECIAL CONSIDERATIONS
Rhinovirus infection, respiratory		
Adults • Respiratory secretions may be infective.	• None	• Dispose of respiratory secretions carefully.
Infants and young children • Respiratory secretions	• Private room • Gown, if soiling is likely	• Take precautions throughout illness.
Rickettsial fever, tick-borne (Rocky Mountain spotted fever, tick-borne typhus fever) • Blood may be infective.	• None	• Handle blood specimens carefully.
Ringworm (dermatophytosis, dermatomycosis tinea) • No infective material	• None	• None
Ritter's disease (staphylococcal scalded skin syndrome) • Lesion drainage	• Private room • Gown, if soiling is likely • Gloves for touching infective material	• Take precautions throughout illness.
Rocky Mountain spotted fever See *Rickettsial fever, tick-borne*.		
Roseola infantum (exanthema subitum) • No infective material	• None	• None
Rotavirus infection See *Gastroenteritis*.		
Rubella (German measles)		
Regular • Respiratory secretions	• Private room • Mask for those who are susceptible and must be close to the patient	• Take precautions for 7 days after rash develops. • Keep susceptible people—especially pregnant women—out of the room, if possible.
Congenital • Urine • Respiratory secretions	• Private room • Gown, if soiling is likely • Gloves for touching infective material	• Take precautions during any admission up to age 1, unless nasopharyngeal and urine cultures are negative for rubella virus and the child is over 3 months old. • Keep susceptible people—especially pregnant women—out of the patient's room, if possible.

(continued)

NURSE'S GUIDE TO ISOLATION PRECAUTIONS
FOR SPECIFIC DISEASES *(continued)*

DISORDER AND INFECTIVE MATERIAL	PRECAUTIONS NEEDED	SPECIAL CONSIDERATIONS
Salmonellosis See *Food poisoning.*		
Scabies • Infested area	• Private room, if patient has poor hygiene • Gown for close contact • Gloves for close contact	• Take precautions for 24 hours after starting therapy.
Scalded skin syndrome, staphylococcal See *Ritter's disease.*		
Schistosomiasis (bilharziasis) • No infective material	• None	• None
Shigellosis (including bacillary dysentery) See *Food poisoning.*		
Smallpox (variola) • Respiratory secretions • Lesion secretions	• Private room with special ventilation • Mask • Gown • Gloves	• Take precautions throughout illness. • Call the state health department and the CDC for further advice. • Smallpox can occur if smallpox virus is stocked in laboratories.

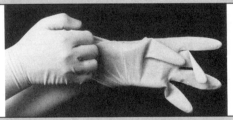

***Spirillum minus* disease** See *Rat-bite fever.*		
Sporotrichosis • No infective material	• None	• None
Staphylococcal *(S. aureus)* disease Skin, wound, or burn infection Major* • Pus	• Private room • Gown, if soiling is likely • Gloves for touching infective material	• Take precautions throughout illness.

*Major refers to draining with no dressing or with a dressing that doesn't contain the pus.

NURSE'S GUIDE TO ISOLATION PRECAUTIONS
FOR SPECIFIC DISEASES (continued)

DISORDER AND INFECTIVE MATERIAL	PRECAUTIONS NEEDED	SPECIAL CONSIDERATIONS
Staphylococcal (S. aureus) disease (continued)		
Skin, wound, or burn infection (continued)		
Minor or limited**		
• Pus	• Gown, if soiling is likely • Gloves for touching infective material	• Take precautions throughout illness.
Toxic shock syndrome • Vaginal discharge • Pus	• Gown, if soiling is likely • Gloves for touching infective material	• Take precautions throughout illness.
See also *Enterocolitis, Pneumonia,* and *Ritter's disease.*		
Streptobacillus moniliformis disease See *Rat-bite fever.*		
Streptococcal disease (group A *Streptococcus*)		
Pharyngitis • Respiratory secretions	• Private room, if patient has poor hygiene	• Take precautions for 24 hours after starting therapy.
Scarlet fever • Respiratory secretions	• Private room, if patient has poor hygiene	• Take precautions for 24 hours after starting therapy.

Skin, wound, or burn infection
   Major*
    • Pus
	• Private room
	• Gown, if soiling is likely
	• Gloves for touching infective material
		• Take precautions for 24 hours after starting therapy.

Minor or limited** • Pus	• Gown, if soiling is likely • Gloves for touching infective material	• Take precautions for 24 hours after starting therapy.
See also *Endometritis* and *Pneumonia.*		
Streptococcal disease (group B *Streptococcus*)		
Neonatal • Feces may be infective.	• Gown during nursery outbreak • Gloves during nursery outbreak	• Have ill and colonized infants share rooms during a nursery outbreak, if needed.

*Major refers to draining with no dressing or with a dressing that doesn't contain the pus.

**Minor or limited refers to draining with a dressing that controls or contains the pus, or to draining from a very small infected area.

(continued)

NURSE'S GUIDE TO ISOLATION PRECAUTIONS FOR SPECIFIC DISEASES *(continued)*

DISORDER AND INFECTIVE MATERIAL	PRECAUTIONS NEEDED	SPECIAL CONSIDERATIONS
Streptococcal disease (not group A or B), unless covered elsewhere		
• No infective material	• None	• None
Strongyloidiasis		
• Feces may be infective.	• None	• Dispose of feces and respiratory secretions carefully.
• Respiratory secretions may be infective in an immunocompromised patient with pneumonia or disseminated disease.		
Syphilis		
Latent (tertiary) and seropositive without lesions		
• No infective material	• None	• None
Skin and mucous membrane, including congenital, primary, and secondary		
• Lesion secretions	• Gloves for touching infective material	• Take precautions for 24 hours after starting therapy.
• Blood		• Be especially careful with the highly infective skin lesions of primary and secondary syphilis.
Tapeworm disease		
Hymenolepis nana and *Taenia solium* (pork)		
• Feces may be infective.	• None	• Dispose of feces carefully.
Other		
• No infective material	• None	• None
Tetanus No infective material	• None	• None

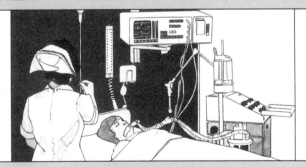

Tinea
See *Ringworm.*

NURSE'S GUIDE TO ISOLATION PRECAUTIONS
FOR SPECIFIC DISEASES (continued)

DISORDER AND INFECTIVE MATERIAL	PRECAUTIONS NEEDED	SPECIAL CONSIDERATIONS
TORCH syndrome See *Toxoplasmosis, Rubella, Cytomegalovirus, Herpes,* and *Syphilis.*		
Toxoplasmosis • No infective material	• None	• None
Toxic shock syndrome See *Staphylococcal disease.*		
Trachoma, acute • Purulent exudate	• Gloves for touching infective material	• Take precautions throughout illness.
Trench mouth See *Vincent's angina.*		
Trichinosis • No infective material	• None	• None
Trichomoniasis • No infective material	• None	• None
Trichuriasis (whipworm disease) • No infective material	• None	• None
Tuberculosis Extrapulmonary, draining lesions (including scrofula) • Pus	• Private room for children • Gloves for touching infective material	• Take precautions until drainage stops.
Extrapulmonary, meningitis • No infective material	• None	• None
Positive skin test with negative sputum smear and X-rays • No infective material	• None	• None
Pulmonary • Airborne droplet nuclei	• Private room with special ventilation • Mask, if patient coughs without covering his mouth • Gown, if gross contamination of clothing is likely	• Take precautions until the number of TB organisms on sputum smears decreases and the patient improves. • Administer antituberculosis drugs, as ordered, to limit transmission. • Infants and young children rarely need isolation precautions because they cough less and have fewer organisms in their sputum than adults.

(continued)

NURSE'S GUIDE TO ISOLATION PRECAUTIONS
FOR SPECIFIC DISEASES *(continued)*

DISORDER AND INFECTIVE MATERIAL	PRECAUTIONS NEEDED	SPECIAL CONSIDERATIONS
Tularemia		
Draining lesion		
• Pus may be infective.	• Gown, if soiling is likely • Gloves for touching infective material	• Take precautions throughout illness.
Pulmonary		
• Respiratory secretions may be infective.	• None	• Dispose of respiratory secretions carefully.
Typhoid fever		
• Feces	• Private room, if patient has poor hygiene • Gown, if soiling is likely • Gloves for touching infective material	• Take precautions throughout illness.
Typhus, endemic and epidemic		
• Blood may be infective.	• None	• Handle blood specimens carefully.
Urinary tract infection, including pyelonephritis		
• None	• None	• Take precautions for infections with multiply resistant organisms, if applicable. • Separate infected patients from uninfected patients who have indwelling catheters.
Vaccinia		
At vaccination site		
• Lesion secretions	• Gown, if soiling is likely • Gloves for touching infective material	• Take precautions throughout illness.
Generalized progressive eczema vaccinatum		
• Lesion secretions	• Private room • Gown, if soiling is likely • Gloves for touching infective material	• Take precautions throughout illness.
Varicella See *Chicken pox.*		
Variola See *Smallpox.*		
Vibrio parahaemolyticus See *Gastroenteritis.*		
Vincent's angina		
• No infective material	• None	• None

NURSE'S GUIDE TO ISOLATION PRECAUTIONS
FOR SPECIFIC DISEASES *(continued)*

DISORDER AND INFECTIVE MATERIAL	PRECAUTIONS NEEDED	SPECIAL CONSIDERATIONS
Viral diseases		
Pericarditis, myocarditis, or meningitis • Feces • Respiratory secretions may be infective.	• Private room, if patient has poor hygiene • Gown, if soiling is likely • Gloves for touching infective material	• Take precautions for 7 days after onset. • Enteroviruses often cause these infections.
Respiratory (not covered elsewhere) Adults • Respiratory secretions may be infective.	• None	• Dispose of respiratory secretions carefully.
Infants and young children • Respiratory secretions	• Private room • Gown, if soiling is likely	• Take precautions throughout illness. • Take precautions to prevent spread of respiratory syncytial virus, adenoviruses, and parainfluenza and influenza viruses.
Whooping cough See *Pertussis.*		
Wound infections		
Major* • Pus	• Private room • Gown, if soiling is likely • Gloves for touching infective material	• Take precautions throughout illness.
Minor or limited** • Pus	• Gown, if soiling is likely • Gloves for touching infective material	• Take precautions throughout illness.
Yersinia enterocolitica See *Gastroenteritis.*		
Zoster (varicella zoster) See *Herpes zoster.*		
Zygomycosis (phycomycosis, mucormycosis) • No infective material	• None	• None

*Major refers to draining with no dressing or with a dressing that doesn't contain the pus.

**Minor or limited refers to draining with a dressing that controls or contains the pus, or to draining from a very small infected area.

Patient-teaching guidelines for common home therapies

Under the new prospective payment system, pressure to limit hospitalization is leading to earlier discharge, often of patients who need continuing medical care. This situation is causing a significant shift to home health care. This shift increases your responsibilities for patient teaching. You must teach patients how to use complex equipment and continue special treatments to make the transition from the hospital to the home as smooth as possible.

You can expect to teach patients about total parenteral nutrition (TPN), intravenous (I.V.) antibiotic therapy, and enteral nutrition quite often. Technologic advances in equipment for these home therapies have made them common *and* cost-effective. Such "high tech" equipment as Hickman® and Broviac® catheters, implantable infusion ports, and smaller bore feeding tubes has put home care within the reach of many patients and improved the quality of their lives. The following guidelines will help you prepare patients for safe, effective home care.

Selecting patients for home therapy

Many hospitals have criteria for selecting home therapy candidates. Patient selection may be based on positive answers to questions, such as:
• Is the patient stable enough to be sent home?
• Can the patient take care of himself? If not, does he have a primary care giver who can care for him?
• Are the patient and his primary care giver motivated?
• Can they learn and carry out the necessary procedures?
• Do they cope well psychologically with the responsibility of home care?

• Is the home a safe environment?
• Do good support systems exist at home?
• Is storage available for equipment and supplies? If not, can the patient arrange for it?
• Is the patient covered by insurance?
• If his insurance pays less than 100%, can the patient pay the balance?
• If the patient has no resources, can other payment arrangements be made, as with charitable funds?

Planning for discharge and patient teaching

As the patient's primary nurse, you may assist with the discharge planning and develop a teaching plan with a multidisciplinary team. Typically, this team also includes the doctor, pharmacist, dietitian, I.V. team, nutritional support team, discharge planner, social worker, home health nurse, equipment supplier, and possibly a company nurse provided by the supplier. Since the home health nurse or the company nurse will continue the patient's care at home, they may assist with discharge planning and preparatory patient teaching. In addition, the company nurse can order supplies and ensure on-time delivery of necessary equipment to the patient's home.

Short, frequent training sessions seem most effective. You may use a variety of teaching tools, such as workbooks, videos, mannequin chests, and resource manuals, but be sure to use the exact equipment that the patient will be using at home. The patient may be afraid that he can't grasp all that he needs to know. But if you describe, then demonstrate, each step of the procedure and have him return the demonstration, he should become confident in his ability to do it. Be sure to give the patient enough time to understand the information and to practice the procedures under your supervision before discharge. Also give him a 24-hour emergency phone number to use after he goes home, and provide a Medic Alert bracelet, if needed.

Preparation for home TPN

Before the patient can be discharged, the doctor must implant a vascular access device, such as a silicone rubber catheter (Hickman or Broviac). An implantable infusion port (Port-A-Cath or Infus-A-Port) can also provide access, but reseach is incomplete on its use in long-term home TPN. Discuss the TPN schedule—usually an overnight, 12- to 14-hour infusion—with the patient. After the infusion cycle, he coils the catheter, tapes it to his chest, and covers the site with a dressing.

Standard TPN equipment

Antimicrobial cleansing agent; 70% isopropyl alcohol; alcohol swabs; antimicrobial swabs; gauze or transparent dressings; tape; TPN solution; TPN solution additives; I.V. pole; unvented administration set with filter; volumetric infusion pump with a three-prong adapter; Luer Loc rubber injection caps; padded clamps; fat emulsions, as ordered; vented administration set; heparin flush solution syringe and needle; blood or urine glucose reagent strips; lancets; scale; thermometer.

Essential steps

Be sure to describe the following essential steps to your patient in detail:

Changing the dressing

• Wash your hands with an antimicrobial cleansing agent.
• Clean a nonporous work area with isopropyl alcohol.
• Gather supplies.
• Remove the old dressing carefully.
• Wash your hands again.
• Check the infusion site for signs of infection, such as redness, swelling, tenderness, or drainage.
• Clean the site with alcohol or antimicrobial swabs, as ordered.
• Apply a dressing, as ordered. Change gauze dressings two to three times per week; transparent dressings, once a week. Change any dressing that gets wet, soiled, or loose.
• Loop catheter and tape to chest.

Infusing the solution

• Remove TPN solution from refrigerator 3 to 4 hours before infusion.
• Perform the first three steps listed under "Changing the dressing," and then wash your hands again. Use sterile technique throughout the procedure.
• Add medications to TPN solution just before hanging it on the I.V. pole.
• Prime the administration set and filter according to instructions.
• Prime the volumetric infusion pump according to the manufacturer's instructions, and set the infusion rate.
• Using sterile technique, connect the administration set to the catheter by Luer-locking the male end of the tubing into the female end of the catheter or by inserting a needle and tubing into the rubber injection cap at the end of the catheter. Note: Whenever the catheter is open to the air, apply a padded clamp.
• Begin the infusion.
• Infuse fat emulsions, as ordered, but never infuse fats with a filter.

Irrigating the catheter

• Flush the catheter after each infusion or after each time blood is drawn.
• Perform the first three steps listed under "Changing the dressing," and then wash your hands again.
• Draw heparin flush solution, as ordered, into a syringe.
• Swab the connection between the catheter and the cap with an alcohol or antimicrobial swab.
• Remove and discard the old rubber injection cap at the end of the catheter. Change this end cap daily if you use a Luer Loc or weekly if you use a needle to connect the tubing.
• Put a new rubber injection cap on the end of the catheter.
• Inject the heparin flush solution.

Self-monitoring

• Check glucose levels by sticking your finger with a lancet and testing a few drops of blood with a reagent strip. Test urine with a urine glucose reagent strip. Do tests as often as ordered.

• Check and record your temperature and weight every day.
• Expect your nurse to draw blood samples periodically.
• Return to your doctor for follow-up, as ordered.

Complications

Review the possible complications of these procedures with your patient, stressing the importance of prevention and intervention. (See *Complications of Home Therapies*, pages 220 to 223.)

Preparation for I.V. antibiotic therapy

If a patient needs I.V. antibiotic therapy, he may have an intermittent infusion device, such as a heparin lock, or a silicone rubber catheter, such as a Hickman catheter. Because gravity infusion with an intermittent infusion device is more common than pump infusion with a central venous catheter, instructions for the former are shown below. For patients who need pump infusion through a central venous catheter, see the equipment and essential steps for TPN.

Standard equipment for I.V. antibiotic therapy

Antimicrobial cleansing agent; 70% isopropyl alcohol; alcohol swabs; antimicrobial swabs; gauze or transparent dressings; tape; premixed or unmixed medications; I.V. solution; I.V. filter; I.V. pole; administration set; heparin solution; needle and syringe.

Essential steps

Be sure to describe the following essential steps to your patient in detail:

Changing the dressing

Expect the nurse or other trained care giver to change the dressing, using these steps:
• Wash hands with an antimicrobial cleansing agent.
• Clean a nonporous work area with isopropyl alcohol.
• Gather supplies.

COMPARING VENOUS ACCESS DEVICES

INTERMITTENT INFUSION DEVICE

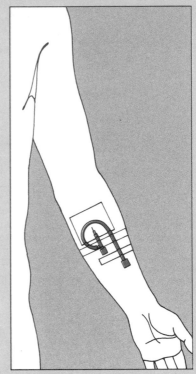

A nurse can insert an intermittent infusion device, which is typically used for antibiotic therapy. This device is most practical for short-term I.V. therapy. It must be filled with a heparin solution to maintain venous access between drug administrations and requires a gauze or transparent dressing. Barring complications, an intermittent infusion device can stay in place for 72 hours.

When a patient needs intravenous therapy at home, he'll require some type of long-term venous access. Three kinds of devices, which may be used for long-term I.V. antibiotic therapy or total parenteral nutrition (TPN), allow access and spare the patient the ordeal of repeated venipunctures.

INDWELLING CATHETER

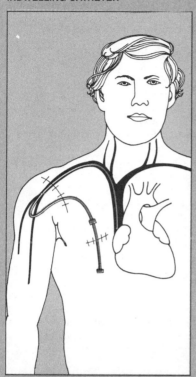

IMPLANTED INFUSION PORT

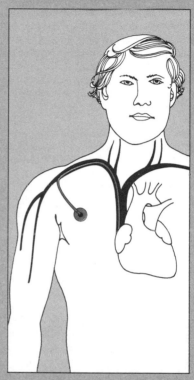

An indwelling catheter can maintain venous access for TPN, I.V. antibiotic therapy, and drawing blood. A surgeon inserts the catheter while the patient is under local anesthesia. Usually, the catheter terminates at the right atrium and passes through the superior vena cava, the cephalic vein, and a subcutaneous tunnel before it exits the body between the clavicle and the nipple. The indwelling catheter requires irrigation with heparin between infusions and special dressing changes to prevent infection. Although an indwelling catheter isn't permanent, it does provide long-term venous access.

For a patient who is at risk for, or who has, damaged veins, an implanted infusion port can provide venous access for TPN, drawing blood, and sometimes I.V. antibiotic therapy. Usually, a surgeon implants the port and its Silastic catheter, which is tunneled to a central vein. The port itself fits in a subcutaneous pocket over a bony prominence, such as the distal third of the clavicle. Because the infusion port is implanted under the skin, it reduces the risk of infection and minimizes changes in body image. It can last indefinitely, requires irrigation with heparin intermittently, and never needs a dressing. However, it's harder to manipulate than the indwelling catheter and requires the patient to insert a needle through his skin to administer drugs or fluids.

- Remove the old dressing carefully.
- Wash hands again.
- Check the infusion site for signs of infection, such as redness, swelling, tenderness, or drainage.
- Clean the site with alcohol or antimicrobial swabs, as ordered.

Expect a dressing change on your intermittent infusion device whenever your nurse inserts a new one (once every 2 to 3 days) or whenever the dressing becomes wet, soiled, or loose. Change gauze or transparent dressings for Hickman or Broviac catheters as described on page 215.

Infusing the I.V. antibiotics
- Perform the first three steps listed under "Changing the dressing," and then wash your hands again.
- Prepare the antibiotic according to the manufacturer's instructions. Check it for the correct name, dosage, and expiration date. Look for leaks in the bag or cracks in the vial or rubber stopper; if you find any, do not use the drug.
- Prime the administration set according to the manufacturer's instructions. Then attach a sterile needle with protective cover to the end of the tubing.
- Inject the needle into the latex part of the injection cap, using sterile technique.
- Adjust the flow rate according to the health care team's instructions.
- Change the administration set once a day. Most patients do this with the first dose of the day.

Irrigating the catheter
- Flush the catheter with heparin at the end of every dose.
- Perform the first three steps listed under "Changing the dressing," and then wash your hands again.
- Draw the prescribed amount of heparin solution into the syringe. Then flush the intermittent infusion device.
- If you're using an implanted catheter, irrigate it according to procedures listed under "Irrigating the catheter" in home TPN on page 215.

Complications
Review the possible complications of these procedures with your patient, emphasizing prevention and intervention. (See *Complications of Home Therapies,* pages 220 to 223.) If the patient has an implanted catheter, review catheter-related complications listed in the TPN section on page 220.

Preparation for enteral therapy
Several options exist for a patient who will have enteral therapy at home. He may have a nasogastric (NG), nasointestinal (NI), gastrostomy (G), or jejunostomy (J) feeding tube. He may administer his feedings by bolus, gravity, or continuous infusion, which is the best-tolerated method and prevents occlusion and formula backup.

Standard equipment for enteral therapy
Antimicrobial cleansing agent; 70% isopropyl alcohol; dressing change supplies; gauze or transparent dressings; tape; formula, as ordered; measuring cup; feeding tube; stethoscope; I.V. pole; feeding bag with administration set; enteral feeding pump, as ordered, with three-prong adapter; adapters or connectors; catheter tip syringe; blood or urine glucose reagent strips; lancets; scale; thermometer.

Essential steps
Be sure to describe the following essential steps to your patient in detail:

Changing the dressing (for G tube or J tube only)
- Wash your hands with an antimicrobial cleansing agent.
- Clean a nonporous work area with isopropyl alcohol.
- Gather supplies.
- Remove the old dressing carefully.
- Wash your hands again.
- Check for signs of infection, such as redness, swelling, or drainage.
- Clean the site, as ordered.
- Apply a new gauze or transparent dressing, as ordered or whenever the old one becomes wet, soiled, or loose.

Infusing the formula
• Perform the first three steps listed under "Changing the dressing," and then wash your hands again.
• Clean all equipment thoroughly with water.
• Assess for correct tube placement by inspecting it visually, by injecting air while listening to the left upper quadrant with a stethoscope, and by checking for gastric residuals. (J-tube placement can be checked *only* by visual inspection.) Once the tube is in place, mark and tape it for future reference.
• Prepare the formula, as instructed. Use a measuring cup to get the prescribed amount of formula. Allow refrigerated formula to come to room temperature, but don't leave it at room temperature for longer than 6 to 8 hours.
• Prepare the feeding bag according to the manufacturer's instructions. Add the formula, and prime the administration set.
• Plug in the feeding pump, using the three-prong adapter, and prime the pump according to manufacturer's instructions.
• Connect the administration set to the feeding tube using adapters or connectors. Reinforce connections with tape.
• Regulate the flow by adjusting the flow rate according to instructions or by starting the pump, if used.
• Use a catheter tip syringe to administer formula by bolus.
• Flush the feeding tube with water after you finish the infusion.
• Change the administration set every 24 hours to avoid bacterial contamination.

Self-monitoring
• Check glucose levels by sticking your finger with a lancet and testing a few drops of blood with a reagent strip. Test urine with a urine glucose reagent strip. Do tests as often as ordered.
• Check and record your temperature and weight every day.
• Expect your nurse to draw blood samples periodically.
• Return to your doctor for follow-up, as ordered.

Complications
Review the possible complications of these procedures with your patient, stressing the importance of prevention and intervention. (See *Complications of Home Therapies*, pages 220 to 223.)

Special Considerations
The prospect of home therapy can overwhelm a patient and make him anxious. But your teaching methods can make him more comfortable with it. Remember to give your patient enough time to understand everything he needs to know. Never hurry through patient teaching—he needs your patience and *time* most of all.

A patient or his care giver may fear causing harm. To allay his fears, discuss potential complications and ways to troubleshoot them. Be sure the patient knows which problems he can handle himself and which ones need medical attention. During your teaching sessions, simulate complications to give the patient a chance to practice solving problems that may occur at home.

Even a patient who's looking forward to going home may suffer depression before and after discharge. So provide emotional support and discuss his concerns to help him cope.

Documentation is crucial to a successful transition from hospital to home care. The doctor must provide written orders for this "high tech" home therapy. You'll have to document your teaching plan, patient-teaching activities, and results of teaching in your nurses' notes. During visits, the home health nurse will need to record her actions and observations. Finally, the patient will have to document his temperature, weight, and other self-monitoring activities. You can make this easier for him by developing a chart to meet his needs.

MARY ANN H. GARDINER, RN, BSN

COMPLICATIONS OF HOME THERAPIES

Total parenteral nutrition (TPN)

PROBLEM AND ITS SIGNS/SYMPTOMS	INTERVENTION	PREVENTION
MECHANICAL		
Air embolus • Cyanosis • Tachycardia • Tachypnea • Dyspnea	• Immediately clamp catheter or tubing as close to body as possible. • Lie on your left side with your chin on your chest. Stay in this position. Have someone call the emergency number.	• Tape all catheter connections and use Luer Locs. • Always clamp catheter before opening it. • Always remove air from tubing, filters, and syringes.
Broken or leaking catheter system • Obvious break or crack in catheter • Leakage from catheter or tubing	• Immediately clamp catheter as close to the chest as possible. • Check all connection points. • If catheter is damaged, go to the emergency room for catheter repair.	• Tighten and tape all connections. • Use approved clamps only. • Never use scissors near catheter.
Occlusion • Inability to irrigate catheter • Inability to infuse fluid	• Check roller clamp on I.V. tubing. • Check catheter clamps. • Check for kinks in system. • Don't force fluid. This could rupture the catheter. • Call the doctor or home health nurse if occlusion persists.	• Heparinize catheter, as instructed. • Secure tubing properly to prevent kinking. • Handle all flow interruptions immediately.
Bleeding • Blood backed up in catheter • Bleeding from disconnected catheter	• Check pump function. • Check system for loose areas or connections. • Clamp catheter if it's open.	• Operate pump according to instructions. • Clamp catheter when opening system. • Tighten all connections.
Pump malfunction • Pump alarm rings	• Check operator's manual. • Call 24-hour company number.	• Follow pump operator's manual. • Clean and maintain pump. • Keep battery charged.
SEPTIC		
Local infection • Redness, swelling, tenderness, or drainage at exit site • Fever over 101° F.	• Call the doctor immediately. • Save all infusion equipment if symptoms are sudden.	• Always follow strict aseptic technique. • Use good hand washing technique.

COMPLICATIONS OF HOME THERAPIES *(continued)*

Total parenteral nutrition (TPN)

PROBLEM AND ITS SIGNS/SYMPTOMS	INTERVENTION	PREVENTION
SEPTIC *(continued)*		
General infection • Fever • Chills • Sweating	• Call the doctor.	• Inspect catheter site during each dressing change. • Use strict aseptic technique in all procedures.
METABOLIC		
Hypoglycemia • Weakness • Diaphoresis • Nervousness	• Eat or drink high carbohydrate food. • Call the doctor.	• Taper off infusions. • Infuse at prescribed rate. • Monitor blood and urine glucose.
Hyperglycemia • Increased urine glucose • Increased urine output • Confusion • Increased thirst	• Call the doctor.	• Taper off infusions. • Infuse at prescribed rate. • Monitor blood and urine glucose. • Avoid infections.
Dehydration • Weight loss • Thirst • Dry tongue and mouth	• Call the doctor.	• Infuse at prescribed rate. • Do not skip infusion. • Report any conditions that may lead to dehydration, such as diarrhea or vomiting.
Electrolyte imbalance • Muscle weakness • Cramps • Tingling • Palpitations	• Call the doctor.	• Keep appointments for follow-up and blood work. • Keep accurate daily records.

I.V. antibiotic therapy

MECHANICAL AND SEPTIC (same as complications of TPN)

OTHER		
Extravasation/Infiltration • Redness • Pain, stinging, burning • Swelling • Warmth	• Stop infusion immediately. • Call the doctor or home health nurse. • Discontinue I.V., as instructed.	• Immobilize area near catheter as much as possible. • Avoid bumping site.
Phlebitis/cellulitis • Redness along path of vein • Swelling • Warmth	• Call the doctor or home health nurse. • Apply warm pack to area, as instructed.	• Prevent rapid drug infusion. • Irrigate catheter, as instructed. *(continued)*

COMPLICATIONS OF HOME THERAPIES *(continued)*

I.V. antibiotic therapy

PROBLEM AND ITS SIGNS/SYMPTOMS	INTERVENTION	PREVENTION
OTHER *(continued)*		
Allergic reaction/ anaphylaxis • Edema • Dyspnea • Generalized or local rash	• Stop infusion immediately. • Call the doctor. • Call the emergency squad if reaction is severe.	• Report any known drug sensitivities. • Expect to receive your first dose of any drug in a controlled environment. Report any side effects, at once.

Enteral nutrition

MECHANICAL		
Broken or leaking tube • Obvious break or crack • Leaking from or around tube or connection • Wet dressing	• Clamp catheter if it's damaged. • Check all connection points. • Call the doctor or home health nurse.	• Secure feeding tube. • Avoid tension on tube. • Avoid using scissors around the tube.
Occlusion • Inability to flush catheter • Inability to infuse formula • Occlusion alarm on pump rings	• Check roller clamp on tubing. • Check clamp on feeding tube. • Check for pump malfunctions. • Irrigate catheter.	• Flush tube with water, as instructed. • Thoroughly mix formulas. • If taking medicine, get liquid form. • Assess for proper pump functioning.
Dislodged tube • Coughing • Gagging • Cyanosis	• Stop formula immediately. • Call the doctor.	• Secure feeding tube. • Avoid tension on tube. • Elevate head of bed 30° to 45° during feedings.
Pump malfunction • Pump alarm rings	• Check operator's manual. • Call 24-hour company number.	• Follow pump operating instructions. • Clean and maintain pump. • Recharge battery.
SEPTIC		
Local infection • Redness, swelling, or tenderness at catheter site	• Call the doctor.	• Wash hands thoroughly. • Clean catheter site.
General infection • Fever • Shaking chills • Sweating • Malaise	• Call the doctor.	• Inspect catheter site during each dressing change for signs of local infection, which may become generalized.

COMPLICATIONS OF HOME THERAPIES *(continued)*

Enteral nutrition

PROBLEM AND ITS SIGNS/SYMPTOMS	INTERVENTION	PREVENTION
SEPTIC *(continued)*		
Aspiration • Fever • Chills • Dyspnea or noisy breathing • Frothy sputum	• Stop infusion. • Call emergency number.	• Check tube placement before each feeding. • Elevate head of bed during feeding.
METABOLIC (same as complications of TPN, plus those listed below)		
Constipation • Infrequent, hard stools • Abdominal pain and distention	• Call the doctor or home health nurse.	• Drink plenty of water. • Monitor fluid loss from such things as an ostomy or fistula.
Diarrhea • Frequent, watery, loose stools • Fever • Malaise	• Call the doctor or home health nurse.	• Increase formula strength and infusion rate slowly. • Never try to "catch up" if you get behind in feedings. • Store and prepare formula, as instructed.

Providing information about organ donation

When a patient dies or is declared brain dead, his family may be asked to consider organ donation. If so, they'll probably turn to you for information and sensitive support. Even if a patient has already signed a uniform donor card, if the family refuses donation, their wishes are usually upheld. So discussing organ donation with the patient's family is vitally important. While supporting a patient's family in their time of loss and grief, you can help them make an important decision that could save another person's life.

If the patient is eligible for organ donation (no history of chronic hypertension, diabetes mellitus, septicemia, or cancer), follow these guidelines when discussing organ donation with the patient's family:

• Help the family make an informed decision by providing objective information. Explain that if they consent to liver, heart, or kidney donation, the patient's vital functions will be maintained until the organ is removed. Emphasize that removing the internal organ won't disfigure the patient or delay burial plans.

• Give the family time to discuss organ donation, yet make yourself available to answer their questions.

• Arrange for a medical social worker or a clergyman to counsel family members if they want to discuss emotional, religious, or ethical questions about organ donation.

• If the family decides on organ donation, have the next of kin sign a written consent form. Inform the family that the attending doctor will probably declare the patient dead, but that a transplant surgeon will remove and transplant the organs. Tell them that they can receive information about the recipient's progress if they wish.

After the next of kin signs the consent form, the doctor will order tests to check organ function, such as liver enzymes or an EKG, and tests to measure the organ's size, such as X-rays and scans.

As ordered, obtain blood, sputum, and urine samples for culture; help obtain tissue specimens for analysis; and maintain the patient's vital functions with I.V. fluids and drugs and by caring for the patient on a respirator.

The following chart reviews specific nursing considerations for the organs now commonly donated.

SANDRA LUDWIG NETTINA, RN, BSN

WHAT YOU NEED TO KNOW ABOUT ORGAN TRANSPLANTS

ORGAN AND INDICATIONS FOR TRANSPLANT	PROCEDURE	NURSING CONSIDERATIONS
Cornea To replace a cornea that's damaged by such things as keratoconus, keratitis, and corneal trauma	The coroner or eye bank technician removes the entire eye within 6 hours of the donor's death. Then the cornea is processed under sterile conditions and can be stored for up to 48 hours.	• Determine if the donor had a history of corneal disease, eye surgery, rabies, or an infectious disease, such as AIDS or syphilis. Any of these conditions may make him ineligible. • Remove any debris from the donor's eyes. Then close his eyelids and cover them with saline compresses to prevent drying. • Notify the eye bank or the doctor who will remove the eyes. • Arrange for prompt donor transportation, if the eyes will be removed in the morgue.
Heart To replace a heart in end-stage heart disease caused by coronary artery disease, cardiomyopathy, congenital heart disease, posttraumatic aneurysm, or nonmalignant cardiac tumor	The donor may be put on life-support devices during transportation to the recipient's hospital. There the transplant team can remove the heart and place it directly in the recipient. Or the transplant team may go to the donor's hospital, remove the organ, store it in a cool cardioplegia bath, and return to the recipient for transplantation within 4 hours.	• Determine if the donor had a history of cardiovascular disease or prolonged hypotension. Either condition may make him ineligible. • Maintain the donor's vital functions until the heart can be removed. Use sterile technique in his care. • Arrange for donor transportation to the recipient's hospital or prepare for surgery, as ordered. • Inform the patient's family that both the heart and lungs may be removed for transplant into a patient with pulmonary hypertension due to heart disease. • Weigh the patient accurately on a bed scale.

WHAT YOU NEED TO KNOW ABOUT ORGAN TRANSPLANTS *(continued)*

ORGAN AND INDICATIONS FOR TRANSPLANT	PROCEDURE	NURSING CONSIDERATIONS
Kidney To replace a kidney in end-stage renal disease caused by glomerulonephritis, pyelonephritis, or nephrotoxic injury	The transplant surgeon removes the kidney at the donor's hospital. He places it in a preservation machine, which pumps plasma and oxygen through the kidney to keep it viable for 72 hours. Or he may place it in an icy slush bath to preserve it.	• Determine if the donor had a history of renal disease or prolonged hypotension. Either condition may make him ineligible. • Tell the donor's family that the recipient's chance of responding to the transplant is as high as 70%. • Maintain the donor's vital functions until the kidney is harvested. Use sterile technique for all procedures. • Prepare the donor for surgery, as ordered.
Liver To replace a liver in end-stage liver disease caused by biliary atresia, chronic active hepatitis, primary biliary cirrhosis, hepatic vein thrombosis, or genetic disorders, such as Wilson's disease and alpha$_1$-antitrypsin deficiency	The transplant team travels to the donor's hospital. They harvest the liver, preserve it, and transplant it in the recipient at the transplant center within 8 to 12 hours.	• Determine if the patient had a history of hepatobiliary disease or prolonged hypotension. Either condition may make him ineligible. • Measure the donor's abdominal girth, and weigh him accurately to estimate his liver's size. • Maintain the donor's vital functions, as ordered, until the liver can be harvested. • Prepare the donor for surgery, as ordered.
Skin To provide temporary skin grafts for patients who are severely burned	Usually, the doctor removes the skin from the donor's trunk and legs within 18 hours of his death. The skin is then processed, frozen, and stored in a skin bank.	• Wash the donor's trunk and legs. Then wrap his body according to hospital protocol. • Notify the skin bank or the doctor who will harvest the skin. • Arrange for prompt transportation of the donor to the morgue.

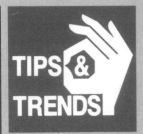

TIPS & TRENDS

Noninvasive techniques relieve pain

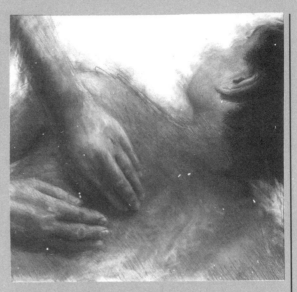

Some centers are now relieving pain with therapeutic touch, a modern version of "laying on of hands." With this pain relief technique, the care giver (or healer) uses his hands to detect areas of excess tension—an indication of pain—in the patient's energy field. Then the healer's hands "channel" the tension out of the field.

This three-phase process begins with *centering.* First, the healer meditates, focusing all of his thoughts on the patient's condition. Next, he begins *assessment,* passing his hands over the patient's body to assess his energy field and detect changes in the energy's rhythm and flow. These changes may feel like heat, a tingling sensation, or pressure. Finally, during *energy transfer,* the healer passes his hands over the tense areas and transfers energy from himself to the patient in a process called "electron transfer resonance."

Other noninvasive methods

A specially trained nurse can perform therapeutic touch to relieve pain for some patients. But *every* nurse can alleviate pain with one or more of these noninvasive techniques:

• *Cutaneous stimulation.* Several common types of cutaneous stimulation provide pain relief, including massage, acupressure, vibration, and application of heat, cold, or a lotion or ointment. A more sophisticated method—transcutaneous electrical nerve stimulation—relieves pain by transmitting electrical impulses that cause a pleasant tingling, massaging, or tapping sensation.

• *Relaxation.* Such techniques as yoga, meditation, and deep breathing can increase the effectiveness of other pain relief measures by decreasing muscle tension and increasing blood flow.

• *Distraction.* This method works by focusing the patient's attention on something other than his pain, such as a TV show, an electronic game, or music.

• *Guided imagery.* Like distraction, guided imagery takes the patient's mind off his pain. In this case, the distraction is a pleasant mental image that uses most of the senses.

Benefits of noninvasive pain relief

By themselves, noninvasive techniques can alleviate mild to moderate pain. When combined with drug therapy, they can help control severe pain. But whenever you use them, you reduce the risk of complications and side effects as you help ease the patient's distress.

NEW PROGRAMMABLE INSULIN PUMPS

CSII regulates blood glucose

Some patients with Type I diabetes mellitus can now benefit from a new type of insulin infusion pump that's continuous, programmable, *and* portable. Continous subcutaneous insulin infusion (CSII) is particularly helpful for pregnant diabetics, patients with poorly controlled diabetes, and those whose life-styles demand frequent changes in insulin dosage.

CSII controls blood glucose more closely than traditional insulin injections. It mimics the normal pancreas by delivering at least a basal amount of insulin continuously and by adjusting the amount of insulin, as needed. In addition, the patient can program it to deliver an insulin bolus before meals.

How it works
A computerized insulin pump and infusion set provide CSII, yet are small enough to fit in a shirt pocket or hang from a belt. Typically, the pump has a display screen, control panel, alarm, battery chamber, motor, and insulin reservoir.

The patient fills the reservoir with regular insulin and uses the control panel to program the basal rates and bolus doses for the pump. Using the display screen, he can verify the information he has inputted. A special battery fits into the back of the pump and runs its motor. The pump primes the infusion set, which is connected to the insulin reservoir. Insulin travels through the infusion set tubing to a subcutaneous needle that's taped in place after priming.

Your role
A doctor or nurse clinician may have taught the patient already about the pump's operation, his insulin requirements, diet and exercise therapy, and self-monitoring for blood glucose. Your job is to reinforce this teaching, answer the patient's questions about his treatment,

and assess his self-care skills and response to treatment. Here are some tips to make this easier.
• When the patient must change the basal rate of insulin infusion, help him make the change. Then assist him as he rechecks the entire basal rate program.
• Ask the patient to report his blood glucose levels before meals and at bedtime, the times when he administered boluses of insulin, and the amount of food he ate at meals.
• Document this information in the patient's chart. Also record any signs of *hypoglycemia* (headache, diaphoresis, lethargy, tremors, pallor, nervousness, and tachycardia) or *hyperglycemia* (nausea, vomiting, polyuria, polydipsia, abdominal pain, and flushed, dry skin).
• Remind the patient to change the battery and recharge it according to instructions.
• Help the patient change and fill the insulin reservoir each day.
• Aid the patient in changing the infusion set at least every 2 days. He should select a new insertion site that's at least 1" away from the old one. If you see redness, swelling, or drainage at the site, change the infusion set and the site.
• If the pump alarm sounds, troubleshoot with the patient by checking the pump, battery, reservoir, infusion set, and tubing.

INSULIN INFUSION PUMP

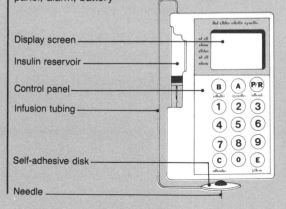

Display screen

Insulin reservoir

Control panel

Infusion tubing

Self-adhesive disk

Needle

Glossary

The terms listed below were selected from three areas of rapid change in and significant influence on health care: immunology, computer technology, and the federal prospective payment system.

A

Ad hoc report. A report printed upon special request and not normally distributed routinely.

Aeroallergens. Airborne particles, such as pollen or house dust, that cause respiratory, cutaneous, or conjunctival allergy.

Agglutination. The clumping together of antigens due to their interactions with specific antibodies (agglutinins).

Agglutinin. An antibody that promotes antigen agglutination.

Aggressin. A diffusible substance produced by a bacterium that interferes with normal defense mechanisms and enhances the organism's ability to establish itself in host tissues. Also known as a virulence factor.

Allele. One of a pair of genes, or of multiple forms of a gene, occupying the same locus on homologous chromosomes and controlling a particular characteristic.

Allergen. An antigenic substance capable of inducing an allergic response.

Allergy. An alteration in immune reactivity resulting in an untoward physiologic response.

Alloantigen. An antigen obtained from different individuals or an inbred line of the same species, such as histocompatibility antigens.

Allogenic. Of the same species but not genetically identical.

Allograft. A tissue or organ graft between two genetically different members of the same species. Also known as a homograft.

Alternative complement pathway. A complement activation pathway involving factor B, factor D, and C3b interaction, eventually leading to C3 activation and C5 cleavage, then progressing as in the classical complement pathway.

Anaphylatoxin. A substance produced by complement activation that functions in inflammation.

Anaphylaxis. An immediate hypersensitivity reaction resulting from sensitization of tissue-fixed mast cells by certain antibodies to a previously encountered antigen.

Ancillary services. Hospital services other than room and board and professional services. These may include X-ray, drug, laboratory, or other services not itemized separately (See Routine inpatient services).

Anergy. A diminished or absent reaction to an antigen or panel of antigens.

Antibody. A protein that is produced in response to an antigen and that has the ability to combine with that antigen.

Antigen. A substance that elicits a specific immune response.

Antigen presenting cell (APC). A cell, such as a macrophage, that captures, processes, and presents the antigen to immunocompetent B and T cells, thus activating them.

Antiserum. Animal or human serum containing antibodies against a specific antigen.

Arthus reaction. An acute, local antigen-antibody reaction to injection of an antigen into a previously immunized host. This reaction may progress to a lesion marked by edema, hemorrhage, and necrosis.

Atopic allergy. A hereditary tendency to develop a hypersensitivity reaction to commonly encountered antigens.

Autoantibody. An antibody that reacts with an antigen that is a normal constituent of the body (a self-antigen).

Autoantigen. A normal body constituent that stimulates autoantibody production. Also known as a self-antigen.

Autograft. A tissue transplanted from one part to another part of the same body.

Autoimmunity. Immunity to autoantigens.

B

Bacteriolysis. Destruction of bacteria induced by antibody and complement in the absence of cells.

Bacteriophage. Any virus that destroys bacteria in the host.

Base year. The 12-month cost-reporting period from which Medicare's prospective payment rates are determined. For the federal portion of the prospective payment rates, the base year was derived from reporting periods ending in 1981. For the hospital-specific portion of these rates, the base year was derived from the hospital's cost-reporting period that ended on or after September 30, 1982, and before September 30, 1983.

BASIC (beginner's all-purpose symbolic instruction code). A language used to provide instructions to most microcomputers.

Baud. A unit of measurement describing the speed at which information is transferred from one device to another, such as from the file to the computer's memory.

B cells. A class of lymphocytes derived from a stem cell and believed to mature in the bone marrow. When activated, they differentiate into plasma cells (which produce antibodies) and memory cells.

Bit. The smallest amount of information that can be used by a computer; 8 bits equals 1 byte.

Blast cell. A large, immature cell with a nucleus containing loosely packed chromatin, a large nucleolus, and a large amount of cytoplasm.

Bradykinin. A 9-amino-acid peptide that causes contraction of smooth muscle, increased vascular permeability, and increased mucous gland secretion.

Bug. A mistake in a computer program that prevents the computer from operating properly.

Bulla. A vesicle on the skin or mucous membranes greater than 1 cm in diameter.

Byte. A unit of information equivalent to one letter or number; for example, the word "ball" is equivalent to 4 bytes.

C

Case mix. The diagnosis-specific makeup of a hospital's patients. Case mix directly influences lengths of stay (LOS), intensity, cost, and scope of hospital services.

Cassette (tape). The slowest and least expensive method of storing information in microcomputers. Cassettes are impractical for computer systems that require rapid data retrieval.

Cell-mediated immunity. The specific immune response that occurs when T cells react to antigens.

Charges. Prices assigned to units of medical services, such as a doctor's visit or a day in the hospital. Charges for services may not be related to the actual cost of providing the services.

Chemotaxis. A process in which phagocytes are attracted to the pathogenic invasion site.

Chip. A tiny component made of silicon that contains computer circuitry. Chips act as the computer's memory and enable it to perform certain arithmetic functions.

Claim. A request to an insurer by an insured person or his assignee for payment of benefits under an insurance policy.

Classical complement pathway. A complement activation pathway involving various enzymes and proteins that cause cleavage of C3 and C5 and ultimately, with binding of other components, cause cell lysis.

Cleavage. The act of splitting a complex molecule into two or more simpler molecules.

Clinical outlier. Cases that cannot adequately be assigned to an appropriate DRG due to unique combinations of diagnoses and surgeries, very rare conditions, or other unique clinical reasons. Such cases are grouped together into "clinical outlier" DRGs.

Clone. A group of cells derived from a single ancestral cell.

Cold agglutinin. An antibody that agglutinates bacteria or erythrocytes better at temperatures below 37° C. (98.6° F.).

Comorbidity. A preexisting condition that will, because of its presence with a specific principal diagnosis, cause an increase in LOS by at least 1 day in approximately 75% of cases. Also referred to as "substantial comorbidity."

Complement. The primary humoral mediator of inflammation, consisting of approximately 20 proteins that interact with each other, with antibodies, and with cell membranes. Complement plays a role in various biologic mechanisms, including lysis, opsonization, and inflammation.

230

Complication. A condition that arises during the hospital stay that prolongs the LOS by at least 1 day in 75% of cases. Also referred to as "substantial complication."

Concurrent review. The monitoring, during the time a patient is hospitalized, of the delivery of care provided. When effective, concurrent review may prevent unnecessary delays and services, improve quality of care, and avoid Medicare payment loss by reevaluating treatment plans when deviations from norms occur.

Costs. Expenses incurred in the provision of a service.

Costs allowable. Items or elements of an institution's costs that are reimbursable under a payment formula.

Cost sharing. Provisions of a health insurance policy that require insured persons to pay some portion of covered medical expenses. The most common forms of cost sharing are deductibles, coinsurance, and copayments. A deductible is a set amount the insured person must pay before payment of benefits. Coinsurance is payment of a set portion of the cost of each service. A copayment is a fixed amount to be paid for each service. Cost sharing doesn't refer to or include the amount paid in premiums for the coverage.

Cost shifting. The passing along of the costs of providing care for indigent patients to Blue Cross or private plans, causing a rate increase for the payers.

Cross subsidization. Professional nursing staff providing ancillary services; for example, nurses mixing I.V. fluids to decrease the number of pharmacy staff members needed.

CRT (cathode ray tube). A computer monitor that resembles a television screen and displays stored information.

Cryoglobulin. An abnormal plasma protein that forms a gel or a precipitate at low temperatures.

D

Data. Information that is entered into or taken out of a computer.

Data base. A stored collection of information.

Delayed hypersensitivity. A delayed inflammatory reaction mediated by T cells and macrophages.

Desktop computer. A microcomputer.

Diagnosis. The commonly accepted term used to describe a disease.

Diagnosis-related groups (DRGs). A system of classifying patients according to type of disease. It was developed by researchers at Yale University and contains 467 disease categories or groups. Medicare's prospective payment system is based on DRGs.

Downsizing. A reduction in the supply of providers.

Downtime. Time in which the computer or one of its devices is inoperable, such as during repairs or a power failure.

DRG cost weight. A number that reflects each DRG's resource utilization. The weight is multiplied by the average cost for a Medicare discharge to derive the payment for the particular DRG.

DRG creep. The deliberate and systematic upgrading of a patient's diagnosis to a disease category that pays higher reimbursement.

DRG rate. A fixed-dollar amount based on the averaging of all patients in a particular DRG in the base year, adjusted for inflation, economic factors, and bad debts.

DRGs 468, 469, 470. Three administrative DRGs. DRG 468 includes all patients who had a surgical procedure that was unrelated to their major diagnostic category. DRG 469 is a discharge assigned to a diagnosis other than the principal diagnosis. DRG 470 is a discharge with invalid data.

E

Endotoxin. A lipopolysaccharide present in the cell walls of some microorganisms (primarily gram-negative bacteria) that has toxic and pyrogenic effects.

Enhancement. The improved survival of tumor cells in animals that have been previously immunized with the tumor antigens. This may occur because these antigens are coated with antibodies that protect them from lymphocytes.

Excluded hospitals. Hospitals excluded from prospective payment systems that will continue to receive payments from Medicare on the basis of reasonable cost subject to the target rate of increase limits. The following hospitals are excluded: psychiatric hospitals, rehabilitation hospitals, children's hospitals, hospitals that have an average inpatient stay greater than 25 days, and distinct parts of hospitals that serve as psychiatric or rehabilitation units of hospitals.

Exotoxin. A diffusible toxin formed by certain gram-positive and -negative microorganisms.

F

File. A collection of related data treated as a unit or stored in one area.

Floppy disk. A device similar in appearance to a 45 rpm record that's used to store information or programs in microcomputers. "Floppies" store more data and retrieve information faster than cassettes.

Function key. A special key on the computer's keyboard that's designed to perform a specific job, such as a "store" key that "tells" the computer to store information in its permanent memory.

G

Gammopathy. An immune disorder characterized by abnormalities of immunoglobulins.

Gene. The biologic unit of heredity.

Genome. The complete set of hereditary units in the chromosomes of a cell.

Genotype. The total genetic composition of an organism.

Granulocytes. Polymorphonuclear leukocytes (includes neutrophils, eosinophils, and basophils) that are derived from the stem cell and participate in immune reactions.

Grouper. Computer software that assigns DRGs.

H

Haplotype. One half of the genotype (each person has a maternal haplotype and a paternal haplotype).

Hapten. Substances of small molecular weight (less than 10,000 daltons) that are incapable of eliciting an immune response except after combining with a carrier molecule, usually a serum protein, to form a hapten-carrier complex.

Hard copy. Computer data printed onto paper.

Hardware. The physical parts of the computer, such as CRTs and printers.

Hemolysin. A substance capable of lysing red blood cells.

Heterograft. A tissue graft transplanted from one species to another. Also called a xenograft.

Histamine. A vasoactive amine that is an important mediator in anaphylactic reactions. Found in mast cell and basophil granules and platelets, histamine causes increased capillary permeability, smooth muscle contraction, and increased secretion by nasal and bronchial mucous glands.

Histocompatibility antigens. The genetically determined cell-surface antigens that stimulate graft rejection in organ transplantation.

Homograft. An allograft.

Hospital insurance. An insurance program (also known as Medicare Part A) that provides basic protection against the costs of hospital and related posthospital services for: persons age 65 and older who are eligible for benefits under the Social Security or Railroad Retirement system; persons under age 65 entitled for not less than 24 months to benefits under the Social Security or Railroad Retirement system on the basis of disability; and certain other persons, medically determined to have end-stage renal disease and covered by the Social Security or Railroad Retirement system.

Hospital-specific prospective payment amount. The portion of a hospital's payment that's based on the hospital's base year costs per discharge, divided by the case mix index, updated for inflation, and adjusted for the specific DRG. In the first year of the system, 75% of the payment is based on the hospital-specific rate; in the second year, 50%; and in the third year, 25%. This rate is adjusted at the beginning of each hospital's fiscal year.

Human leukocyte antigen (HLA). The major histocompatibility complex.

Humoral immunity. The specific immune response that occurs when B cells react to antigens by producing antibodies.

Hypogammaglobulinemia. An immunodeficiency characterized by a decrease in all of the major classes of serum immunoglobulins.

I

Immediate hypersensitivity. An immune response to an antigen that occurs within minutes after the antigen combines with the specific antibody.

Immune complexes. Antigen-antibody complexes.

Immune response genes. Genes within the major histocompatibility complex that control immune responses to specific antigens.

Immunity. Resistance to possible invasion by an infectious agent.

Immunoelectrophoresis. A test that combines electrophoresis and immunodiffusion techniques to distinguish between proteins and other materials.

Immunofluorescence. A technique used to identify an antigen by observing its antigen-antibody reaction with known antibodies tagged with fluorescent dye.

Immunoglobulin. A protein molecule composed of light and heavy polypeptide chains, linked together by disulfide bonds. All antibodies are immunoglobulins.

Indirect medical education costs. The higher costs of patient care incurred by institutions sponsoring approved educational programs (other than the cost of such items as trainee stipends, teacher compensation, supplies, and materials directly attributable to the approved educational program itself). Examples of the indirect costs of medical education include added tests and procedures ordered by residents and such intangible factors as the socioeconomic status and the severity of patients treated. Under the new prospective payment system, hospitals will receive an 11.59% increase in the DRG payment rate for each 0.1 increment in the hospital's ratio of interns and residents per hospital bed.

Inflammation. The complex of protective responses caused by infection, injury, or intrusion of foreign substances. These responses help to eliminate dead tissue, toxins, microbes, and inactive foreign substances.

Information systems department. The hospital department responsible for the hospital's shared data base system computer and for storage and retrieval of data.

Input. Information—either data or programs—that's entered into computers.

Interferon. A class of small, soluble proteins, produced by infected host cells, that interfere with viral multiplication.

International classification of diseases. A system developed by the World Health Organization for classifying diseases and procedures for purposes of indexing hospital records.

Isograft. A graft between genetically identical individuals, such as monozygotic twins.

K

K. An abbreviation for kilo or 1,000, used to calculate a computer's memory. One K actually equals 1,024 characters of information, so a computer with 64K of memory is capable of storing 65,536 characters of information.

Keyboard. The part of a computer that resembles a typewriter, used to input data.

L

Length of stay (LOS). Duration of hospitalization, reported as the number of days spent in a facility per admission or discharge. A hospital's overall average LOS is calculated as the total number of days in the facility for all discharges occurring during a given period, divided by the number of discharges during the same period.

Lymphokine. A soluble mediator, produced by lymphocytes, that regulates macrophage, lymphocyte, and nonlymphoid cell interactions.

Lysosomes. Granules, occurring in the cytoplasm of many cells, that contain hydrolytic enzymes and participate in localized intracellular digestion.

M

Macrophage. The chief cell of the mononuclear phagocyte system, derived from the stem cell. Primarily engaged in phagocytosis, this cell also plays a role in antigen processing and presentation, the release of various mediators, and the production of fever. Macrophages are also known as mononuclear phagocytes.

Main frame. A large computer capable of storing massive amounts of data and retrieving it rapidly; it's the fastest and most expensive type of computer.

Major diagnostic category (MDC). One of 23 broad clinical categories, based on body system involvement and disease etiology, used to develop and organize the DRGs developed at Yale University.

Major histocompatibility complex (MHC). A group of genes, located on the short arm of chromosome 6, that code for cell-surface antigens. The MHC is critical in the recognition of self versus nonself, since it defines what is self. Also known as human leukocyte antigen.

Mast cell. A tissue cell, resembling a basophil, with granules containing serotonin and histamine. Mast cells are essential for the antibody (IgE) response, important in anaphylactic reactions.

Medically unnecessary services and custodial care. Custodial days of care or noncovered services incurred when a doctor discharges a patient but the patient chooses not to leave the hospital. The beneficiary must be notified in writing that he will be billed for these days or services, and the Medicare fiscal intermediary must concur with the hospital's determination that the services aren't covered by the Medicare program.

Medical meaningfulness. The concept that patients in the same DRG can be expected to evoke a set of clinical responses that result in a similar pattern of resource use.

Medical review agent. A peer review organization (PRO), professional standards review organization (PSRO), or a fiscal intermediary that has an agreement with the U.S. Department of Health and Human Services to review the quality and appropriateness of services covered by Medicare, Medicaid, or the Maternal and Child Health Program.

Memory. The section of the computer where data and programs are stored.

Microcomputer. The smallest and least expensive type of computer, often referred to as a personal or desktop computer.

Microfiche. Greatly reduced film records of documents that require a special viewer for reading; microfiche eliminates bulky hard copy for long-term recordkeeping.

Modem. A device that enables a computer to receive or transmit information over telephone lines.

Monitor. A television-like device used to display data from the computer's storage or keyboard input.

Monoclonal antibody. A homogeneous group of a single type of antibody made against a specific antigen.

Mononuclear phagocyte. A macrophage.

Mononuclear phagocyte system. The reticuloendothelial system.

Morbidity. The rate of disease or proportion of diseased persons.

Mortality. Death or death rate.

N

Neutralization. The interaction in which an antibody or an antibody in complement counteracts the infectivity of a pathogen.

Nursing resources. For billing purposes, the amount of nursing care provided to a patient, calculated in minutes.

O

Oncogene. An altered version of a normal gene.

Opsonin. A substance that enhances phagocytosis.

Opsonization. The coating of foreign particles with opsonins, making them more susceptible to phagocytosis.

Other diagnosis. All conditions that exist at the time of admission or develop subsequently that affect the treatment received and/or the LOS. Diagnoses that relate to an earlier episode or have no bearing on the current hospital stay are excluded.

Outliers. Cases assigned to a particular DRG that differ from the average cases within that DRG by either unusually long or short LOS or unusually high or low resource consumption. Cases with shorter than average LOS or lower than average costs will be paid the regular DRG prospective rate; additional payments will be made to supplement the regular DRG rate for cases that exceed the average LOS or cost limits for the DRG to which they are assigned.

Output. Information from the computer's internal storage area that can be transmitted to a monitor, printer, cassette, floppy disk, or another computer.

P

Pass-through costs. Capital-related costs and direct medical education costs reimbursed on a cost basis; this practice will continue until the federal government devises a formula to include reimbursment for these expenditures in prospective payment.

Peer review organization (PRO). An entity composed of licensed doctors of medicine or osteopathy representative of the practicing physicians in a particular geographic area and judged by the Secretary of the U.S. Department of Health and Human Services to be capable of assessing the acceptability and adequacy of medical practice in that area. PROs are responsible for determining whether the care furnished by providers, physicians, and other health practitioners under Medicare is reasonable and medically necessary, meets professional quality standards, and could, when provided on an inpatient basis, be more economically provided on an outpatient basis or in a different type of inpatient facility.

Peripherals. Hardware accessories for a computer, such as a printer or modem.

Phagocytes. Cells that are able to ingest particulate matter. Examples of phagocytes are macrophages and neutrophils.

Phagocytosis. Engulfment and ingestion of bacteria, fungi, dead tissue, antigen-antibody complexes, and tumor cells by macrophages and neutrophils.

Phenotype. The sum total of physical, physiologic, and biochemical makeup of an individual as determined by genetic and environmental factors.

Plasma cell. A cell derived from B cells that secrete large amounts of immunoglobulin.

Preadmission planning. Determining a patient's treatment plan and progress goals according to predetermined standards.

Precipitation. Formation of interlocking aggregates caused by interactions between soluble antigens and antibodies.

Preferred provider organizations. A payment arrangement whereby insurers contract with hospitals or doctors to provide health care services on a negotiated fee-for-service basis. Subscribers can select any provider but have economic or other incentives to use the designated (preferred) hospitals or doctors.

Prevailing charge. The charge that would cover 75% of the customary charges made for similar services in the same locality. It is the maximum amount Medicare will recognize as a reasonable charge for reimbursement purposes, and its rate of increase is controlled by an economic index.

Primary diagnosis. The medical condition that required the greatest resource consumption during the period of hospitalization.

Principal diagnosis. The condition chiefly responsible for a patient's hospital admission.

Principal procedure. The procedure most related to the principal diagnosis and which was performed for definitive treatment, rather than for diagnostic or exploratory purposes, or for treatment of a complication.

Program. A detailed and explicit set of directions, expressed in a computer language (such as BASIC), that instruct the computer to carry out certain functions.

Prospective payment. The method of paying hospitals in which full amounts or rates of payment are established in advance for a designated period of time. Hospitals receive such payment regardless of actual costs incurred.

R

Radioallergosorbent test (RAST). A test that measures IgE antibodies in serum that are directed at specific allergens.

RAM (random access memory). A section of the computer where data is filed; data in RAM can be viewed and changed on command.

Rejection. An immune response directed against transplanted tissue. Rejection can be classified according to the time span between transplantation and rejection; namely, hyperacute (occurring within minutes to hours); accelerated (occurring after about 5 days); acute (occurring within days to months); and chronic (occurring 6 months to years later).

Resolution. The clarity of the picture on a computer monitor; the higher the resolution, the clearer the picture.

Reticuloendothelial system (RES). The system of cells distributed throughout the body that removes microorganisms from the blood and tissues and responds to activated lymphocytes to participate in immune responses. The chief cell is the macrophage. Also known as the mononuclear phagocyte system.

Retrospective review. The monitoring of admission and treatment pattern after discharge.

Rheumatoid factor (RF). Anti-immunoglobulin antibodies formed in response to altered IgG. RF is often found in the serum of patients with rheumatoid arthritis and other rheumatoid disorders.

ROM (read only memory). Memory that's permanently entered into the computer by the manufacturer; information stored in ROM can be read by a user but not altered or deleted.

Routine inpatient services. Hospital room and board and related professional services for which there is generally no separate charge (*See* Ancillary services).

S

Secondary diagnoses. Problems and important symptoms, both related and unrelated to the principal diagnosis, which either exist at admission or develop and are treated during hospitalization.

Sensitization. Immunologic activation of cells in response to an antigen.

Shared data base. A computerized filing system that combines data from different applications; for example, in a hospital, a shared data base may contain a patient's financial and medical data.

Skimming. The practice of giving priority admission to patients whose disease categories will bring in the highest payments.

Soft copy. Information not printed on paper, such as information displayed on a computer monitor.

Software. Computer programs.

Sole community hospital (SCH). A hospital that, because of such factors as isolated location, weather conditions, or absence of other hospitals, is the sole source of inpatient hospital services reasonably available to Medicare beneficiaries in a geographic area. A provider that qualifies as an SCH may qualify for an exception or adjustment to the prospective payment rates. To be classified as an SCH, a rural hospital must meet one of the following criteria:
• located more than 50 miles from another similar hospital
• located between 25 and 50 miles from other, like hospitals and either no more than 25% of the residents in the hospital's service are admitted to other or like hospitals for care, or, because of local topography or weather, the other hospitals generally aren't accessible for more than 1 month during a 12-month period
• located between 15 and 25 miles of other, like hospitals and, because of local topography or weather, the other hospitals generally aren't accessible for more than 1 month during a 12-month period.

Supplemental security income (SSI). A program of income support for low-income, aged, blind, and disabled persons, established by Title XVI of the Social Security Act.

Supplementary medical insurance (SMI). The voluntary portion of the Medicare program (also known as Medicare Part B) in which all persons entitled to the Hospital Insurance Program (Part A) may enroll. After the deductible has been met, it pays for 80% of the reasonable charge for most covered services. Covered services include physician services; home health care, medical and other health services; outpatient hospital services; and laboratory, pathology, and radiologic services. The SMI program is financed by monthly premiums paid by persons insured under Medicare, and by matching federal payments.

Syngraft. An isograft.

T

T cells. A class of lymphocytes that is derived from the stem cell and matures in the thymus. When activated, they differentiate into various cells, including helper cells, suppressor cells, lymphokine-producing cells, cytotoxic cells, and memory cells.

Toxoid. A toxin altered to reduce toxicity but retain antigenic properties.

Transfer factor. An extract of sensitized lymphocytes that transfers cell-mediated immunity from one individual to another.

Trim points. The length of stay or cost cutoff points that separate patients with unusually long lengths of stay or unusually high costs from "normal" cases within each DRG. Patients who exceed these cutoff or "trim" points are classified as outliers and are eligible for additional Medicare payments.

U

Unbundling. The transfer of ancillary services from the hospital to outside contractors.

Uniform bill-patient summary. A document that combines a patient's billing information and medical data.

User friendly. A term referring to a computer that's easy to use; user-friendly computers may "prompt" the user through the program that's being run.

Utilization review. The monitoring of activities involved in the treatment of patients. Medicare requires utilization review to ensure that services provided to beneficiaries are covered, reasonable, and necessary. Under PPS, utilization reviews are performed by PROs.

V W X

Vaccination. Immunization with antigens to prevent infectious diseases.

Virulence factor. Aggressin.

Wage index. An index representing local hospital wages that's used to figure the labor-related portion of a hospital's federal payment rates.

Word processor. Software that enables the user to write and edit information in text form, and to enter the text into the computer's memory for future recall.

Xenograft. A heterograft.

Selected references and acknowledgments

Selected references

Blackburn, G.L., and Baptista, R.J., "Home TPN: State of the Art," *American Journal of Intravenous Therapy and Clinical Nutrition* 11(2):20-31, February 1984.

Eaves, D. "Radiation Alert," *Nursing Times* 80(32):46-49, August 8-14, 1984.

Emergencies. Nurse's Reference Library. Springhouse, Pa.: Springhouse Corp., 1985.

Fairbanks, D. "Snoring: Not Funny—Not Hopeless," *Hospital Medicine* 20(3):173-89, March 1984.

Fromme, L.R., and Kaplow, R. "High Frequency Jet Ventilation," *American Journal of Nursing* 84(11):1380-83, November 1984.

Gallico, Gregory. "Permanent Coverage of Large Burn Wounds with Autologous Cultured Human Epithelium," *New England Journal of Medicine* 311(7):448-51, August 16, 1984.

Garner, J., and Simmons, B. *CDC Guidelines for Isolation Precautions in Hospitals.* Bethesda, Md.: U.S. Dept. of Health and Human Services, Public Health Service, 1983.

DeCrosta, T., ed. "Megatrends in Nursing: Ten New Directions That Are Changing Your Profession," *NursingLife* 5(3):17-21, May/June 1985.

Mensher, J.H. "Laser Therapy for Eye Disorders," *Postgraduate Medicine* 76(7):51-56, November 15, 1984.

"Morbidity and Mortality Weekly Report. Update: Lyme Disease—United States," *U.S. Dept. of Health and Human Services* 33(19):268-70, 1984.

Newberg, L.A. "Cerebral Resuscitation: Advances and Controversies," *Annals of Emergency Medicine* 13(9):853-56, September 1984.

Perry, Anne G., and Potter, Patricia A. *Fundamentals of Nursing.* St. Louis: C.V. Mosby Co., 1985.

Recommendations for the Safe Handling of Parenteral Antineoplastic Drugs. Bethesda, Md.: U.S. Dept. of Health and Human Services, Public Health Service, National Institutes of Health, 1983.

Rehncrona, S. "Brain Acidosis," *Annals of Emergency Medicine* 14(8):770-76, August 1985.

Shoemaker, William C., et al. *The Society of Critical Care Medicine: Textbook of Critical Care.* Philadelphia: W.B. Saunders Co., 1984.

Skelley, L. "Practical Issues in Obtaining Organs for Transplantation," *Law, Medicine, and Health Care* 13(1):35-37, February 1985.

Stites, Daniel P., ed. *Basic and Clinical Immunology,* 5th ed. Los Altos, Calif.: Lange Medical Pubns., 1984.

"Screening for AIDS," *The Medical Letter* 27(684):29-30, March 29, 1985.

Whitney, F. "Alzheimer's Disease: Toward Understanding and Management," *The Nurse Practitioner* 10(9):25-36, September 1985.

Acknowledgments

p. 10 Photos courtesy of Dosimeter Corp., Cincinnati

p. 29 Photo courtesy of S. Warren Gross, MD, Chairman, Department of Radiology, Warminster (Pa.) General Hospital

p. 49 Photo courtesy of Thomas J. Brady, MD, Associate Professor of Radiology, Harvard University Medical School; Assistant Radiologist, Massachusetts General Hospital, Boston

p. 56 Photo courtesy of Abass Alavi, MD, Professor of Radiology and Neurology, and Chief, Division of Nuclear Medicine, Hospital of the University of Pennsylvania, Philadelphia

p. 68 Photos courtesy of Marc S. Lapayowker, MD, Department of Radiology, Abington (Pa.) Memorial Hospital

p. 78 Adapted from Lixi Imaging Scope information provided by Lixi, Inc., Downers Grove, Ill.

p. 154 Adapted from cochlear implant information provided by 3M/Otologic Products, St. Paul

p. 155 Adapted from information about the ventricular assist device provided by Novacor Medical Corp., Oakland, Calif.

p. 155 Adapted from information about the ventricular assist device provided by Thermedics Inc., Woburn, Mass.

p. 220-223 Guidelines on home therapies provided by Travenol Laboratories, Inc., Home Nutrition and Intravenous Therapy, Morton Grove, Ill.

p. 227 Adapted from Eugly Insulin Pump information provided by Travenol Laboratories, Inc., Travenol Home Diabetes Therapy, Deerfield, Ill.

Index

Boldface page numbers indicate major entries; i refers to an illustration, t to a table.

Boldface page numbers indicate major entries; i refers to an illustration, t to a table.

How to cut out frustration, burnout, and the blues.

Yearbook86/87

JULY

21-8/15
Nursing Program in London. Contact: Office of Overseas Study, Michigan State University, (517) 353-8920.

AUGUST

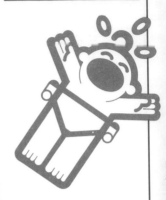

14-15
"Advanced Trauma Life Support for Nurses." University of Maryland at Baltimore. Contact: Maryland Institute for Emergency Medical Services Systems, (301) 528-6846.

SEPTEMBER

17-19
"Neonatology—The Sick Newborn." Desoto Hilton Hotel, Savannah, Ga. Contact: Medical College of Georgia, (404) 828-3967.

24-28
Emergency Nurses Association Annual Conference. Sheraton Waikiki Hotel, Honolulu. Contact: ENA Meeting Services Division, (312) 649-0297.

26-28
American Association of Occupational Health Nurses Conference of Presidents. Hyatt Regency Hotel, Dallas. Contact: AAOHN Dept. of Professional Affairs, (404) 262-1162.

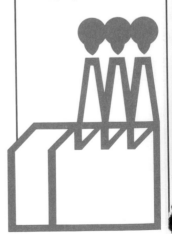